The
Psychoanalytic
Study
of the Child

VOLUME FIFTY-FOUR

Kindly submit seven copies of new manuscripts to

Albert J. Solnit, M.D.
Yale Child Study Center
230 South Frontage Road
P.O. Box 207900
New Haven, CT 06520-7900
Phone: (203) 785-2518

The
Psychoanalytic
Study
of the Child

VOLUME FIFTY-FOUR

New Haven and London
Yale University Press
1999

Designed by Sally Harris
and set in Baskerville type.
Printed in the United States of America by
Vail-Ballou Press, Inc., Binghamton, N.Y.

Library of Congress catalog card number: 45-11304
International standard book number: 0-300-08004-2
A catalogue record for this book is available from the British Library.

The paper in this book meets the guidelines for
permanence and durability of the Committee on
Production Guidelines for Book Longevity of the
Council on Library Resources.
2 4 6 8 10 9 7 5 3 1

*This volume is dedicated to Gladys Topkis, who has retired from
her full-time position as a senior editor at Yale University Press.
The editors of* The Psychoanalytic Study of the Child *feel fortunate
that Gladys Topkis—an astute, generous, conscientious editor—
will continue her association with this annual.
In the first paper of this volume, presented at a 1998 symposium honoring
her more than fifteen years of zestful editing at Yale University Press,
Ethel Spector Person captures the extraordinary talent
and contributions of Gladys Topkis.*

Contents

ETHEL S. PERSON
Creative Collaborations: Writers and Editors   1

DEVELOPMENT AND TECHNIQUE

SAMUEL ABRAMS, PETER B. NEUBAUER, AND ALBERT J. SOLNIT
Coordinating the Developmental and Psychoanalytic
Processes: Three Case Reports—Introduction   19
WENDY OLESKER
Treatment of a Boy with Atypical Ego Development   25
ANITA G. SCHMUKLER
Detours in Adolescent Development: Implications
for Technique   47
ALAN B. ZIENTS
The Psychoanalytic Treatment of a Child with Deviational
Development   68
SAMUEL ABRAMS, PETER B. NEUBAUER, AND ALBERT J. SOLNIT
Coordinating the Developmental and Psychoanalytic
Processes: Three Case Reports—Discussion   87

THEORY

LEON BALTER
Constant Mental Change and Unknowability
in Psychoanalysis   93
ARTHUR S. COUCH
Therapeutic Functions of the Real Relationship
in Psychoanalysis   130
LINDA C. MAYES
Clocks, Engines, and Quarks—Love, Dreams, and Genes:
What Makes Development Happen?   169
RONNIE SOLAN
The Interaction between Self and Others: A Different
Perspective on Narcissism   193

vii

CLINICAL PAPERS

JUDITH FINGERT CHUSED
   Obsessional Manifestations in Children   219
DONALD J. COLEMAN
   Narrative Performance Mode (NPM) of Discourse   233
OSCAR F. HILLS
   Ego Erection: Regressive Perceptual Phenomena
   in Relation to Psychic Growth   259
M. A. TALLANDINI
   The Dread of Integration: Integrative Processes
   in a Chronically Ill Borderline Patient   289

ADOLESCENCE

DEBRA S. ROSENBLUM, PETER DANIOLOS, NEAL KASS,
AND ANDRES MARTIN
   Adolescents and Popular Culture: A Psychodynamic
   Overview   319
ANITA G. SCHMUKLER
   Use of Insight in Child Analysis   339

Creative Collaborations

Writers and Editors

ETHEL S. PERSON

Creativity, which the culture often depicts as a solitary enterprise, is almost always impacted or even dependent upon one or another aspect of a real relationship or an internalized object relationship. This paper utilizes the example of creative collaborations between writers and editors to illustrate aspects of co-creativity, co-construction, and mutual influence. It draws on Howard Gardner's observation, based on a series of biographical studies, that a creator during a time of artistic or intellectual breakthrough requires both an affective support system and a cognitive one. His observation echoes that of child researchers who emphasize that the contour of developmental lines depends not only on an internal dynamic but on interactions with significant others and on cultural and social influences as well. This paper describes both successful and problematic collaborations between writers and editors and demonstrates the strengths of such collaborations and some of their potential faultlines as well.

Professor of clinical psychiatry at Columbia University and a training and supervising analyst at the Columbia University Center for Psychoanalytic Training and Research. She is currently a vice president for North America of the International Psychoanalytical Association.

This paper is dedicated to one of the great psychoanalytic editors, Gladys Topkis, whose authors have included such psychoanalytic luminaries as Peter Gay, Otto Kernberg, Leonard Shengold, and the late Robert Stoller. It was presented at a symposium in her honor, sponsored by Yale University Press, on October 10, 1998, on the occasion of her retirement.
The Psychoanalytic Study of the Child 54, ed. Albert J. Solnit, Peter B. Neubauer, Samuel Abrams, and A. Scott Dowling (Yale University Press, copyright © 1999 by Albert J. Solnit, Peter B. Neubauer, Samuel Abrams, and A. Scott Dowling).

ALL OF US AT ONE TIME OR ANOTHER EXPERIENCE PAINFUL FEELINGS OF powerlessness. Such feelings may be constant or intermittent, conscious or preconscious; they may be due to our awareness of our own mortality, some aspect of our current life situation, or the dependency of our earliest days. To counteract them and achieve a countervailing sense of power we may invoke one or more of four strategies.

The first strategy, reliance on or surrender to a greater power, often takes the form of religious conviction. A comparable "transference," though perhaps to a lesser degree, occurs in the relationship of patient to psychoanalyst, mentee to mentor, or lover to beloved (Becker, 1973; Person, 1988).

The second basic strategy, the exertion of power vis-à-vis another person, can find expression through the tactics of the strong, which may be negative—punishment or the threat of some kind of punishment or withholding—or positive, via the promise of certain advantages or benefits. Alternately, we can invoke the tactics of the weak, such as ingratiation, submissiveness, or slavishness. The interaction on the dominant-submissive axis is not always negative. For example, it may be nurturant, as in the case of mother and child, teacher and student, and sometimes it may be mutually sustaining, as it is in a number of creative collaborations.

The third strategy consists of achieving self-regulation, self-control, and autonomy, colloquially referred to as "will-power." Will-power is to self-control and self-determination what the will-to-power is to the control of other people. Paradoxically, even when the goal is autonomy, another person or an internalized object relationship is generally implicated. Positive identification with an autonomous figure, whether it's someone we know, have observed from afar, or merely read about or seen in a movie, for example, facilitates the achievement of a sustained sense of self-control and autonomy.[1]

The fourth strategy involves the exercise of creativity. Like will, creativity is an expression of our deepest nature and leads to its own kind of exhilaration. Some people are authentically creative and gifted in ways that automatically bring a feeling of empowerment into their lives. They express themselves through the music they play, the poetry they write, the pictures they paint, or through other modes of artistic expression. But this strategy, too, often involves another person in either a fantasized or a real relationship that encourages or catalyzes creativity. In fact, sometimes a full-fledged partnership is required. Thus,

---

1. Sometimes the need to assert command as a response to a dependent parent is another route to autonomy or pseudo-autonomy.

creativity, which we think of as a solitary enterprise, can at various times be impacted upon or can even rely on one or another of the interpersonal aspects of the other strategies for transcending powerlessness—transference; a relationship of either dominance or submission to another person or of nurturance; or identification with another person.[2]

Even when there is no real "Other" involved in the expression of creativity, I believe that there may be an internalized other. Consider, for example, a vignette in May Sarton's journal *At Seventy* (1984), in which she catches the sense of creativity as a form of personal power. In the course of a talk she gave on old age, she told the audience: "This is the best time of my life. I love being old." Someone from the audience inquired: "Why is it good to be old?" Sensing what she described as incredulity in the question, Sarton notes in her journal how she responded: "'Because I am more myself than I have ever been there is less conflict. I am happier, more balanced, and' (I heard myself say rather aggressively) 'more powerful.' I felt it was rather an odd word, 'powerful,' but I think it is true. It might have been more accurate to say 'I am better able to use my powers.' I am sure of what my life is about, have less self-doubt to conquer" (p. 10).

Here Sarton is speaking of a kind of power that has little or nothing to do with the domination or control of another person and does not depend on our subjugation of someone else. However, when she talks about the self-doubt she has conquered, I believe she is writing about the silencing of an internal critic. Until such an internal critic is silenced, or at least brought under control, one's creative voice will be stifled. Only when it is unencumbered by fear or timidity can *creativity* find natural expression as the unified product of our physical, mental, and emotional makeup, stemming from deep sources within our psyches.

What I have observed of creativity among psychoanalysts is similar: Several of the most intelligent psychoanalysts of my acquaintance—certainly gifted enough to have been major contributors to the psychoanalytic literature—have failed to do so because they seem incapable of suspending their critical standards. As a result, they stifle all those little shoots of intuition—as yet illogical, non-linear, unsubstantiated—that can sometimes flower into important new insights and ideas. Intimidated by their own powers of logic, they squelch their creative insights for fear that inconsistencies in their ideas might embarrass them. Sarton speaks as one who has overcome her internal critic and is thus able to use her powers of creativity to the full.

2. Sometimes, too, the creative person uses consciousness of mortality as a spur—to transcend mortality by creating something enduring.

Of course, one's own self-doubts are often intensified by the comments of external critics—friends or professionals. For writers, criticism can be devastating to the point of paralysis. One editor at a major publishing house stopped requesting critiques on book submissions from a brilliant but critical reader whom she came to call "Dr. No." Nothing she showed him did he deem fit to publish.[3] Unfortunately, the brilliant person who sees too quickly the flaws and gaps in someone else's early drafts will miss the kernel of genuine insight or originality that may be there and will not be able to provide useful input to his colleagues, no matter how insightful his criticisms are, because only the most self-confident can surmount such unmitigated negativity. This kind of assault on the creative impulse can be deadly, not just on the personal but on the institutional level. In psychoanalytic circles, for example, there have been decades when the organizational pressure to adhere to one or another theory has stifled many potentially creative people because of their fear of being marginalized. This is the external critic writ large.

There are other ways in which both internal and external forces may stifle creativity. Some of us are so fearful of not being good enough that we maintain our good opinion of our own potential only by never putting it to the test. Others are so inhibited by the potential envy of others that they obey the internal injunction not to stand out from the crowd. Only when we negotiate a sufficient degree of self-confidence and independent judgment are we able to express our creative powers fully, those powers that have been freed from our internal fear of finding ourselves wanting, our fear of someone else's criticism, our fear of exclusion.

The task of freeing ourselves is often made easier by encouragement from a supportive friend, or by deep intellectual or creative connection to someone who may serve to give us courage, spark an insight, or engage in a full-fledged collaboration. In addition, some creative individuals utilize the evocation of a muse. In all those roles the Other may serve as a transference object.

Freud drew a parallel between the child at play, the adult daydreamer, and the creative artist: "Might we not say that every child at play behaves like a creative writer, in that he creates a world of his own, or rather, rearranges the things of his world in a new way which pleases him? . . . The creative writer does the same as the child at play. He creates a world of phantasy which he takes very seriously—that is, which he invests with

3. And Dr. No's own creativity was stifled.

large amounts of emotion—while separating it sharply from reality" (1908, pp. 143–144). Here Freud evokes the artist as the person he is culturally depicted to be—a solitary genius whose brilliant work springs forth full-blown.

For some, play, fantasy, and creativity do feel solitary. But more often than not there is an interpersonal component to creativity. Even in the nursery, children spark each other's creativity in imaginative play. Vivian Gussin Paley, in *The Boy Who Would Be a Helicopter: The Uses of Storytelling in the Classroom* (1990), posits play acting and storytelling as the primary reality for preschoolers and kindergartners and their jointly authored stories as the vehicle for their bonding. Children invoke friendship and what I call shared fantasy (as expressed in their joint play) to avoid fear and loneliness, to find a comfortable relationship with people and events, and to address current concerns and future dreads. Friendship and fantasy are the braided paths that lead children into an imaginative world of expanded possibilities (Person, 1995).

For many of us, it is the support and input from our interpersonal world that allow us to more fully express our creative possibilities throughout the life cycle. During the 1970s and 1980s, a number of analysts observed that certain artists required a supportive and often intense relationship with another person, particularly during a period of creativity (e.g., Kligerman's report on Buddy Meyer's concept of the "Secret Sharer," 1972).

Co-creativity, co-construction, and mutual influence remain important areas of current inquiry into creativity. In his studies on seven extremely creative minds,[4] Howard Gardner (1993) found that during the period in which "a creator made his or her most important breakthrough. . . . Not only did the creators have some kind of significant support system at that time, but this support system appeared to have a number of defining components. First, the creator required both affective support from someone with whom he or she felt comfortable and cognitive support from someone who could understand the nature of the breakthrough. In some situations the same person could supply both needs, while on other occasions, such double-duty was unsuccessful or impossible" (pp. 43–44). Gardner confesses that he was surprised by the discovery of the social forces surrounding the emergence of creative insights. He compared the relationship between

4. In addition to Freud, Gardner presents "an anatomy of creativity seen through the lives" of Einstein, Picasso, Stravinsky, T. S. Eliot, Martha Graham, and Gandhi.

artist and those who made up the artist's support system to critical relationships earlier in life: between caregiver and child, for example, or between a youngster and peer group.

As a general proposition, Robert Emde suggests that "development today is understood in terms of a biology of increasingly organized complexity. Developmental processes occur throughout life, are enabled by transactions with significant others, and are immersed in cultural influence" (1995, p. 157). This is as true of the support system for creativity as it is for any other developmental process.

Freud is the first of the creative geniuses Gardner describes. It is an oft-told tale that several emotionally charged alliances were critical in Sigmund Freud's creative breakthroughs (see, e.g., Shengold, 1993, chap. 6; Coen, 1994, chap. 4), but it is largely Gardner's account that I draw on here. Freud was his mother's first-born. Not only did she shower special attention on him, but she had the good grace to live until he was over 70. In addition, his nurse doted on him and is believed to have reinforced the idea that he was special. Freud was, of course, extremely gifted, and this was evident even in his earliest life. He chose to study medicine but he immersed himself in a wide variety of other subjects and even taught himself several languages in order to read important works in their original language.

From early life, he found people in whom to confide his interests and his ideas. These included his great friend Eduard Silberstein and later on his fiancée, Martha Bernays, and still later his friend Wilhelm Fliess and his sister-in-law, Minna. Many commentators have noted that in his early letters he already expressed great ambition and extreme confidence in his ability to achieve greatness. At 17 years of age, Freud wrote his friend Emil Fluss: "You have been exchanging letters with a German stylist. And now I advise you as a friend, not as an interested party, to preserve them—have them bound—take good care of them—one never knows" (S. Freud, ed. E. L. Freud, 1960, p. 4).

Undertaking the study of medicine, Freud worked in the laboratory of Ernst Bruecke and wrote articles on neuroanatomy. His correspondence shows that he remained infatuated with the quest for fame and with experiments he hoped would win it for him. But his experiment with cocaine, which he dispensed to his friends for medical purposes, nearly ended in disaster when one of his colleagues became addicted to it. Although cocaine did in fact prove to have medicinal powers, it was Carl Koller, not Freud, who achieved recognition for discovering the usefulness of cocaine as an anesthetic for eye surgery.

The year after the cocaine debacle, Freud went to Paris to study with

Charcot, and it was there, Gardner suggests, that Freud shifted "his 'ego ideal' from the precise and rigorous neuroanatomical investigator Bruecke to the more expansive, charismatic, and psychologically oriented Charcot" (p. 57). Returning to Vienna, Freud attached himself to Breuer, through whom he began to see hysterical patients.

Together Breuer and Freud wrote about the "talking cure," a term coined by one of Breuer's patients, and jointly published their *Studies in Hysteria* (1900). Not only was Breuer uneasy with their hypotheses, but Freud's presentation of "The Etiology of Hysteria" to the Vienna Society in 1896 was not well received. The sexologist Krafft-Ebing declared it a "scientific fairy tale." As Freud commented later, "The development of psychoanalysis afterwards cost me his [Breuer's] friendship. It was not easy for me to pay such a price but I could not escape it" (1935, p. 34).

Gardner presents Freud's plight at that time very poignantly: "Once an individual who had been virtually canonized by his own family, appreciated and admired by peers and mentors, and able to master vast bodies of information in a veritable library of subjects, Freud had evolved to a most unhappy situation: one where his closest colleagues, like Breuer, were no longer willing to stand with him, while his closest family members, like his wife, could not possibly understand what he was claiming" (pp. 60–61).

It was during this time of stress and in this vacuum that Freud's friendship with Wilhelm Fliess flowered. For over ten years they corresponded. Even though Fliess's ideas may seem eccentric and marginal today, he was valuable to Freud as someone who was intellectually interested in his theories and hunches as well as emotionally supportive. Although Freud refers to this period as a time of "splendid isolation," Fliess was for him a major transference figure and even a necessary one. Given Fliess's intellectual limitations, the fact that their interaction was chiefly via letter was probably a critical factor in Freud's ability to sustain his idealization of Fliess as long as he did.

Gardner writes that Freud's sharing of "The Project" with Fliess illustrates a theme that he encountered repeatedly in his study of creativity: "At times when creators are on the verge of a radical breakthrough, they feel the need to try out their new language on a trusted other individual—perhaps to confirm that they themselves are not totally mad and may even be on to something new and important. . . . I suggest that this desperate effort to communicate may harken back in some ways to the initial communication link between mother and child and to youthful links between peers" (pp. 68–69).

After his success, Freud himself became the transference object for idealization and inspiration, and his problems with "father figures" gave way to his problems with rivals and disciples.

While Gardner is describing world-class creative geniuses, what both he and Emde point to has relevance to creativity at all levels. For most of us, the sense of a strong independent self emerges only slowly, with the accumulation of small successes. Though we may appear autonomous and creative to others, it takes a while before we ourselves can incorporate such a self-concept. In her autobiography, Edith Wharton (1933) writes about her feelings just after the publication of her first two short stories: "Both attracted attention, and gave me the pleasant flutter incidental to first seeing one's self in print; but they brought me no nearer to other workers in the same field. I continued to live my old life, for my husband was as fond of society as ever, and I knew of no other existence except in our annual escapes to Italy. I had as yet no real personality of my own, and was not to acquire one till my first book of short stories was published—and that was not until 1899" (p. 112). When that first book, *The Greater Inclination,* was published (she was already 37), she writes of her unbelieving response: "*I* had written short stories that were thought worthy of preservation! Was it the same insignificant *I* that *I* had always known?" (p. 113).

Edith Wharton, like Freud, found strength through a friend, the lawyer Walter Berry. She described Berry as "born with an exceptionally sensitive literary instinct, but also with a critical sense so far outweighing his creative gift that he had early renounced the gift of writing" (p. 108). But because Berry had found personal fulfillment in another field, he had both the sympathy and the instinct to help her. He knew how to help silence her internal critic. Wharton says that she would begin to write something in a "burst of lyric rapture" and then lose the path. Berry advised her just to write down everything she felt like telling. Once she was finished with the manuscript, "how meticulously he studied it from the point of view of language, marking down faulty syntax and false metaphors, smiling away over-emphasis and unnecessary repetitions, helping [me] patiently through the beginner's perplexities, yet never laying his hand on what he considered sacred: the *soul* of the novel, which is (or should be) the writer's own soul" (p. 115). Clearly, he served many roles, both as the object of emotional support and as the ideal editor. Wharton experienced Berry as the instrument for her expansion of herself.[5]

5. Wharton says that Berry followed her "literary steps with the same patient interest" until his death 27 years later (pp. 112–113).

Perhaps less attention has been paid to the collaboration between writer and editor than has been lavished on other kinds of creative partnerships—choreographer and ballerina, playwright and actor, composer and musician. I turn now to the formal writer-editor relationship. Burroughs Mitchell, an editor at Scribner's who overlapped with the legendary Maxwell Perkins for one or two years before Perkins died, writes that "in the act of writing a book the writer is very much alone. Various people interest themselves in what he is doing—such people as wives and husbands, editors, literary agents, critics, and, now and then, a psychotherapist; but for the most part they remain quite outside the work that holds the writer absorbed." He believes that Perkins was a great editor because he had "the ability to go inside, to enter into the writer's solitary enterprise without intruding" (p. 25). This is exactly what Berry did for Wharton.

Many writer-editor collaborations operate this way. Some are so famous that the public couples the name of a writer with his or her editor, and some collaborations work out very well. In recent years, such a successful partnership appears to exist between writer Pat Conroy and editor Nan Talese. "[Conway's] method is to write 'full-out,' as Talese describes it, 'frequently setting down all the thoughts that occur to him rather than just one or two.' What emerges is a manuscript with a meandering narrative and an overabundance of scenes, characters, subplots, and insights. The paring down and restructuring come afterward with the help of his editor. 'Nan is one of the great editors in the world and she has a great sense of structure,' says Conroy. 'I write the manuscript, then she helps me find the book that's in there'" (Berendt, 1995, p. 140). This was the *modus operandi* for both *The Prince of Tides* and *Beach Music* (Berendt, 1995; Feldman, 1995).

While the Talese-Conroy collaboration seems to work well for both, internal tensions often result in the break-up of such partnerships. Just as the Greeks warn us to "count no man happy until he is dead," there are faultlines that ultimately prove destructive to many kinds of creative collaborations, whether artistic, romantic, commercial, or psychoanalytic, and writer-editor collaborations are no exception.[6] The fol-

---

6. Often the writer is unable to credit the full role of the editor, and the editor, in turn, does not provide a holding environment for the writer. It was by chance that early in my career I saw in treatment a writer who was famous on the basis of his first novel. We had what I thought of as a rather successful treatment. Because of a curious coincidence that was to occur some years afterward, I later realized that he had spoken relatively little of his relationship with his editor. In fact, I didn't even know—or perhaps I had forgotten—his editor's name. That is how it came about that I ended up taking into treatment the person who had been the novelist's editor—the kind of situation I would

lowing brief vignettes describe how dissatisfaction may arise on the part of the author, the editor, or both.

One of the most famous writer-editor collaborations in recent literary history is that of Thomas Wolfe and Maxwell Perkins. Perkins worked with other famous writers as well, including Ernest Hemingway and F. Scott Fitzgerald, but the Wolfe-Perkins collaboration is the legendary one. Wolfe eventually dumped Perkins to seek a different editor. The irony is that their break was a result of their colossal success.

In his "Introduction" to the 1957 edition of *Look Homeward Angel*,[7] Perkins says, "The first time I heard of Thomas Wolfe I had a sense of foreboding. I who loved the man say this. Every good thing that comes is accompanied by trouble. It was in 1928 when Madeline Boyd, the literary agent, came in. She talked of several manuscripts which did not much interest me, but frequently interrupted herself to tell of a wonderful novel about an American boy. I several times said to her, 'why don't you bring it in here, Madeline?' and she seemed to evade the question. But finally she said, 'I will bring it in if you promise to read every word of it.' I did promise but she told me other things that made me realize that Wolfe was a turbulent spirit and that we were in for turbulence. When the manuscript came, I was fascinated by the scene where Eugene's father, Oliver W. Gant, with his brother, two little boys, stood by a roadside in Pennsylvania and saw a division of Lee's army on the march to Gettysburg" (Perkins, 1957, pp. viii–ix).

But then came what Perkins deemed to be some 90 irrelevant pages about Gant's life in Newport News. Turned off, Perkins gave the manuscript to his colleague Wallace Meyer to read. Meyer found still another wonderful scene, and the two of them agreed that *Look Homeward Angel* was to be an important book. Perkins cut out the first wonderful scene and the 90 or so pages that followed, to unify the story through the boy's memories.[8]

---

normally avoid. (By the time I made the connection, it was too late.) And so it was that I heard something of the collaboration from the point of view of the editor. Though the novel was a huge success, there were ego conflicts between author and editor that were never resolved. Though both derived benefits from their therapies, and each maintained a successful career, I think it a literary tragedy that they never worked together again insofar as neither of them ever again reached the pinnacle they had achieved in their joint venture.

7. The publisher received the Introduction (originally published separately in the *Harvard Library Bulletin*, Vol. 1, No. 3, Autumn 1947) from Perkins's secretary two days after the editor's death.

8. Perkins says that for years it was on his conscience that he "had persuaded Tom to cut out the first scene of the two little boys on the roadside with Gettysburg impend-

Perkins believed that the trouble between them arose when Wolfe dedicated his next novel, *Of Time and the River,* to his editor in the most extravagant terms: "I never saw the dedication until the book was published and though I was most grateful for it, I had forebodings when I heard of his intention. I think it was the dedication that threw him off his stride and broke his magnificent scheme. It gave shallow people the impression that Wolfe could not function as a writer without collaboration, and one critic even used some such phrase as 'Wolfe and Perkins—Perkins and Wolfe, what way is that to write a novel'" (p. xi).[9] Wolfe switched both editor and publisher.

According to Perkins's biographer, Scott Berg (1979), "At the base of all Wolfe's anger was the general belief that without Perkins, Wolfe was unpublishable—a writer manqué" (p. 315). Perkins, too, thought this was the basis of their rupture. My own reading is that Wolfe had depended on Perkins in too many other ways and had revealed too much to him. The very closeness of their relationship appeared to prove threatening. Not only had Perkins edited Wolfe and dissected out two viable novels, but he mentored Wolfe, nursed him, wrote and talked him through his crises, including the prolonged rupture with his mistress and benefactor, Aline Bernstein, and urged upon him (as he did upon his other authors) certain of his own favorite books, in particular *War and Peace.* In the end, the break may have come over Perkins and Scribner's settlement of a lawsuit against Wolfe, which conceded that he had appropriated someone else's life story without adequate disguise and inserted it into his novel.

But Perkins believed the switch in publishers did not serve Wolfe well,[10] and many critics concurred. In the end it appears that Wolfe, too, agreed. Dead at age 38, Wolfe made Perkins his literary executor.

An even more problematical writer-editor partnership is described by D. T. Max in a recent article about Raymond Carver and Gordon Lish ("The Carver Chronicles," *The New York Times Magazine,* 1998). In

---

ing." But he need not have fretted, because, as he later discovered, Wolfe incorporated the scene into *Of Time and the River,* and to greater effect. Perkins "began then to realize that nothing Wolfe wrote was ever lost, that omissions from one book were restored in a later one" (Perkins, p. ix).

9. As Perkins saw it, "Nobody with the slightest comprehension of the nature of a writer could accept such an assumption. No writer could possibly tolerate the assumption, which perhaps Tom almost himself did, that he was dependent as a writer on anyone else. He had to prove to himself and to the world that this was not so" (p. xi).

10. Perkins believed that as a result of switching editors, Wolfe broke "his own great plan by distorting Eugene Gant into George Webber. That was a horrible mistake" (Perkins, p. ix).

contrast to Perkins, who gave full credit to Wolfe's literary genius and saw his own role more or less the way we ideally think of an editor's role, Lish presented a very different view of what he contributed to the early works of Raymond Carver:

"For much of the past 20 years, Gordon Lish, an editor at *Esquire* and then at Alfred A. Knopf, who is now retired, has been quietly telling friends that he played a crucial role in the early short stories of Raymond Carver. The tales vary from telling to telling, but the basic idea was that he had changed some of the stories so much that they were more his than Carver's. No one knew quite what to make of his statements. Carver, who died ten years ago this month, never responded in public to them. Basically it was Lish's word against common sense. Lish had written fiction, too: If he was such a great talent why did so few people care about his own work? As the years passed, Lish became reluctant to discuss the subject" (Max, p. 34).[11] There are often such difficulties when the editor desires nothing more than to be a writer.

Because Lish sold his papers to the Lilly Library at Indiana University, a few Carver scholars have been able to look at them. On the basis of a careful examination of various stages of Carver's manuscripts and a close reading of the published works, Max has concluded, somewhat to his own surprise, that Carver's first two collections, which Lish edited heavily, differ considerably from the later two collections, which Lish did not edit. The stories that went through Lish's hands were "minimalist in style with an almost abstract feel" (p. 36). Max is of two minds. He says, "Overall, Lish's editorial changes generally struck me as for the better. . . . His additions gave the stories new dimensions, bringing out moments that I was sure Carver must have loved to see. Other changes . . . struck me as bullying and competitive. Lish was redirecting Carver's vision in the service of his own fictional goals. . . . In all cases, however, I had one sustained reaction: for better or worse, Lish was in there" (p. 38).

Max interviewed Lish, who "was still embittered . . . by the biting ingratitude of 'this mediocrity' he had plucked from obscurity." But Max points out that as Carver grew more confident, "collision was inevitable" (p. 39). Carver rebelled, in part, Max suggests, because friends had seen first drafts of the stories for his second collection, and he was afraid that in looking at the published work, post-Lish, they would note the extent of the edit. However, Carver caved in to Lish's insistence on his edit, and the book received raves. Afterwards, Carver

11. Max goes on to say, "Maybe he was choosing silence over people's doubts. Maybe he had rethought what his contribution had been—or simply moved on" (p. 34).

wrote to Lish, "I can't undergo [that] kind of surgical amputation and transplantation. . . . Please help me with this book as a good editor, the best . . . not as my ghost" (p. 40). And Lish, whatever his feelings about the limits being placed on him, accepted his new role. Although he thought of going public, he was advised against it. Carver's new book, *Cathedral*, became his most celebrated work to date.

Some of Carver's friends feel that Lish overedited as a result of unconscious jealousy. Max, though ultimately ambivalent about Lish's claims, brings to light the problems when the editor is someone whose primary ambitions to be a great writer are thwarted; usually the complementarity of the writer-editor relationship will be compromised in some way. But there are exceptions; for example, Pound's edit of T. S. Eliot. And those who have once held but ultimately renounced their writerly ambitions are often brilliant editors, the late William Shawn of *The New Yorker* being a prime example (Ross, 1998). In general, however, the Perkins-Wolfe and Carver-Lish travails catch some of the essential tension in the collaborations between writers and editors: feelings of not "owning" one's own work and fear of dependency on the part of the writer, and envy and desire for glory on the part of the editor.[12]

Carol Posegrove, a professor at Indiana University, suggests that one's opinion about the Carver/Lish question depends in part on how one regards the creative person: "If you exalt the individual writer as a romantic figure who brings out these things from the depths of his soul, then, yes, the awareness of Lish's role diminishes Carver's work somewhat. But if you look at writing and publishing as a social act, which I think it is, the stories are the stories that they are" (quoted in Max, p. 56).[13]

Lish was not the only editor infamous for overstepping editorial boundaries—insisting that the author adopt his view, overediting to the point where the book reads differently from the author's intention, and in general setting up in competition with the author. Why should this be so? Sometimes it's only the writer who is considered to be creative by the outside world, and some editors may suffer from a sense of

12. It's much the same, though perhaps to different degrees, in all genres of writing, whether fictional, biographical, historical, scientific, or psychoanalytic.

13. Max ends his essay with Carver's answer to a query from one of his students about the editor-writer relationship, listing "the famous examples of heavy editing: F. Scott Fitzgerald's cutting of Hemingway's *The Sun Also Rises*, Perkins and Wolfe, Pound and Eliot" (p. 57). Carver quotes Pound's explanation of the process: "It's immensely important that great poems be written, but it makes not a jot of difference who writes them" (p. 51).

diminishment. Yet the editor is creative in his or her own right and has a specific gift of his or her own. In fact, the best editors have no wish to take over the author's role but find gratification in their creative role as *editor.* While no work can be truly fine unless the basic ingredients are already present, in many instances it takes a brilliant edit to showcase or frame those ingredients.

Good editing is transparent, which means that the editor may help to sharpen ideas or, in fiction, help facilitate pace or the emotional flow while preserving, through transparency, the underlying integrity of the work. The editor who can read the meaning and innovativeness embedded in the work functions much as an analyst who "reads" a dream. Joel Spingarn, an editor/essayist from the early nineteen hundreds, reportedly said that the function of the editor is "to dream the poet's dream."

Thus, the editor-writer dyad is in some ways analogous to the psychoanalyst-patient dyad. The primary transference may be writer to editor or editor to writer or sometimes both, as it appeared to be with Gordon Lish and Raymond Carver. In most instances the major transference probably goes from writer to editor, where the editor starts to loom rather large in the writer's world and to assume a variety of guises/functions in his or her imagination—not exactly muse or parent figure or therapist, but bits of all—and more. But editor-to-writer transferences frequently do exist, particularly in reference to major literary figures or in the editor's dream of "hatching" a major talent.

In the most successful writer-editor collaborations there is probably always some mutual transference between writer and editor, which is analogous to the transference-countertransference in patient-analyst dyads. What this means is that it's almost inevitable that there be an emotional interaction and some degree of conflict, just as there is in therapeutic interactions.[14] I've already described the writer's resent-

---

14. I would perhaps be remiss not to mention how the process I have been describing differs from what occurs in psychoanalytic writing for journals. The strength of a journal is blind peer review, generally by three different readers, and this is presumed to guarantee the relevance and scientific scrupulousness of the paper. Often enough the paper is strengthened by incorporating ideas from the three psychoanalytic readers. But this system has its problems. I had occasion to reread a paper I had reviewed after the author had revised it in order to have it reconsidered for publication. It is customary at that stage for the reviewer to see the other prior reviews of the paper. It was startling to me that my review and one other review that were sent to the author were so diametrically opposite that the author could not incorporate both critiques. The author had been asked to include such conceptually different frameworks that his own idea, whatever its merit, was lost in the conflicting demands being made on him. The revised article was not nearly so good as the earlier one. (continued)

ment at his or her reliance on an editor and an editor's hostility toward the writer when the editor lacks a sense of his or her own creative input. One editor friend tells me that the mark of a good copy editor is sometimes extreme but sublimated hostility, so that the incorrect use of a piece of punctuation is the occasion for rage. The problems between editor and writer arise when one or the other's envy and resentment are not sublimated or resolved but enter into the relationship. In general, conflict is not the problem; the problem is the incapacity of one or the other to address the conflict and work it out or work it through—sometimes explicitly but more often preconsciously.

In the best-case scenario, the editor often senses the deeper meaning and preconscious reverberations of what the writer has produced, even when they are unknown to the writer—the editor is able to "dream the poet's dream." The editor is often able to contextualize the text and thus strengthen its overall conception. The editor may also combine, as did Edith Wharton's friend Walter Berry, emotional support with literary expertise, which in Wharton's case helped her hone her language in such a way as to carry the *soul* of her novel. How like the analyst, who provides the holding environment while helping the patient recover and/or recreate the narrative of his life. But the writer must also be appreciative of the editor, as Wharton was of Berry. This attitude parallels the response of the patient in psychoanalysis whose therapy is successful and who is able to feel gratitude to the analyst.

In many ways, then, the great editor is to the creative writer as the best analyst is to his or her patient—she lends her support to her authors and uses her own creative instincts to serve as the facilitator of the creativity and the full potential that resides within them.

BIBLIOGRAPHY

BECKER, E. 1973. *The Denial of Death*. New York: Free Press.
BERENDT, JOHN. 1995. *Vanity Fair,* July, 1995, pp. 108–141.

Writing for psychoanalytic books and writing for journals do not entail the same kind of writer-editor collaboration. In writing for journals there is less often the kind of supportive writer-editor relationship that may ideally occur for the writer of a book. This is not to say that I believe there's a fundamental problem with journal writing. Journals carry much of the forward thinking in the field. But a book sometimes has the advantage of permitting an author to look at an idea from all angles without needing to worry about quoting from *all* those who have written about the subject, but whose ideas would detract from the thesis being developed.

BERG, A. S. 1978. *Max Perkins: Editor of Genius.* New York: Thomas Congdon Books, E. P. Dutton.

BREUER, JOSEF & FREUD, SIGMUND. 1900. Studies on Hysteria. *S.E.* 2:1–309.

COEN, S. 1994. *Between Author and Reader: A Psychoanalytic Approach to Writing and Reading.* New York: Columbia University Press.

EMDE, R. 1995. Fantasy and beyond: A current developmental perspective on Freud's "Creative Writers and Day-Dreaming." In *On Freud's "Creative Writers and Day-Dreaming,"* eds. E. Person, P. Fonagy, and S. Figueira, 113–163. New Haven: Yale University Press.

FELDMAN, GAYLE. 1995. A conversation with Nan Talese. In *Publishers Weekly,* September 25, 1995, pp. 22–23.

FREUD, S. 1908. Creative writers and day-dreaming. *S.E.* 9:141–153.

———— 1935. *An Autobiographical Study.* New York: W. W. Norton.

———— 1960. *Letters of Sigmund Freud,* ed. E. L. Freud. New York: Basic Books.

GARDNER, HOWARD. 1993. *Creating Minds.* New York: Basic Books.

KLIGERMAN, C. 1972. Panel report on "Creativity" (from the 27th annual Psycho-Analytic Congress, Vienna, 1971) *Int. J. Psycho-Anal.* 54:1–30.

MAX, D. T. 1998. The Carver Chronicles. *The New York Times Magazine,* August 9, 1998, pp. 34–40, 51, 56–57.

MITCHELL, BURROUGHS. 1980. *The Education of an Editor.* Garden City, N.Y.: Doubleday.

PALEY, V. G. 1990. *The Boy Who Would Be a Helicopter: The Uses of Storytelling in the Classroom.* Cambridge, Mass.: Harvard University Press.

PERKINS, M. 1957. Introduction. In T. Wolfe. *Look Homeward, Angel.* New York: Scribner Paperback Fiction: Simon and Schuster.

PERSON, E. 1988. *Dreams of Love and Fateful Encounters: The Power of Romantic Passion.* New York: W. W. Norton.

————. 1995. *By Force of Fantasy: How We Make Our Lives.* New York: Basic Books.

ROSS, L. 1998. *Here But Not Here: My Life with William Shawn and The New Yorker.* New York: Random House.

SARTON, M. 1984. *At Seventy: A Journal.* New York: W. W. Norton.

SHENGOLD, L. 1993. *"The Boy Will Come to Nothing!": Freud's Ego Ideal and Freud as Ego Ideal.* New Haven: Yale University Press.

WHARTON, E. 1933. *A Backward Glance.* New York: Macmillan (1964).

WHEELOCK, J. H. ed. *The Letters of Maxwell E. Perkins.* New York: Charles Scribner's Sons.

DEVELOPMENT AND TECHNIQUE

Coordinating the Developmental and Psychoanalytic Processes: Three Case Reports

Introduction

SAMUEL ABRAMS, PETER B. NEUBAUER, AND ALBERT J. SOLNIT

THE PSYCHOANALYTIC RESEARCH AND DEVELOPMENT FUND SPONSORED a five-year study group on coordinating the psychoanalytic and developmental processes in children and adolescents. Some of the methods and aims of the study were described in a previous publication (Abrams and Solnit, 1998).

Early in the course of the project, it was recognized that there are significant controversies and ambiguities about the terms "psychoanalytic process" and "developmental process." Consequently, it was important to come to some consensus as to how each would be understood.

Psychoanalysis was seen as a method of inquiry that leads to the revival of past conflicts and impaired relationships within the treatment interaction. Engagement of the pathologic past through the vehicle of transferences and countertransferences leads to a specific mode of therapeutic action that entails integrating the discovered antecedent pathogens into a new view of the self and the world. The developmental process, on the other hand, was seen as a conceptual model of normal growth consisting of a sequence of anticipated organizational hierarchies that arise over time. The new developmental organizations are a complex product of maturation and the stimuli arising from the social and familial surround. They bring in transformations of earlier conflicts and antecedent phases, thereby creating changing views of the self and of the world.

19

While analysts who treat adults have found the model of the psycho-analytic process (and some of its recent variants) quite congenial for their work, child analysts have always been required to deal directly with the vicissitudes of ongoing development. One goal of the five-year study group was to sort out some of the encountered difficulties and begin to address ways to manage them. A second goal was to consider additional techniques that might assist the needs of development without necessarily compromising fundamental analytic approaches.

The method of psychoanalytic inquiry characteristically accesses un-recognized conflicts. Attempts to undo fixations and regressions and to overcome the attendant conflicts are expected aims of the treatment setting. However, with children and adolescents, the method of inquiry also accesses data about the developmental process, the emergence of new hierarchies that usher in different needs, and fresh defensive and adaptive strategies. When development has gone awry, the expected transformations of earlier conflicts and modes of relating are ob-structed. The group wondered if it was possible to identify different kinds of impairments in the developmental process and ways in which each might be addressed.

For example, it has long been known that conflicts can interfere with development. Earlier pathological conditions may be carried forth into succeeding developmental organizations without being resolved and either co-exist with maturationally induced changes or obstruct the entire process altogether. Resolution of these earlier conflicts, preferably through analysis, is necessary to free the developmental process from the severe consequent constraints.

The study group acknowledged that kind of impediment, but over time the members highlighted at least two other forms of obstruction to the progressive hierarchies as well. In one the pull forward in the process was itself weakened. This limited the opportunity for the mat-urational potential to interact with the stimuli provided by the sur-round in order to promote advanced structures. In the other, specific ego functions were so impoverished that the abilities to cull features from within and without that might provide a nucleus for the new hi-erarchies were badly burdened. In these two pathological situations, the transformational opportunities of the developmental process were sorely impaired. At the same time the opportunities for customary an-alytic work were also limited because of the unstable nature of the avail-able psychological organization. Was it possible to introduce addi-tional techniques to encourage the pull forward or to improve the impaired ego functions so as to promote the developmental process and perhaps even make conventional analytic approaches possible?

The first report of the study group concluded that developmental assists were possible and that, at least in some instances, those assists could be coordinated with the customary technical approaches that characterize analytic work. Those conclusions, however, were leveraged by logical arguments and brief anecdotes and lacked extensive clinical data that would have made them more convincing.

This chapter attempts to redress that lack.

What follows are extensive reports of three cases treated by experienced and talented child analysts. They reflect productive differences of opinion generated within a study group over many years about what might be learned about development and what the word "developmental" may mean; about the technique of child and adolescent analysis; and about unique difficulties encountered with particular kinds of children. The reports also reflect how each analyst processed the treatment of the individual child. Each freely integrated what he or she had learned into customary approaches and each formulated a unique perspective about developmental considerations and ways of bringing those considerations into clinical work.

To be sure, their approaches were influenced by the kinds of issues the group had discussed over the years, including the value of recognizing different deviations in development. Deviations arise from different determinants and may appear in different forms. Consequently, careful attention to the source and form was required in order to provide the specific kind of assistance needed to enhance development.

In general such assistance is intended to support the organization and integrative functions of the developmental process, but those functions may become burdened in different ways. Some pathology can be characterized as a primary deviation in development—e.g., a limitation of the inherent pull forward. Other interferences can be classified as secondary—i.e., consequences of impaired ego equipment or results of fixation or regression inducing pathological transformations of earlier preoedipal disorders. Etiologically different disorders may present themselves in similar ways; but, as is evident in the case reports, they require different technical approaches. The treating analysts recognized that they were required not only to be alert to such distinctions but also to acknowledge the status of the prevailing phases of the children they were treating. Children and adolescents are in the midst of growth patterns. Attending to the specifics of shifts and changes in psychic organization inspired by maturation is not generally a required part of an adult analyst's orientation. However, the prevailing phase of a distressed child and the anticipated new one very much influence the stance that child analysts assume.

Dr. Schmukler's approach is implied in her title, "Use of Insight in Child Analysis." Her patient's adolescence has been interfered with—a detour has occurred—and the analytic work she introduces is an attempt to understand the dynamic conflicts that have encumbered the anticipated progression. She illustrates a useful approach that child and adolescent analysts can implement when conflict is the principal obstruction to development.

She balances the needs of the analytic process and the developmental process in several ways. For example, one pathogenic target lies in the area of separation-individuation. Problems derived from the early mother-child relationship have interfered with the movement toward autonomy—thereby detouring the ordinary developmental expectations. As these problems are revived and dealt with in the emerging transference, the issues become less burdensome and her patient is freed to resume development.

Dr. Schmukler also recognizes that to coordinate the needs of development and analysis, there are times when the relationship can provide a "real" object as well as the vehicle to a past one. For example, Dr. Schmukler notes that adolescents need to develop the capacities to tolerate contradictions and contain fantasies instead of acting upon them. She explains that different dynamic issues (bisexuality, aggression, faulty identifications) have impaired her patient's tolerance. She assists in promoting that capacity partly by offering a model for identification and partly by helping her patient deal with the dynamic conflicts.

In an even more complex setting, Dr. Schmukler addresses the patient's emerging idealization of her. She recognizes that this idealization is necessary for the adolescent's need for object removal but that it is also a defense against aggressive trends revived within the mother-transference. She skillfully moves between these positions, putting off the engagement of the idealization to a later time in deference to the developmental need. In these and other ways, Dr. Schmukler's contribution addresses the needs of the analytic process and coordinates them with developmental assistance.

Dr. Zients's paper is more specific about therapeutic modes and outcome, partly because his patient suffers from something far more serious than dynamic conflicts. In his title, "The Psychoanalytic Treatment of a Child with Deviational Development," he describes his child as a patient with a developmental deviation. Apparently he means several things by this. He suggests, first, that the expected pull forward in development is not strong; and secondly, that certain inherent weaknesses in ego functions interfere with expectable new organizations.

Those weaknesses include synthetic capacity, engagement (he calls this the "gluing" function), and problems in internalization (probably related to those gluing difficulties). As the work moves forward, Dr. Zients notes that a great many interpretations were offered while he attempted to sustain the customary attitude that might promote transferences. In the course of the technical approach of interpreting, however, Dr. Zients concluded that some if not many of his attempts served another function—the creation of formative narratives around which new psychological emergences might organize. He notes that this was useful in helping to create a more coherent sense of self and also contributed to his patient's ability to assimilate new experiences and thereby further promote new organizations. The inherent pull forward toward more advanced organizations was facilitated as well. Interpretations and articulation of affects and ideas assisted the needs of development, not by accessing dynamic conflicts and resolving them, but by offering coherent narratives to build structures. As Dr. Zients notes, as these structures evolved, words could be attached to past conflicts, giving rise to new chances to engage the infantile struggles. In a sense, this is reciprocal to the work described by Dr. Schmukler. Dr. Schmukler understood that her work with the dynamic freed the developmental process to move forward; Dr. Zients explains that his assisting the developmental process permitted the dynamic issues to become more coherent and more readily accessible.

Dr. Olesker's case is of a boy with ego deviations. She comes to understand that her patient's developmental progression is secondarily impaired because of serious difficulties in several ego functions. She makes an important distinction between oedipal content and oedipal organization, meaning that even the most disordered youngster might experience oedipal feelings but that an oedipal organization requires that the triadic exchange be placed within an emerging coherent organization. Children with intact, albeit conflicted, oedipal organizations can be approached by way of interpretations of drives and defenses. However, the presence of oedipal content alone is not sufficient to ensure the presence of an oedipal organization.

As her work moves forward, she comes to understand that her "interpretations" are not accessing unconscious oedipal fantasies but rather are providing coherence and narrative scaffolding in a boy suffused with chaotic primitive demons that populate his world. A moving example is how Dr. Olesker works with his inability to feel in control by buttressing his capacity to be the boss of his own feelings and actions. Repetitions within the sessions serve to reinforce his sense of control. Dr. Olesker also offers examples of how she facilitated integration by taking a series of events and making them sequential for her patient in terms of cause and effect. Control functions are further promoted by clarifying neologisms and placing anger into a hierarchical order. In these and other ways, Dr. Olesker assists in his refashioning of his inner world and of his view of himself as not entirely human.

In reviewing her work, Dr. Olesker notes her shift from conventional approaches that deal with reviving past narratives to an approach of integrating, stabilizing, and organizing inner representations. Such work entails titrating the affect level so that it is strong enough to assure that it is represented but not so strong as to be disorganizing. The affect-regulation problem in this instance was also aided by her attention to her patient's unique language and how his words conveyed gradients of meanings. She also sought to build a social-interaction scaffolding through the medium of the therapeutic interaction. Dr. Olesker concludes that these assists all led to an improved object constancy, permitting growth through identifications rather than primitive introjective processes. Furthermore, they brought together the original scattered components of conflict into a more coherent form. Her work illustrates techniques that assist in the growth of ego functions and structures even in seriously disordered youngsters.

As suggested by these brief summaries, the cases that follow are rich in descriptive details and conceptual proposals. They will also provide the reader with opportunities to consider additional or even alternative approaches to the data. The growth of our discipline depends upon making available the kinds of extensive, meticulously prepared, and carefully detailed case reports such as these.

BIBLIOGRAPHY

ABRAMS, S. & SOLNIT, A. J. (1998). Coordinating developmental and psycho-analytic processes: Conceptualizing technique. *JAPA* 46, 85–103.

Treatment of a Boy with Atypical Ego Development

WENDY OLESKER, Ph.D.

A multifaceted mode of therapeutic action is delineated as the complex neuropsychological and psychogenic factors in the development and functioning of an unusual four-year-old boy became elucidated. In addition to standard technique, the author developed a variety of psychoanalytically informed ways to facilitate his growth and ameliorate deviational aspects, especially his difficulties in appreciating and responding to the social-emotional world and establishing stable, integrated mental representations of self and other. The evolving treatment process is presented as well as attempts to coordinate and harmonize analytic and developmental goals.

I DESCRIBE HERE A MULTIFACETED MODE OF THERAPEUTIC INTERVENtion, necessitated by neuropsychological and psychogenic factors in the development and functioning of an unusual child. In addition to the standard technique of interpreting conflict and compromise for-

---

Training and supervising analyst at the New York Psychoanalytic Institute; assistant clinical professor in Psychiatry (Psychology), Albert Einstein College of Medicine; adjunct professor, New York University Postdoctoral Program in Psychoanalysis and Psychotherapy.

I wish to acknowledge and thank the members of the Study Group on Coordinating Analytic and Developmental Goals, whose comments made a major contribution to my thinking. Co-Chairmen: Sam Abrams and Al Solnit; Members: Judith Chused, Donald Cohen, Alice Colonna, Theodore Jacobs, Laurie Levinson, Roy Lilleskov, Steven Marans, Peter Neubauer, Mortimer Ostow, Anita Schmukler, Anna Wolf, and Alan Zients. I especially would like to thank Anita Schmukler for her thoughtful editorial comments.

The Psychoanalytic Study of the Child 54, ed. Albert J. Solnit, Peter B. Neubauer, Samuel Abrams, and A. Scott Dowling (Yale University Press, copyright © 1999 by Albert J. Solnit, Peter B. Neubauer, Samuel Abrams, and A. Scott Dowling).

mation and of reviving and understanding unrecognized narrative meanings and structures, I created psychoanalytically informed ways of facilitating growth in my attempts to ameliorate the patient's developmental deviations.

Anna Freud (1978) distinguished primary developmental disturbances due to imbalance in the unfolding of development from neurotic disturbances initiated by frustrations at higher levels of development and characterized by the regressive search for drive satisfaction at an earlier mental level. Fonagy and Moran (1991) suggested that the greater the unevenness in development, the less effective is technique that relies solely on interpretation of conflict. We must devise strategies of analytically informed intervention to support and strengthen the child's capacities to tolerate conflict. In the following material, I specify those aspects of ego functioning that account for Don's disturbances, and I describe my ways of working with him. I then discuss my attempts to coordinate and harmonize analytic and developmental goals as they evolved in the course of his treatment and their consequences. Although one cannot generalize from one case, I hope that others may profit from what I have learned in their work with children with a wide range of deviational as well as neurotic components.

INITIAL PICTURE

Don was an attractive but extremely inhibited and withdrawn three-and-three-quarter-year-old boy when he was first brought for a psychological evaluation at the suggestion of his nursery school director. He was reportedly unable to relate to the other children, spent his time pulling erasers off pencils, and when frustrated howled and bit himself. He had not improved over the course of the school year.

HISTORY

Mother had a normal pregnancy. At a birthweight of five pounds one ounce, Don spent his first six days in an incubator. He showed unusual sensitivities to auditory and visual stimuli. The parents recalled the first year as difficult. They spent a great deal of time trying to keep Don from screaming. He was up for three hours every night and did not differentiate day from night until nine months, showing prolonged asynchrony and problems in internal regulation and organization.

The parents' differences produced so much tension between them that they eventually separated when Don was aged 15 months. Both came from divorced Jewish families. Mother had become very observant in her religious practices; she was stoic and contained and saw Don's problems as neurologically based. Father was religiously nonobservant and participated in a Reform Jewish community; he was volatile and intense and saw Don's difficulties as entirely emotionally based, a response to what the father perceived as the mother's emotional deadness and limited responsiveness.

At age two Don attended a full-day nursery school twice a week. The director of the school thought Don showed major social problems in that he treated other children as furniture and seemed oblivious to their presence. By age three the social problems had worsened: Don had withdrawn even more from social interaction, refused eye contact, made flapping, fan-like motions with his hands, and had many fears— of strangers, cats, horses. He was preoccupied with mechanical and electrical devices in which repetitive motion was prominent. He was clumsy and had always been delayed motorically. Psychological testing done later (at age ten) revealed superior functioning on the verbal level, a 150 Verbal I.Q. (98th percentile), a 105 Performance I.Q. (50th percentile), a significant 45-point discrepancy between verbal and nonverbal functioning, and delayed functioning (below the fifth percentile) in two areas. One was social judgment on a nonverbal level, in which the task is to observe a sequence of pictures and tell a sensible story. Unable to use facial cues to guide his behavior, Don was caught by unimportant irrelevant details, leading to a disjointed, unintegrated description of details with no narrative. The other area of difficulty was perceptual organization, assessed by putting together puzzle pieces of familiar objects (face, hand, car, horse). Don had difficulty identifying the object and putting the puzzle together when no model was provided, yet he functioned on the superior level when a model was provided.

Don initially seemed to show interference with the preconditions necessary for awareness of his own and others' mental life (Mayes and Cohen, 1996). He did not appear to understand that his parents had thoughts, feelings, and desires that guided their actions toward him and others or that others had thoughts, feelings, and desires different from his. He displayed impaired selective attention and could not process social stimuli; emotional stimuli lacked salience for him. Thus, he had difficulty making sense of the world of people and responding to and making sense of social information, leading to limited efforts at social engagement. In his one-sided monologues he was blind to others' reactions and did not associate their reactions with his own behavior. His attention appeared to be directed to objects engaged in repetitive motion—e.g., helicopters, revolving doors—and he could not flexibly attend to incoming stimuli. His language, although quite developed, was used not to communicate but rather to express his own thoughts and interests, with little intentional interchange and with a flat atonal pattern. He was often flooded with anxiety, unable to quiet himself. He saw the world as a frightening place, fraught with dangers. He seemed to prefer things to people. He did not attend to the implications of others' gestures and affects. Don's basic difficulties convey a limitation in establishing integrated, stable mental representations of self and other. Using DSM-IV terminology, my diagnostic impression of Don was that of Asperger's Syndrome (Asperger, 1991).

Don initially resembled an autistic child in his preoccupation with numbers and control switches, moving toward contact with doll play. During the initial evaluation he avoided eye contact and focused only on turning my space heater and lights on and off. When it was clear he could be in charge of the "on and off," he relaxed and showed enlivened affect.

Early on he displayed his unusual sensitivities. He claimed to hear a distant stereo playing music; when I listened very carefully and screened out all else, I could hear it faintly. He was overwhelmed by visual stimuli, covering his eyes when shown a design on a card. He had difficulty shifting sets, was slow to process transitions, and readily acted self-destructively, hitting and biting himself when he tried to do something and couldn't or when he was interrupted.

TREATMENT

I will report on the first four years of a four-time-a-week treatment with Don. The initial work focused on clarifying anger, the most prominent early theme, in a variety of situations. It was in this context that Don evinced obsessive-compulsive behavior by relying on letters and reciting the alphabet to give himself a sense of control when his world seemed unmanageable.

In response to my indicating that our time was up, Don began a boat game (he loved waterways and could map each one on every continent) in which he was the tour guide and called out all the stops a boat would make as it sailed around the Mediterranean Sea, for example. Asserting this pseudo-control, he seemed oblivious to my presence. He used this play when he later bumped himself. At first upset, he said that a cat had broken open, a "bad" cat, and that chemicals flowed out into the street. He then returned to the boat play but was greatly distressed when he broke an umbrella and reverted to the alphabet. Attempting to interpret his defensive response, I said that reciting the alphabet seemed to take his mind off the idea of getting broken. He stopped, smiled, and went back to the alphabet. When this failed to bring the desired relief, he invited mother in, bumped his head, bit himself, said "ate Mommy," and started to bite her. He said he "ate her all up," then put her on a chair, turned out the lights, and said he was "spinning Mommy away." I again attempted an organizing comment and said it seemed he got confused about what could happen to people, especially if they got him mad; mom got him mad when he felt she didn't pay attention to him. He seemed to think eating her up would keep her close, and saying the alphabet took his mind off the whole thing. Don agreed.

Over several sessions he worked on the theme of getting hurt, with feelings about his mother's going away being linked to his doing naughty things. When I suggested a cause and effect by saying he worried that if he did something naughty Mommy would go away or he could get hurt, he seemed to relax. He turned out the lights and said, "I'm scared at night." In an apparent attempt at mastery, he hid in the toy chest, then popped out, turned the light on, and said, "It's morning." When I once turned on the light, thinking I was helping him, he howled and bit himself. I said he got angry at me for turning on the light and showed me by howling and biting himself, but he could just tell me, I wouldn't go away or hurt him. Aided by this encouragement to verbalize, he said loud and clear, "I'm angry." I added that I thought he was afraid to get angry because he was afraid Mommy might disappear (I had been told she cleans the bathrooms when angry). He continued to work toward mastery through repetitive play by pretending to be angry at his teachers and his mother. Following this work, he seemed to dare to move closer to mother, wanted to be with her, and asked for her instead of father at times. In school, instead of withdrawing, he said to his teacher, "I'm lonely. I want you to sit with me." She readily joined him.

As Don continued to work on themes of hurt and anger, allowing my interpretive and clarifying comments, we saw improvement in his integrative capacity. Six months into the treatment he asked mother in, shot at her hat, then hid next to the refrigerator. I said he was asking mother if it was O.K. to be angry. Mother said, "It's O.K." Don tested his aggression in school by taking his shoes off and throwing them across the room. He threw toys in my office and tried to break a toy tiger's tail; I said he was testing out how much he could do and still feel safe. He brought up his fear of cats; I suggested that he put his biting, angry feelings onto cats because he could run away from cats, but he couldn't run from himself. He announced to me that "Mommy is broken"; I said that I thought he got scared when he shot her, scared that she could get hurt by his anger, she could get broken or go away. That was why he was scared to get angry at her. At home when Mother was angry, he asked her, "Did you break?" When she left the room, Don said, "Now everyone will break." He talked of wanting to "eat Mommy up" but feared that "then she'd be gone."

Following eight months of treatment Don revealed the vulnerability of his gains and the fragility of his boundaries and his sense of others' boundaries. Frustrated when building a log cabin, he turned red in the face, sucked in his cheeks as he gathered his saliva and was about to spit at me when I grabbed a tissue and said, "Hurry, put your spit in the tissue; I know spitting feels good when you feel so angry and frustrated, but this is where it goes." He covered my mouth and said, "Oh, oh . . . there are two Wendys," but couldn't explain further. I said I seemed like two different people, the calm Wendy and the hurry Wendy, which perhaps seemed angry or scary, but I was still the same Wendy. Mother reported that the next day he said to her, "Mom, I'm not you and I'm not Dad; I must be me." Soon thereafter, Mother reported that when she had shown impatience with Don for taking the vacuum cleaner apart, he grew very upset, saying, "It's not a nice day because you're angry. Do I have a hole in my nose, in my head, a hole for ballies [his word for b.m.]? I'm a different boy." I repeated this sequence to him and suggested that he felt like a different boy when he was so angry. He responded, "I won't be Don when I grow up." I clarified that he could be the same boy angry or calm, happy or sad, young or old. He seemed to calm down. That night he told Father, "I'm not an alien, I'm a boy. I feel that way when I'm angry. I'm starting to like Mom now. I used to be very angry at Mom. I'm not angry any more." Nevertheless, the focus on anger and the associated fear of object loss and body dissolution remained central for some time.

A separation from both his teacher and me 15 months into the treatment allowed further interpretation of his obsessional defense of preparing lists and reciting the alphabet to help him forget his worry that leaving would mean to leave forever because it made him so angry. After I had made a link between his fear of anger and the danger of getting hurt, he shed light on this defensive process when he told me, "People can break or leave, but letters and lists are forever."

Showing more affection toward me, he shifted his play to a focus on aggression toward the father figure. When I suggested that he wished to get away from Dad because at times Dad seemed bossy even though at other times Don felt close and safe with Dad, Don gave me a big smile. Elaborate aggressive play toward the Father followed.

After the second summer separation, the parents' divorce was finalized. Don was now just six. Mother kept the family brownstone; Dad took an apartment. The idea of Dad's moving to an apartment produced great anxiety in Don. He told me, "Dad sometimes gets angry and you never know when. You could get killed." (He told me he was scared to visit the new apartment because Dad could turn into a woman. Don wished for the change because "Women are nicer. They don't get angry so much.")

He thought at one point that Dad might break apart. We learned that he wanted Dad to break apart because he thought it was Dad's fault that Mom and Dad were now apart. He initiated a conversation in the waiting room with Dad and me, asking him who was responsible for the divorce, and adding that he thought it was the husband because he screams. Father explained that both parents made the decision after a long time of wondering what would be best for Don and for the grownups, too. He and I explained that even if the parents don't get along, they will always be Don's Mom and Dad even if they don't live in the same house.

Later on Don worried that Dad would kill him, eat him up, make him a slave, or turn him into a girl; he perceived his father's move as a threat to his sense of integrity and integration. He couldn't separate his father from the surround, fearing that his Dad would be a stranger because he was in a strange place.

After he pretended that he had built a beautiful house for Mom, he talked of Dad's getting killed. When he then verbalized his fear that Dad was going to kill him, and I suggested that he sometimes feels like killing Dad because part of him wanted Mom all to himself, he said, "Yes, but which part of me wants to get rid of Dad? My feet? My heart is medium. My lips love Dad." His focus on the literal yielded evidence of his unintegrated sense of self. Later he added, "I can't have Mom. Mom is a grownup and likes to be with other grownups."

Further fantasies with oedipal content (but not oedipal organization) emerged a number of months before the second summer vacation but intensified after his father moved out of the brownstone. I was a lizard, he was "Charging Horse," we got married, I had 17 lizard babies, he was a protective father, getting the babies food. When the babies were scared of the rain, we calmed them down. A tiger came and scared everyone, but we called the police, who came and locked the tiger up.

The therapeutic work thus far had centered on interpreting defenses against frightening impulses, which led to some calming but did not address Don's problems with integrating the chaotic, primitive, unrepressed demons that populated his world and had begun to emerge.

An added therapeutic focus was finding a middle ground between intense affect and defense, establishing a meaningful relationship, and facilitating Don's recognition and repair of some of his ego deviations, especially in the sphere of affect modulation, signal anxiety, integration of self and object mental representations, integration of affects into his world, and appreciation of how others thought and felt. I aimed to help him organize defenses in part by clarifying inner versus outer reality and by acting as an adult who could represent a reliable reality and its description.

At age six-and-a-half, he came in with a sprained ankle (which made him angry), cut up some toy money, stepped on a toy chair, which hurt his foot, and began to howl, repeatedly stepping on the chair and cutting the money. I said that when something happens that he didn't expect, he gets so angry because he doesn't feel like the boss of his feelings; he does it again and again to try to feel that he is the boss. I made a toy rabbit jump and told him the rabbit was like his feelings, jumping around, and he wanted very much for them to stop jumping. He connected with the idea. I also reminded him of earlier games of being the boss of the transatlantic ship and of the lights, by turning them on and off. Now he was being boss of his feelings. He told me that he sometimes gets stuck on making lists, especially when they have more than fifty items. I said it was important to know about what got him stuck so that he could get unstuck, and that being stuck seemed to feel like being the jumpiest person in the world. He asked me if it was more embarrassing or more scary to get stuck; I said that he seemed to worry about both and added that when he makes lists or plays the boat/geography game, he knows what's coming next, so he doesn't get stuck, that being stuck happens with things he didn't expect, like stepping on the chair. Don now laughed and stepped on a toy chair, saying, "I didn't get stuck because I made it happen, I was the boss of it. Loud noises take me to 'stuck' automatically. The day you go on vacation is the end of the world, year 3000." He later added that he didn't like to play with other kids because they did things he didn't expect and didn't do what he liked.

Fears of death, rats, tigers, bats, poison, and going to boarding school surfaced before my Christmas vacation. In his fantasy play lizards were taken to a museum of poisonous animals. They made their own poisonous animals, deadly crabs that exploded all over the house. I became an eel baby and my mother, who protected me from crabs, died. Another eel killed me, ate me, and pooped me out, so I became a turd. A grizzly bear bit my arm and killed me; I got bitten by a spider and died; a ferret ate its babies. Don became a poisonous snake. I died and he ate me.

In an effort to help Don with integration, I said that he was so angry at me for going away he wanted to destroy me, put his poop into me, give me all the things he feels are so terrible about him, see if I could take it, and eat me up so I could never leave him again. Don then turned passive to active by taking trips and leaving me. I said I could see how he felt about my leaving. He started to pick his nose and said, "I do this when I'm angry. I used to feel like I was going to fall apart, but not my whole body now, just my feelings get jumpy like the toy rabbit." He crawled under the desk and told me he was getting away. When I asked what he was getting away from, he told me he was getting away from "sad." Later he said he was afraid his angry feelings would make me disappear. He recalled the calm Wendy and the hurry, angry Wendy and talked of Mom and Dad being the at-home Mom and the executive Mom, Dad the hurry Dad and the calm Dad. After my return it took some time for Don to reconnect. He told me that it felt as if the whole world had fallen down when I was away. He had wanted to stay with me in a hotel for eternity.

Tension between the parents escalated while they were deciding on the appropriate school for Don. Don was now seven-and-a-half. He said he and a classmate were under threat of floating out of the classroom and that, once in space, meteorites go very fast. He grew omnipotent in the face of his anxiety and anger, telling me that he could turn lead into tin and people into meteors. When I suggested that he put his angry feelings onto the meteors to get rid of the anger inside him, but then grew scared of the meteors so it didn't really help him to feel better, he told me he was scared, got onto my lap, and genuinely turned to me for comfort.

A somewhat more organized period followed, centered around feelings toward Father. When I acknowledged his perception of his father's intense and difficult anger, Don told me it was bad to feel angry. When I said that everyone feels angry some of the time, he said he had an anger meter inside him and that "ploook" was the loudest; sometimes there were whispers that he couldn't even hear. He explained further: "Mom goes 'verwonk' if I eat ham. It is 'verwink' if I spill juice on the table. 'Ploook' is the angriest you can get when you want to kill someone." Then, "Dad put me in my tornado room when I asked if dinner was going to last forever. Dad went 'ploook.' A murderer followed Dad." I said that when Dad punishes him, it sometimes makes him furious, like a storm inside; he felt so angry he felt like killing Dad. Don replied that it scared him that Dad turned into a tyrant, making him afraid he'd never turn back. Mom could be bossy too. Sometimes he was afraid Dad would turn into a scary lady in a black dress, a witch.

With my help, he made a chart of the different levels of anger, assigning numerical values to "verwink," "verwonk," and "ploook" and to "jumpy 'toy rabbit' feelings" (anxiety): "tidar"—least scared; "casub"—being in the dark; "maratick"—scary movies; "sacara"—Halloween; and the jumpiest, "bukartack"—a nuclear explosion. At the end of the session he told me, "This session should go down in history." Don's language system helped make his feelings less frightening and more playful and manageable, and it aided communication by allowing him to make careful distinction between feelings. With this language he shared his private world with me and felt understood, a great help when he is very angry or anxious in that he feels less alone and overwhelmed by his feelings. By using the terms "bukartack" or "ploook" when appropriate, he or I have facilitated the control function. That day he told me he went "verwink" because it was the end of the session. I could increase his attentiveness by alerting him that I was going to say something that might make him "bukartack" but only for a short time. He could laugh and listen rather than tune me out, feeling prepared and confident he could handle what I had to say (See Katan, 1961; Pine, 1976).

Now I learned a good deal more about Don's inner life, which at first had seemed populated by unreal, other-worldly characters to whom overwhelming things happened for no apparent reason. No one was safe. People were devoid of feelings, wishes, and intentions. Things just happened. He was in the sub-basement, changing elevators; it went down to the Haunted Huxley, a scary cave with ghosts. There was a nuclear plant with toxic wastes; a witch caught a kid, Frank (who teases him). He elaborated a fantasy with red vultures and Draculas who set fire to anything with red on it. He told of a rat giving birth to a vampire and marrying a vampire. After much repetition, I learned to find the affect triggering the overwhelming visual imagery of his inner world.

By age seven-and-three-quarters the story of himself as universal soldier took center stage after his father had set a limit about candy: "If you saw it, you would think I was part man and part machine." I remarked that part of what makes it hard to tell what is real and what is not is that when he is angry, as at Mom's or Dad's limit-setting, he tries to get so far away from what he feels that he no longer feels real and alive. He replied that sometimes when Dad got angry, he didn't seem human, but like a mechanical man; he hadn't put his raincoat on and Dad got so angry. Later on he told a story of a woman who had a robot come to her house; she liked it so much she called it her husband. Initially he'd experienced himself as a computer, with no feelings. Loud noises made him "escape" right away. Over time he felt less need to push "escape" so immediately, began to feel more real and alive, and grew to understand his use of depersonalization—"I used to get so far from my feelings, especially my killing feelings, that I didn't feel like a real boy."

As I familiarized myself with Don's inner world, his images seemed to be translatable into emotions and meanings. Some examples convey his concreteness vividly. They also underscore his literal interpretations, his visual thinking, as well as the instability of his mental representations (or inability to integrate positive and negative feelings toward the same person). People are transformed into different beings when he is angry but are changed back when his anger subsides. One day in school he was hungry, talked loudly, and was asked to sit in the hall. He described his experience: "I heard a clap of thunder and a flash of lightning. My teacher turned into a cobra, a costume flicked on." Angry at his teacher when he was told to do some extra work because of his poor handwriting, he said the teacher had turned into a werewolf; she would still be a werewolf in June, but in the fall she would be back to being Mrs. Goldberg.

Another deviation in Don's functioning was taking a word out of context and turning it into a thing. When I was empathizing with his disappointment in his parents' divorce, he fixed (stuck) on the word "disappointed," took it out of context, and claimed I was saying he had a pointy head. When someone called him a snot-head, he got furious because "that's as if I am only a head."

Don presented me with a range of fantasies, some about shy dogs that get eaten by vultures, many about tyrants and battles. I tried to extract a coherent story that addressed his emotional concerns. Slowly, by age seven-and-three-quarters, a tale emerged about an iguana egg being put into a woman. Maxwell Jackson was born and then came Sam, an iguana. Sam could have turned human if he took his blood out, but he didn't want to. Maxwell had a wife, Meg, and eleven children—six boys and five girls. It took twenty years for Maxwell to learn Sam's signals. Sam felt lonely; his only friend was Maxwell. He was an alien.

I enthusiastically helped nurture the development of this story, not only for its transference implications, but also because it captured something so fundamental about Don and his experience of the object world, his sense of alienation and labored connection. I helped Don connect with the emotional essence of the story, organize and develop it, develop empathy for Sam and the family members, and return to the story when he was caught by superfluous details about letters, outer space, or whatever. We followed the adventures of the Jackson family for years. Constructing and playing with this narrative helped

Don make sense of his own family in a more coherent way, allowed us to explore his feelings of alienation and then his growing pleasure in feeling intimate and understood, and provided a vehicle for the expression of the gains in inner organization.

Details of his work on his parents' divorce provide a sense of our interaction. An argument between the parents in front of Don, now almost eight, seemed to catch his attention, and his response revealed the process he engaged in as he attempted to master what seemed incapable of integration. He told me that he had had other parents from California, who left him in child care when he was three days old. Their plane crashed, and a neighbor heard him and took him into her family. I said he hated it so much when Mom and Dad fought that he wished he had a different family. Don told me he feared that his father was going to kill his mother and he wished to be adopted; this led to much discussion about his feelings about his parents' divorce.

At one point we spoke to Don's mother in the waiting room so he could ask her questions about the divorce. Mother gave an example of why she and Don's father couldn't get along. When Don was a baby, she was working at her potters wheel, and Don began to cry. She expected Father to comfort him since he was closer to Don. Father was enraged at her for not putting down what she was doing. Don now asked her, "It's your fault that you got Dad so angry. Why didn't you stop?" She again explained that Dad was closer to Don. Don responded, "But it's Dad's fault that he can't control himself." To my comment that he seemed to feel each parent bore some of the blame, to my empathy with his wish for a family that would be together, to my reminder that he couldn't control someone else—I jumped the "toy rabbit"—but he could control himself, Don said, "Dad should have come here [to my office] when he was young."

Don's perception of the world as dangerous persisted in many contexts. Meg Jackson, Maxwell's wife, fell in a hole, storms and fires broke out. Mechanical children were built, and Don insisted I not tell the secret that they were not real. I ventured that he was still so angry from thinking about his parents' divorce that he felt like killing both of them; that scared him so much that he got far away from his rage and then didn't have any feelings at all; and this made him feel not real, like a mechanical boy. What helps someone feel real is when they can let themselves know what they feel. Here I was identifying and verbalizing his feelings, using interpretation and serving as an auxiliary ego.

Don talked of insane men and of killing. To my response that his feelings of violence and rage emerged when he was scared of wanting to kill Mom and Dad for getting a divorce, a new, more cohesive story line developed. In it, Maxwell Jackson and his family moved out West and overcame many natural disasters, in part by working together. This was interspersed with thoughts and feelings about his parents' divorce: "Mom didn't follow Churchill and not surrender. Dad gave up trying to work things out with Mom." He became catastrophic: "I feel dead. I don't have a family at all. I am all alone. I hate Mom and Dad. If I don't have a family that lives together, I wish I were never born." Tearfully he said, "Mom and Dad are very bad, but it could be a lot worse."

Don struggled with the wish to find another family. He wanted to be kidnapped; stepfathers were bastards and stepmothers were bitches. He wanted me to be a magician, to bring the family together. If his father had been adopted he would be a different person and would have stayed with Mom. If Mark (Mother's boyfriend) became his stepfather, he would become a bastard and remain one even if Mark and his mother got divorced. He never liked me after the separation; he needed a real magician.

Externalizing his anger, he dumped some grapes on the floor and began squashing them. I took them from him, which made him furious. He asked if I was going to starve him; was it going to be a "grape famine"? I replied that he could have the grapes when he was able to eat them and not step on them; I empathized with his anger at my restricting his activities and the limits of my power and told him I could help him with his feelings about the divorce even if I couldn't change his parents. I added that if he liked Mark now he would probably still like him after he married his mom. Don responded that Mom could have tried to stop the arguments but Dad got too angry and Mom wouldn't stop. Dad could have tried to stop being angry and Mom could have tried to stop the arguments. He reflected that some kids are born divorced and some don't even know who their father or mother is and some are even born without mothers. He couldn't remember his parents ever being together without fighting. Mother had explained to Don that Dad didn't like who she was as he got to know her. His interpretation was that Mom was in disguise, she was wearing a mask. When I remarked that he seemed confused as to whether the disguise was like wearing a costume and noted that what was hidden had to do not with the way she looked but with her ways of doing things and her inner life—her ways of experiencing, thinking, and feeling—Don said that he wanted to start all over again as a tiny baby. He added, "Dad was like a criminal when he got so angry. He lied to Mom. He said he would work it out, but he couldn't take it. Dad exaggerated Mom in a way. He called her a robber. She wanted to try to get along. He had a hard time trying. He wasn't comfortable."

I told him that I thought he had given himself a chance to think over the divorce more and more and that helped him. I even mentioned the idea of giving himself a "time out" as an opportunity to think about things independently—to try to know his own thoughts and not get stuck in a rage storm. I thought this technique might help him develop the capacity for delay, provide a chance for inner reflection before impulsive action, differentiate surface behavior from inner life, and help him retain anxiety as a signal rather than a cue to rush to panic and action. He acted this theme in play with his version of the Titanic disaster. He was going back in history and reworking. The captain was taking a vote with his crew about whether to go ahead full speed and given one minute to make a decision. As part of his fantasy I said, "Think it over, don't just vote. You can't think when the toy rabbit is jumping." Six crew members thought it over but one went to "full speed" automatically. The ship hit an iceberg and sank. When I asked how he might want to change his own history, Don said there was no way to stop the divorce.

DISCUSSION

A multidimensional mode of therapeutic intervention, with an emphasis on promoting development and organization, was needed for this disorganized boy. At first I treated Don predominantly using a traditional conflict pathology model, with a focus on interpreting conflict and compromise formation. I soon realized that my interventions were confusing or didn't reach him and that Don's perceptual oversensitivity, his difficulty perceiving social cues, his restricted thinking, and his very reactive nervous system had resulted in substantial difficulties in processing stimuli. In attending to these issues, I drew upon my knowledge of development to create a variety of psychoanalytically informed ways of working with him in addition to standard technique. My intent was to facilitate workable defenses that would allow him to experience himself as a whole, integrated, real person, able to differentiate inner perceptions from outer reality and to organize his object world. Given his insensitivity to or tremendous difficulty with processing emotional information, especially subtler emotions, the task of integrating, stabilizing, and organizing inner representations was overwhelming. He could not experience people with sufficient clarity to incorporate and integrate images of them—objects could be changed, turn into robots or mechanical men, be blown apart or away before opportunities for comfortable relatedness emerged. This might lead to difficulties with identification and internalization—processes essential to psychic structure formation, affect tolerance, and reality testing. Don couldn't understand his experiences, so together we developed narratives of experience in both the office and his fantasies. This method made his past clearer and more meaningful. (The contribution from his parents, themselves with such different ways of coping, must not be minimized.) The key to our work was dealing with Don's affective life. He did not understand what he felt and often did not perceive cues to what others were feeling, so he had no reliable guide for negotiating relationships. He did not initially understand that the actions and words of others reflected and were motivated by feelings. He did not realize that mental life was different from the sensory perceptual world (Mayes and Cohen, 1996).

Because of Don's difficulty in processing and modulating emotions, I had to help him make his feelings loud enough to be heard and felt, yet soft enough so as not to overwhelm him. I exaggerated feelings as I participated in his play; at other times, when his shame, hurt, depression, anxiety, or anger grew too intense, I helped him process his feelings by facilitating displacement and externalization. In what might be characterized as "the analyst as a developmental object," I was Don's affective memory, reminding him of his positive feelings when he was in a rage at a parent or of his negative feelings when he could not anticipate potential disappointment with a peer who repeatedly treated him with disdain. Through this work, Don was able to synthesize and integrate objects as whole and stable representations.

Our work with Don's unique language ("verwink," "verwonk," "ploook") helped to ameliorate his affect-modulation problem by building in small increments so that Don could function more on a signal basis rather than being overwhelmed by his feelings. My helping him to articulate his deep and complex feelings and to translate his often intense visual imagery into feelings enabled him to modulate, delay, and channel his affects. This led to gains in self-regulation, an improved sense of mastery, and a corresponding reduction in extreme and primitive defensiveness, such as obsessive-compulsive behavior, withdrawal, depersonalization, denial, and splitting. For example, his talk of fires could be translated and modulated by a realistic discussion of what initiated his anxiety (e.g., he was afraid Mother would ignore him when working at her pottery). The image of overwhelming storms that seemed to come out of nowhere—an image that caused Don to obsessively recall the boating report for every date of the year—and his preoccupations with bombs and uranium led to my showing him the personal cause of such thoughts. For example, he felt explosively enraged about my vacation and through projection thought that I wanted him out of my way.

Slowly Don began to associate sharing feelings with me with dissi-
pating his distress. I focused on his feelings toward me and what he
thought mine were toward him to help him maintain a focus on those
feelings, which otherwise would diffuse. Such work helped to stabilize,
buttress, and anchor his representations by imbuing them with more
fused energy, interest, and affect. In a sense I was trying to build in social affective scaffolding for his elaborate cognitive processing, helping him to organize, sequence, and contain affects through verbalization.

Narrative structuring was most important for facilitating psychic integration. We underscored the affectively important aspects of his communications. I had to provide a better frame for order and containment than his obsession with lists and letters. I had to stay with his
experience, clarify his false, distorted perceptions, and help construct
and offer a picture of his experience because he had no picture of his
own that was coherent, meaningful, or stable. Since he could easily fly
off in all directions, owing, in part, to his developmental deviations, I
acted as an auxiliary ego function.

My first steps were to help clarify and contain his perceptions and
then stabilize representations by helping him appreciate how his anxiety over aggression made him feel that he or others were endangered
or destroyed. Next came the task of developing coherent narratives
leading to internal regulatory structure. By extracting a coherent story
from his chain of disorganized associations and affectively registering
with his protagonists by questioning how they felt and why they did
what they did, I helped to integrate coherent representations and a
more understandable narrative, leading to a greater degree of organization. I selected what I felt I could work with, what I felt was most emotionally meaningful and pressing to him: his hopes, wishes, and affects.
In subtitling what he did, reflecting about why, and verbalizing the sequence, I helped him weave together his feelings and ideas in the context of our relationship. I could participate in this process only after
Don had come to integrate me (the two Wendys) as someone he could
trust and relate to and with whom he could talk. Early on, when I tried
to participate by turning on the light when he popped out of the toy
chest, he reacted strongly by howling and biting himself. As I came to
be viewed as a sustaining, containing object, neither too far nor too
close, he could use our life in the office together to better integrate his
world, both inside and outside. We established areas of consensus on
what was happening and how to work things out, which led him to learn
about his feelings with me: "That's not right, but it's close," he indicated with satisfaction. He developed an attachment to me, and, again,

as a child might with a primary object, he internalized aspects of my ways of coping with his feelings rather than holding fast to rigid maneuvers to gain a sense of safety. He could see me with my limitations: no magician but still of help.

I worked with Don's integrative and synthetic difficulties by helping him hold in mind his ambivalence toward me, as evinced in the two Wendys and his punitive teacher, who was a werewolf in June but by fall would be a regular person again. In each case we could talk about the mixed feelings that made it seem that the person changed into something else and how frightening that was. Don's gradually developing object constancy could allow for identifications with the analyst rather than a more primitive introjective process. I helped him integrate his shifting images of me as a tyrant, a witch, by staying calm in the face of his rage, interpreting what precipitated his reactions and why; slowly his sense of my benevolent presence grew more integrated, increasing over time as his drive balance and subsequent available drive fusion improved. By establishing a midground with me, he could separate himself from his parents and look at each of them with their different ways of treating him and viewing the world. He came to see his father as a person with his own likes and dislikes: "Mom didn't stop her pottery when I was crying. Why didn't she? Maybe if she had come from a different family, she could have." Or "Dad said Mom stole something, but he just exaggerated Mom in a way." We paid attention to the confusion he felt given the very different messages he was often getting from his parents. He was able to say what he thought was right or wrong with less fear that either parent would disappear or turn into a something or someone else.

Identification with me and the developmental progress that accompanied it promoted the revival of earlier pathological relationships and the regressive transference. At times I was viewed as a cold, unresponsive mother or a tyrannical father/mother. At other times his images were disorganized, archaic, compelling, fluid creatures: "Those scary monsters in the dream are my parents. I'm so mad at them" (attesting to his ability to connect real-life experience with his representations in his inner world). He may have found for the first time a symbiotic relationship in which I was part of him. At such times his commands were as if to himself. He tried to control me through bullying as he felt his parents at times did to him.

The therapeutic action involved tackling Don's dynamic constellation too. While my work did not often extend to relieving the repressed, interpretation did convey a belief in conflict and an attempt to link or bring together in awareness its various scattered components.

His oral-aggressive fantasies of devouring me and his anal-sadistic desire to put his excrement into me and destroy my body, my office, and even my neighbors had as counterpoint persecutory fears of being poisoned, eaten up, and destroyed for his badness. Initially he tried to control and defend against these fantasies by the use of obsessive-compulsive rituals. In our long path toward a less primitive way of coping, he externalized terrible things within himself and tested my capacity to deal with his direct aggression. I repeatedly showed him how he used his neurocognitive problems in the service of defense. For example, I showed him that his defense of making feelings unreal to control them led him to turn people into weird creatures—robots, universal soldiers; he confirmed his understanding by telling me that when Dad got very angry he seemed like a "mechanical man." When Don's anger was projected and caused the world to appear as a hostile, destructive place, I helped locate the anger in himself, not in meteors or tyrants. I discovered meaning hidden within his hypertrophied, decontextualized knowledge; I suggested to him that fracturing his perceptions and focusing on an out-of-context detail served to avoid the emotion of sadness or anger, as did, for example, his confusion between disappointment and pointed head, or between snothead and being only a head. I showed him how using the intellectual sphere and treating words like things (the opposite of putting words to things) helped protect him from the anger and narcissistic hurt he feared would be so destructive. Don knew of the dangers, but had not known what set them off or his ways of dealing with them.

At the beginning of treatment, because some material suggested a higher level of organization, I spoke too much to his castration anxiety and not enough to his body-dissolution fears. When he fell on top of me and fantasied about cut-off fingers, or when he tried to open my blouse and spoke of a bird getting its wings clipped off, or when he played out building a house for Mom followed by destruction, and I interpreted, either in the transference or in the family, that part of him wanted Mom or me to himself and feared Dad wouldn't like it or that Don might get hurt or punished, he focused on concrete parts: "Which part wants to get rid of Dad—my feet?" He functioned on this concrete and literal level, unable to understand symbolic triadic organization. He was struggling with the basics of feeling real and alive, not with oedipal dynamics, when he had the fantasy of a woman bringing home a robot which she liked, so she decided to call it her husband. Oedipal content was present, but Don's world was one of unstable self and object mental representations: to wish Dad away meant that he would be turned into a different person. While there were fragments of sexual fantasies and behaviors—for example, the birth fantasy—"A spirit goes up and comes down into a woman, and she goes to the hospital to pick out a baby" or "You go up to heaven when you die and get born a girl"—attempts to follow such fantasies early on led to a diffusion rather than a deepening of material and to elaboration of undigested primary-process material that seemed to go nowhere. A "turd" would not be contained as something inside the body that comes out with pleasurable and unpleasurable feelings but devolved quickly into stream-of-consciousness associations of unpleasure. Basic body boundaries and a sense of wholeness needed development before Don could construct, elaborate, and explore more coherent fantasies.

Don contended with superego representatives as well. His growing knowledge that controlling his behavior because it might displease the other or embarrass himself and not because something terrible will cause him to die suggests the beginning of more benign superego development.

There were a number of shifts, maturation-developmental acquisitions guided by me, in the course of treatment: the development of object constancy, empathy, shame, intrapsychic defenses, and the move into latency. At the start of Don's treatment his object relatedness was substantially impaired as was his object constancy; although I was in the room, he did not invest me with interest or attention. By the second summer separation, when Don was five and three quarters, he responded to my absence with a sense of my existence: he asked for me, wrote me a postcard, and called me on the phone once or twice. He could evoke an image of me even when he was angry at me; I was no longer felt to be a "different" Wendy when I was gone. Before he had seemed to have a sense that the world could explode at any point, that anger could break him or another apart, that anyone could easily be killed or made to turn into someone else. He gradually grew better able to organize his representations with integration, clarity, and stability. He had a clearer sense of himself as an "I," felt whole, and professed less intense anxieties—"Now I worry that I could hurt my leg, not my whole self." His splitting diminished, and he tolerated separations more easily. Following much work on his sense that there were two Wendys, two dads, two moms, he announced—very pleased with himself: "Dad, you're you, Mom is Mom, and I'm me." At age six and a half he talked about his differentiation from his father: "Dad doesn't like Mom's family. But I do. He doesn't know them like I do."

Around the same time he showed his first signs of empathy, quite a shift from his previous obliviousness to the feelings of others. Following the accidental loss of his transitional object, a teddy bear, and the

fact that he had been able to stay in my office alone without his father
for a few days, he worried that Father was not O.K. being alone, and
brought him a teddy bear from my office. I don't think this was projection since it appeared that Don's father may have preferred to stay
in the sessions while Don was clearly ready to have him leave. Later on
Don could take another perspective, see himself through the eyes of
others, question the motive for someone else's behavior, and figure out
how to get along in his class. He told me that one boy didn't like him
because he talked too loud. He was upset with his teacher because he
could tell that she preferred two other children to him; this made him
feel jealous, hurt, and angry.

By the middle of the third year of treatment (age six and a half), I
witnessed the emergence of a new affect—shame. Don externalized
his anxiety by playing with a "jumpy" toy rabbit. After an affect storm
because he felt his classmates did not recognize and appreciate his
"boating memory," he asked me despairingly, "Is it shameful to get that
jumpy and feel so stuck?" He was aware of his outburst and of other
people's reactions and hated to feel he couldn't control himself. About
four months later shame followed messing and not having bodily control of urination and defecation. He introduced the topic by referring
to the disgrace of his dog, which made messes; play involving spilling
and wetting became central themes in my office and at home. By playing with messing, he learned to feel more the boss of his "messy" feelings, establishing firm bowel and bladder control.

By the beginning of the fourth year of treatment (age seven), Don
had developed a range of intrapsychic defenses, including intellectual
defenses in which he used language to modulate and titrate his feelings instead of going into a panic or the stereotyped obsessional reciting of the alphabet, making lists, or reciting of boat stops—the beginning of his use of signal affects. He could use his special words
("bukartack," "maratick," "tidar") as an anxiety signal, allowing him to
institute new defenses, coherent fantasies, which stopped the quick
move into panic.

By the fourth year (age eight), Don moved into latency coincident
with feeling more powerful physically. He seemed more in touch with
his bodily feelings and more aware of his body in space. He seemed
more motivated to have relationships with peers. He wanted a friend
to sleep over. The two put a sign on the door of his room: "For Boys
Only." He was interested in team sports, how the Knicks were doing,
and was taking in not only the teacher at school but classmates as well.
He understood the need to negotiate with others. He felt sad because
he was going to a new school and two friends would not be going with

him. He was aware of who could do what well: "Jon is good at painting, but he is one year older than I am"; he didn't like another child in his class, Fred, because he talked about treasures, not feelings. He didn't like to play with a blind girl because she couldn't see him. When I said that sometimes when he plays he doesn't see others, he replied, "Oh, no, I want to play with them. I have to look."

Because I saw Don's developmental deviations and unconscious conflicts as overlapping and not sequential, I buttressed integrations when they were failing and approached the unconscious (or its split-off parts) when the ego was more available. Often there was insufficient repression; I brought into his awareness and linked up the fears and dangers set off by his wishes, his fear of punishment, and his attempts to deal with reality. It did not seem to matter in terms of my work with him whether the drive derivatives were actually unconscious or simply not linked or organized. Don began to experience conflict between his opposing wishes and his fear of punishment in addition to his structural difficulties (i.e., affect tolerance, signal anxiety, object constancy).

At the outset of treatment Don's lack of integrative capacity and his tendency toward fragmentation meant that his compromise formations were of a different order from most others. Dangers were exacerbated by fears of total annihilation and disintegration, unchecked by a stable sense of reality. Punishing components were extreme for anything less than perfection. His defenses were primitive and disruptive, including splitting and depersonalization, and his drive derivatives were experienced as unusually intense. Through treatment, Don was able to find more comfortable compromises, allowing for more pleasure, less fear of punishment, more consideration of reality, and a gradual relinquishing of his sense of omnipotence and maladaptive defenses.

Initially, Don did not have the preconditions necessary to establish oedipal organization: delay capacity, integrative capacity, stable self and object mental representations. His body representation remained chaotic, diffuse, and undifferentiated until well into latency. He had not even traversed some of the earliest and most basic steps on the developmental line as outlined by Yorke and Burgner (1980), from primarily body discharge to internalization and the development of signal anxiety. By magical means Don was trying to achieve a degree of safety and security and to ward off threats of catastrophic disintegration (Sandler and Jaffe, 1965). The internal dynamics first had to be organized into coherent integratable narratives before the signal function of anxiety could be stabilized. Don could then develop a clearer sense of reality and cause-and-effect relationships, leading to the establishment of predominantly secondary-process thinking. With this in better order, interpretation of the transference and work on organization, synthesis, and object stabilization could be complementary and not confusing. I was aware of the role of conflict throughout this treatment as Don struggled to put his world together. Since I could represent both a developmental object and a transference object without one interfering with the other, in time Don has come to know and understand his mental life.

BIBLIOGRAPHY

ASPERGER, H. (1991). Autistic psychopathy in childhood. In U. Frith (ed.) *Autism and Asperger's Syndrome.* New York: Cambridge University Press.
FONAGY, P., & MORAN, G. (1991). Understanding psychic change in child psychoanalysis, *Int. J. Psycho-anal.,* 72:15–22.
FREUD, A. (1978). The principal task of child analysis. *Bull. Hampstead Clinic* 1:11–16.
KATAN, A. (1961). Some thoughts about verbalization in early childhood. *Psychoanal. Study Child,* 16:184–188.
MAYES, L., & COHEN, D. (1996). Children's developing theory of mind, *JAPA,* 44, 1:117–142.
PINE, F. (1976). On therapeutic change: Perspectives from a parent-child model. *Psychoanal. Contemp. Science* 5:537–569.
SANDLER, J., & JOFFE, W. (1965). Notes on obsessional manifestations in children, *Psychoanal. St. Child,* 20:425–438.
YORKE, C., & BURGNER, M. (1980). A developmental approach to the assessment of obsessional phenomena in children, *Dialogue,* 4:38–48.

Detours in Adolescent Development

Implications for Technique

ANITA G. SCHMUKLER

Dora's six-year analysis began when she was sixteen. In presenting this material, I shall focus on coordinating the technical demands of working analytically during a period of intense developmental change. This affords us an opportunity to examine the adolescent's use of analytic interventions both for work with neurotic conflicts and to facilitate development. A central issue in my work with Dora has been to examine her potential for navigating the tumultuous currents of adolescence while maintaining sufficient neutrality and abstinence so that later in the treatment, as the patient approached young adulthood, the analysis could be conducted in a manner consistent with our usual work with adults.

Training and supervising analyst at the Institute of the Philadelphia Association for Psychoanalysis; clinical assistant professor of Psychiatry at the University of Pennsylvania Medical Center; practitioner of both child and adult analysis.

I am grateful to the members of the study group, sponsored by the Psychoanalytic Research and Development Fund, whose cogent inquiries contributed to my thinking about the coordination of development and conflict. Members: Sam Abrams and Albert Solnit (coordinators), Judith Chused, Donald J. Cohen, Alice Colonna, Theodore Jacobs, Laurie Levinson, Roy Lilleskov, Steven Marans, Peter Neubauer, Wendy Olesker, Morton Ostow, Anna Wolff, and Alan Zients. I am also indebted to Denia Barrett and Drs. Walter Troffkin and Martin Silverman, friends and colleagues, for their invaluable editorial suggestions and thoughtful, insightful comments in discussions during the preparation of this paper.

The Psychoanalytic Study of the Child 54, ed. Albert J. Solnit, Peter B. Neubauer, Samuel Abrams, and A. Scott Dowling (Yale University Press, copyright © 1999 by Albert J. Solnit, Peter B. Neubauer, Samuel Abrams, and A. Scott Dowling).

DORA'S PARENTS MOVED THEIR FAMILY FROM BUENOS AIRES WHEN DORA, the youngest of five daughters, was eighteen months old. The purpose of the move was for her father to pursue advanced training at the Mayo Clinic. Ultimately the family remained in the United States; they moved to the Philadelphia area when Dora was thirteen. They consulted with me when Dora, at sixteen, threatened to quit high school and intimated that she might commit suicide.

Dora's acute distress occurred after she had missed two weeks of school following a planned family trip abroad. Upon returning to classes, she felt that she had fallen so far behind in her work that she would be unable to regain her prior academic standing. She appeared terrified of losing the respect of her industrious and academically talented peers. Dora had seemed moody during the preceding year, but her parents felt that her distress during the two weeks preceding their request for consultation was dramatic, frightening, and uncharacteristic of their daughter. Immediately upon return to school, Dora began for the first time to cut classes. Alternatively, she sought unpopulated nooks of the school building in order to read her favorite books undisturbed, an activity in which she had always found solace.

Dora, an attractive sixteen-year-old, appeared very sad when we first met. Tearfully, she said that she couldn't possibly complete all the schoolwork she had missed. She said that she differed from her parents and her four siblings, all of whom were somewhat volatile emotionally and "not so perfectionistic" as she. Dora, in contrast, felt impelled to achieve a very high standard of academic perfection and felt she could not meet that goal now that she had "screwed up." As she spoke, her sadness was quickly replaced by anger. She was furious to have missed so much schoolwork for a family excursion that was "not [her] fault." At the same time she told me that she hated school and any activity in which she felt forced, like studying. Dismissing her earlier intensely motivated goal of pursuing advanced education, Dora decided that she wanted to be an available mother. In this context, Dora assured me that her inward conviction was of greatest import and that a college degree would be, at the very least, superfluous.

Within days of Dora's birth, Mrs. L. became depressed. She longed for her family in Argentina and was especially distressed when she permitted herself to acknowledge that her own mother, who had died immediately after Dora's birth, would never see her youngest grandchild. In spite of her marked sadness, Mrs. L. reported that being with her newborn cheered her. Mrs. L., a professional woman, returned to part-time work on the third month following her delivery and engaged her elderly, somewhat obsessional, widowed aunt, a recent immigrant to the United States, to care for Dora. The aunt introduced toilet training considerably earlier and somewhat more rigidly than Mrs. L. would have preferred. This provided us with clues to understanding Dora's early experiences: obeying, acting reflexively, without negotiation or even thought, and responding with unmodulated aggression over experiencing what she perceived as "feeling forced."

From the time Dora was 18 months old, Mrs. L. interpreted her frowns as "blaming" her mother for "inadequacies." At times Mrs. L. perceived these unhappy facial expressions as a form of punishment by her newborn, which included religious and superstitious elements. From that point on, Mrs. L. viewed Dora as "different," defective. In response to this perception, Mrs. L., with her aunt's spirited, perhaps even zealous, assistance, invested enormous energy in trying to provide Dora with an unusual degree of self-control, an attribute that she imagined would sustain her daughter during adversity and also one that Mrs. L.'s family, originally from Eastern Europe, had valued for generations. In Mrs. L.'s opinion, this characteristic was lacking in children she knew who had been reared in the United States.

Dora at 16 was depressed, and the factors appeared to relate to both developmental issues and neurotic conflicts. With respect to developmental issues, she felt overwhelmed by her feelings of intense episodic anxiety and fury whenever she felt "forced." Early in our work there appeared to be an insufficient barrier between impulse and action, leading her family to form an impression of Dora as a "risk taker," a trait that her mother regarded with alarm and her father with cautious pride. Typically a phenomenon of normal adolescence, Dora's impulse to take particular types of risks (leaving school, engaging with boys who were involved in potentially dangerous situations) appeared to be especially intense, based on both dynamic and developmental factors. Dora's risks involved action, particularly with respect to distancing from parents. Early in our work they did not include what Dora perceived as the "risk" of deep affective engagement. It was notable that Dora displayed an extraordinary ability to assess what risks would be tolerable to her parents and her analyst.

Dora's efforts to negotiate a second individuation of adolescence were encumbered by faults that appeared to have taken place during her separation-individuation phase. One mode in which Dora attempted to disengage from her scholarly parents was by becoming an academic failure. In separating herself from both parents and peers, she lost objects. And Dora seemed to be searching for something that she felt was missing in her very early tie with her mother. While the resurgence of unresolved preoedipal issues is seen regularly in adolescent development (object hunger, for example), Dora's search for an object was particularly intense because of very early difficulties in maintaining deep empathic connections (negotiating separation-individuation and establishing object constancy). In retrospect, I think that Dora sought a relationship in which she and the other felt a profound need for each other. Dora alluded to this by telling me that she wanted to feel completely indispensable to "someone." It was with this imperative search to engage in a relationship of intense mutual need that Dora began treatment.

In view of Dora's intense conflicts, a hint to her parents of suicidal ideas, and her seemingly impulsive wish to abandon school, I saw her frequently from the start. Aware of Dora's marked distress and feelings over her academic future, I asked if she could permit herself some time to think about her feelings so that her decision about school would be her own rather than a response to external pressure. Dora replied that an immediate decision about school was not necessary; yet, in her characteristic manner of turning one aspect of her conflict to action, she formally withdrew from school the following day, announcing this proudly at our next session.

Dora spoke of longing to get "an important job" that would enable her to be totally independent from her parents, yet simultaneously she wanted desperately to have someone take care of her. Her shifting stance of longing for the protection afforded a young child and wishing earnestly to plunge boldly into adulthood was an example of the way in which she experienced intense conflicts, both those of a developmental nature and those representing neurosis.

Following Dora's departure from school, I felt a keen awareness that any offering that took the form of suggestion might be perceived as "pressure," to which Dora might well respond with action. In view of this, I felt it particularly important to attend to Dora's responses to my interventions.

After several meetings, I told Dora that it would take some time for us to understand her troubles, and I recommended that we meet four times weekly. Dora was relieved to hear this, feeling that I had taken her problems seriously; I learned much later that she was quite pleased to think that perhaps I had worried about her.

As Dora began to express her feelings with increasing freedom, she seemed to have a compelling impulse to elicit my opinions. I held fast, explaining how important it was for us to try to understand the meanings of her questions and how, ultimately, this would help her decide for herself. At that juncture, I felt that Dora was inviting me to become involved while warning me of the potential hazards. She both longed for intense involvement (developmental need) and feared close contact (articulated as a fear of betrayal). In maintaining a neutral stance, I wanted to permit Dora the widest opportunity to experience me from whatever transference perspective was most useful to her and, when necessary, to utilize me as a developmental object. Ultimately Dora identified with (and, to some degree internalized) my stance of observing, exploring, and tolerating the anxiety of waiting. She developed a keen interest in examining her behavior and in identifying and examining her feelings, conflicts, and the nature of our evolving relationship.

For at least the first year of our work together, Dora experienced substantive aspects of transference feelings and "real" aspects of our relationship (analyst as developmental object) in displaced form. I did not interpret this material for some time because it was my impression that at this stage Dora required externalizations and displacements for the expression of her intense conflictual feelings. My early interventions were directed primarily toward helping Dora to identify and examine her feelings, to distinguish between her feelings and those of idealized objects, and to delineate defense and conflict, in the context of a therapeutic alliance.

Within weeks of our beginning to work, Dora established a friendship with Carmen, a bright, perceptive young woman who worked feverishly at odd jobs in an effort to save money for college tuition. Carmen represented, in part, a displacement object that Dora needed early in treatment, to defend against emerging positive feelings in the transference. A few days later, Dora met Roberto, with whom she promptly entered into an intense relationship.

Roberto was "a New Yorker who was wonderfully different." He was a twenty-five-year-old, occasionally employed blue-collar worker and compulsive gambler who appeared to be very eager for rehabilitation. When Dora began to inquire with persistence and intensity about what I thought of Roberto, I said, "Dora, generally when you feel pressure to know what I think, there's something that you don't want to acknowledge about your own feelings." She said, "Roberto keeps asking, 'when can we live together?'" To which she replied, "As soon as I learn to use a toilet." While Dora was able to use humor to distance herself from Roberto, she was unable to explore her conflicted feelings and developmental needs about the relationship for many months.

Early in Dora's life, when her mother attended occasional professional meetings abroad, Dora's father helped to provide maternal care. On a couple of occasions, when Mrs. L., to her deep distress, had to be absent for a full week, Dora's father took his younger children to visit relatives in California. These episodes were among Dora's most idyllic memories. From this period, Dora recalled what we eventually understood as an early organizing fantasy, in which she imagined playing on a jetty that extended far out over the Pacific Ocean. From this vantage point, Dora, in fantasy, surveyed endangered species and attempted to feed creatures whose very existence depended on her beneficent nurturance. Dora externalized her helplessness on the needy animals, finding gratification in acting as the rescuer. Much later, she was able to recognize that she found gratification in protesting her helplessness.

Dora's fantasies of rescuing imperiled wildlife symbolized part of her effort to surpass her mother by offering greater support than Dora felt she herself had received at an early stage in her development. Roberto was one of the recipients of this effort. A parallel process emerged: Dora wanted to provide for Roberto as she hoped that I would provide for her. When Dora persistently sought career advice from me, I told her that while she rejected advice from family and friends and appeared to want to decide for herself, somehow she wished that I would offer something that would be exactly right. Dora burst into laughter and said that she wanted to feel sheltered and protected and that was why she had been considering marriage! It seemed to me that Dora felt she needed to create a family to satisfy her wish to belong. And Dora wanted to elicit from me a response of protective intervention. When she demanded that I provide her with immediate direction and advice in order to relieve her feelings of anxiety, I commented on how much she wanted me to rescue her, and I addressed her very special pleasure in finding ways to be, or to feel, rescued. Dora's face brightened, and she expressed her notion of being rescued as an ideal state, one that engendered an incomparable sense of safety, coincident with a lack of indebtedness.

In addition to my role in transference, Dora used her attachment to me to repeat (and repair) aspects of early object relations. One example of the reparative work was directed toward preoedipal experiences of object constancy that were somewhat unstable. This took the form of a persistent, implicit question: At what point might I reject or overwhelm her? Dora's earliest defenses included efforts to protect herself from feared and fantasied rejection by me. As we examined these efforts in the context of transference, we explored her intense fear of deep affective engagement from a wide variety of vantage points. This included oedipal issues (retaliation from Mother), negative oedipal ones (would Father be dismayed over the time that I [mother] spent with her?), and earlier matters involving object constancy—difficulty in being able to hold on to the object.

Dora returned from the first summer break to say that she realized she did not need me and that she was planning to become engaged to Roberto. While her decision seemed like yet another effort to induce me to intervene, it was clear that I could not do so, and Dora's responses to my various trial interventions made it clear that she was not yet ready to deal with her anger over my absence during the summer. At that point, Dora imagined that her direct expression of intense anger at me would create an impassable breach, a malignant rift in our relationship. This related both to projections of her rage and to unstable object representations.

When Dora described her intense worry about Roberto's failure to use his full intellectual potential, I said that her concern about Roberto made me wonder if that was how she wanted people to feel about her. She smiled and spoke of her parents' worries about her academic goals and their profound dismay over her departure from family tradition in leaving school. From her studied assessment of my bookshelf, Dora assumed that I also valued scholarship and might also worry about her. I reminded Dora that, with her deep and abiding interest in Spanish literature, she too reads a lot. She looked rather surprised; she said that was so, but her interests were "not academic." Yet, in contrast to Roberto's family, she recognized that she valued education a great deal, so the issue of returning to school was not simply her family's values or a cultural matter.

While Dora entertained the idea of marriage and family, she acknowledged that she feared having children. She described the "dreadful uncertainty" of childrearing and the possibility of finding that "you raised kids with values that are totally screwed up." This was the beginning of a growing awareness that some of her behavior was determined by her anger and her wishes for revenge on her parents.

Following a vigorous defense of Roberto's disappointing her, Dora mused that her "moodiness" was probably a result of "genes and chromosomes," because many members of her family displayed emotional volatility. I told Dora that she was so afraid of feeling angry at Roberto that she wanted to blame biology. Dora sobbed and said that Roberto was "just too different, not just that he's a 'New Yorker' but in every other way"; he might gamble for the rest of his life and continue to live "below poverty" level. She felt that she had changed very much during the time of our meeting and acknowledged that she had been hoping to accomplish similar changes with Roberto. I interpreted her conflictual identification with me, commenting on her apparent embarrassment about her feelings of wanting to emulate me—in clothing, jewelry, etc. She said that was because sometimes she only wanted to do the opposite of what she thought I wanted, similar to her experience with her parents. This represented, in part, her adolescent development, characterized by efforts to define herself. It also represented a revisiting of preoedipal issues. Part of her adolescent development, it must be noted, took place in the context of the therapeutic relationship, where Dora was increasingly free to express both conflicts within the transference and feelings that appeared linked to her early difficulties in maintaining sustained object relations.

When Dora experienced me as failing to support her relationship with Roberto, she wanted to "deepen the relationship" with him, even though she herself thought it unsuitable. She was surprised by the intensity of her defiance—"like a little kid's feeling," she observed. And it was difficult for her to believe that my feelings about her plans with Roberto were neutral. "You talk in a dispassionate way because you are a doctor and that is your professional responsibility," she asserted, "but it's hard for me to think that any adult with responsibility can hear about my plans to spend my life with Roberto and not feel some objection." Then I asked, "And if I objected?" She said, "I hate to admit this, but I might want to marry him even more."

As Dora continued to try to encourage her parents and me to worry about her academic goals, I helped her to delineate areas of conflict, but expressed little (perhaps "limited" is more accurate) concern about if, or when, she would decide to resume formal education. This left Dora feeling occasionally puzzled and sometimes furious but it enabled her to examine the degree to which she used academic performance both as a weapon in her struggles with her parents and as a way of assessing their concern.

By the conclusion of our second year together, Dora had begun to move from deeply conflictual relations with her parents to a much more flexible interchange with them, openly acknowledging her identification with them—her love of their cultural pursuits and her avid intellectual interests.

Preceding the second summer vacation, Dora was anxious. She explained that while she wanted to work with me to "solve problems," she was terribly worried about a "vague" growing attachment to me. She found this particularly disconcerting because she wanted to be sure to avoid suffering at the conclusion of treatment. Following this exchange, Dora applied to various schools and gained admission to a junior college. She worked, with decorators hired by her parents, at furnishing a luxurious apartment that was the envy of her newly acquired circle of peers. Soon after school began, she reported feeling troubled by her "emotional dependence" on her new college friends and her impulses to control them.

As Dora began to study with unprecedented enthusiasm, she spoke of feeling "stronger," linked associatively to doing damage. About midsemester, Dora dreamed that the front part of her walkway needed repair, and the workman repaired a rear stairway but paid no attention to her original request. She associated to conflicts about femininity and early notions of the inadequacy of the female. At this juncture, a shift took place in which phallic representations emerged more clearly in the material.

Dora's anxiety over uncertainty was multiply determined. It appeared to be linked, in part, to early longings to please her father by becoming like a son, whom she imagined her father would value more than he did her, judging by his relationship with her brothers. "Was this culturally based?" she wondered. Despite the rivalry with her brothers, Dora also longed to be her father's favorite ("and prettiest") daughter. At this juncture, Dora was able to move beyond her earlier emphasis on cultural issues to explore her own conflicts over being a woman. "Can a woman be assertive, certain, and still be desirable to a man?" she mused.

Dora was angry that the treatment took so long and imagined that only a man could have the competence to "really speed this up." As Dora expressed fears of owning her strength, I told her that she seemed to connect feeling strong and independent with worries that somebody will get hurt. Dora felt that Roberto would be hurt if she left him, an action that would be a direct result of her feeling stronger. I underscored her anxieties over her wish to control the other person, and she smiled and expressed her fantasy of demanding that I accommodate the treatment hours to her schedule.

Dora associated to intense conflicts over her feelings of attachment to me. She experienced her tie to me as alternately comforting and threatening, the latter most prominent when it felt fueled by an "external, invisible source." I pointed out that her angry wishes toward me might contribute to her fear of feeling tied to me. In this context, we could examine some frightening objects that populated her inner world and became projected onto the object, an encumbrance to her adolescent development. At this point I served as a developmental object for Dora in her efforts to repair early deficits that appeared to encumber her oedipal conflicts and thus affected the shaping of the transference.

When Dora referred to her gradual disengagement from Roberto, yet added fervently, "I made a promise to marry him and I will keep it,"

I said I wondered whether she was trying to provoke me to say something that she would feel was protective—perhaps recommending restraint. Dora's eyes filled with tears and she said, "I hate to say it, but, in a way, if you tried to stop me, I would hate you, but at least I would know that you care." Following this piece of analysis, Dora expressed anxieties about my well-being with much more ease.

As Dora associated to her conflicts over being a woman, she expressed curiosity about my personal life. At that point she was much more tolerant of our focus on her curiosity as a subject worthy of examination. In beginning to interpret her conflictual wish for identification with me, I told Dora that she wondered what kind of woman I am and what kind of woman she wanted to become.

Dora said that she was terribly disappointed when she first met me because I wore "a suit and high-heeled shoes." She had interpreted this as "too old and too formal," but by the time she related the incident, she felt that I seemed more "casual" and "easy to talk to." When Dora spoke of wanting to be loved for herself, I interpreted her wish for me to love her for herself.

To this point, Dora had exhibited a persistent, prominent defense of explaining every detail of her external life. One day she told me of a new friend at school who described events in minute detail. "It is hard to feel close to her, because she always appears to hold back." With that precious window of opportunity, I told Dora that I wondered if a similar phenomenon might be occurring between us. Dora sobbed and said that if she really allowed herself to feel close to me, I might disappoint her. Perhaps I'd "leave town or die," she reflected. Then she recalled the pain that she had experienced during early childhood over her mother's very occasional professional trips abroad. She linked this to her profound distress when her aunt, an essential caretaker during her childhood, left, in what appeared to be a precipitous manner, for month-long visits to Buenos Aires. This took place at what Dora perceived to be several crucial moments. "It felt like such a betrayal," she said tearfully. "I just couldn't stand it if that happened one more time in my life. I would rather keep you away than trust you and have you decide not to see me."

The material shifted in a substantive way following this sequence. Dora reported an interest in dating classmates, deciding to end her relationship with Roberto. She complained periodically that her relation with Carmen was much more secure than that with me because she could reach Carmen at any moment of the day or night to find solace. Our analytic scrutiny of this material led to her fears of trusting me. Within a week, Dora reached me, through an emergency paging service, at 10 one evening. Roberto, who had been gambling again, had telephoned her in a frenzy, desperate for money. He wanted her to withdraw a large sum of money with her automated bank card and was threatening to visit. Following a careful exploration of her feelings, I told Dora I understood that she felt frightened and wanted support, and it seemed to me that she already had an idea of what she wanted to do. Since her parents were out at a late dinner, she decided to spend the night with a classmate who lived at home with her extended family. Dora experienced my responses to her urgent plea for help as pivotal in her growing trust in me.

At that point, I felt the material demonstrated some of Dora's progress in development, in addition to our beginning work on conflictual issues. Dora's adolescent struggles over tolerating contradictions and entertaining fantasies instead of engaging in immediate action, for example, were burdened by her unresolved difficulties of autonomy and compliance, conflictual aggressive wishes, faulty identifications, and unresolved bisexuality. Activities that brought her near danger represented, in part, an expression of her difficulty in finding gratification in fantasy. Early on, she used action defensively rather than in the interest of sublimation, and I felt uncertain about whether her developmental difficulties might preclude analysis of her conflicts. Yet it seemed to me that Dora gave evidence of substantial strength, and, from the start, I thought that it would be worthwhile to begin to work analytically, delineate conflict where possible, and give development an opportunity to recover its pathway.

During the third year, we were able to trace Dora's concern about whether I really wanted to work with her to explore her early fears that her mother would leave for yet another trip to her own parents. This emerged in the context of Dora's anxieties when I informed her of upcoming interruptions in our work. It provided us with a context for understanding Dora's behavior very early in treatment, when her response to feeling as if she had fallen irretrievably behind in schoolwork was to feel frantic, with threats of suicide and quitting school.

Dora's response to potential failure in competition was another factor in her departure from school. Within the transference, she feared that I (father) would be threatened by such a successful person and abandon her. Her early admiration of her father in an oedipal context was burdened by her profound wish for him as caretaker.

When Dora spoke of warm feelings for her mother after feeling a strong connection with me, I told her that sometimes there was a back-and-forth motion in her feelings. At times she experienced me in some of the ways that she had perceived her mother—rejecting, punishing, or withdrawn. Yet, at other times, she felt very much accepted by me and receptive to her mother's affection.

In tandem with our work on conflictual issues and Dora's recovery of early memories of both her mother's perceived abandonment and support, Dora's relationship with her mother improved considerably. As they increasingly enjoyed each other's company, Dora considered leaving town when she was accepted at a school that, from her perspective, was "the best in the country"; yet she did not want to leave as a response to fears of closeness with me. She struggled a good deal over the meaning of leaving and the potential effects of an interruption of our work. She imagined working with another analyst, and when her anger toward me was intense and prolonged, she felt that this might be a preferred alternative. With minimal intervention, I permitted her to struggle over her dilemma about where to attend school. Her final decision seemed to be based largely on her wish to maintain continuity in treatment.

Dora's emerging idealization of me centered on her view of me as unusually calm, having achieved academically, lusty in bed with my husband, independent yet flexible, and probably a very liberal mother— that is, setting few if any limits on teenagers. She expressed the expectation that I would not be threatened by provocative behavior.

Dora engaged in a series of brief, intense involvements with men whom she described as "from the Latin community," and she complained of rushing into relationships so that she could avoid scary situations, such as the uncertainty of casual dating. I said that it seemed to be part of her wish to feel closure, which might be one way of trying to avoid anxiety; I added that she seemed to leave all the decisions to the men, as if she wanted to be unaware of her own feelings and thoughts.

"That's true," she exclaimed. "It's like if I leave the decisions to them, I won't make a mistake. Wow! I can't believe I really think like that. But I think it has something to do with you too. When I go to bed with guys without thinking, I imagine that you'll think it's wrong. Part of me still gets a mild kick out of that. On the other hand, I think it's wrong, and I myself certainly don't want to do things I don't believe in just because I imagine that you will feel something about it. It would be like you are my mother and I am about fifteen."

Dora reported that her sometimes promiscuous behavior left her feeling "bad," sometimes even "evil." In her associations this was linked to being "dirty," "defective," and "stupid." I pointed out that punishing herself by thinking of herself as "bad" may sometimes substitute for thinking about what she does. Her sense of urgency in establishing liaisons with men appeared to be a defense against intimacy as well as against homosexual impulses, although this was not yet available for interpretation in the material.

As our third summer break approached, Dora became insistent about knowing my thoughts about her gains in treatment. I acknowledged both her worries and her wish to look to me for advice, and I delineated some of her conflicts with respect to autonomy and compliance. Then I asked Dora what she imagined I might think.

Dora feared my viewing her as fully capable, a perception that might bring the treatment to a close before she felt prepared. She wanted me to worry about her even though she had begun to realize that perhaps our working well together was sufficient. One of her sisters was by then among Dora's closest friends, yet Dora felt that her sibling tie was "different" from our relationship.

In anticipating my vacation, Dora sought, in the transference, the "worrying" mother of early childhood. Based on a good deal of associative material, I speculated that she may also have sought the caretaking father, a factor that may have contributed to her promiscuity. Finally, she looked for an object to replace me in my absence. She wanted a piece of me (my advice) as well. Her anxiety over my leaving led to a re-emergence of a state of helplessness, which she observed was different from her (by then) real experiences. In a further shift in the material at that time, there was deeper engagement in the transference of oedipal conflict, and evidence emerged that superego consolidation had begun to take place. Earlier her superego had been so effectively externalized that we dealt with it largely in the form of displacement.

Dora associated to a dream about a frightening monster. She had felt angry with me for failing to give her advice. Yet she appreciated the way we worked, particularly each time that she became aware of feeling like a much stronger person than she had been. She suspected that the monster of the dream might have been her boyfriend or me, a secret not to be revealed to a casual acquaintance. It might also have represented herself, capable of murder. Independence and aggression were linked associatively and were, in Dora's view, incompatible with intimacy.

She dreamed that she was a little girl—happy, confident, and lying in a forbidden bed. A Dutch father whom she recognized as a single parent appeared and behaved seductively. Dora arose abruptly and energetically completed a long-overdue research paper for school. A very handsome young man who seemed to be from Argentina appeared. She thought, "Finally, a man who's just right!" Then the man's appearance altered and he strongly resembled a twenty-five-year-old photograph of Dad that she had re-discovered on the preceding day. She awakened in terror.

The dream occurred just before our interruption for the summer break, and Dora thought, "It's like I wanted to reassure myself that I will soon find a new boyfriend, but I'm scared that he won't be right for me and I won't be able to talk it over with you."

I felt that this was a wonderful example of why her academic efforts—her tie to her father—had to be undone. She had selected academic failure to wrench herself away from her father. Excellence in scholarship had been, in Dora's view, a substantive factor in her father's value of her and her love for him. It seemed to me that this material demonstrated how acting-out behavior is an attempt to forget or deny the connection to the incestuous object. The incestuous wish broke through in the dream, so she woke up. Its occurrence just before my vacation may have been an expression of an effort to avoid awareness of the incestuous tie in the transference and consequent retaliation. When I underscored Dora's attributing traits of her parents to me, she said, "Well, in some ways I wish that you were my mother. I think that I might have grown up healthier. It would be nice if you had strong feelings about what I do, but of course I wouldn't listen anyway." With respect to her career plans, Dora continued, "Most of the time I want to be a rich chief executive officer, maybe of an international firm. Yet a part of me still wants to do work that would drive my parents crazy, whatever it is." Dora reflected upon her growing and changing images of herself, and acknowledged her pride over this.

When Dora's parents telephoned me to arrange a visit to talk about her progress, I suggested that they begin by talking with Dora about her feelings about this. The following day, Dora associated to a dream that related to her initial fury with her parents for "interfering" by telephoning me. Feeling "violated," she was anxious about expressing her anger in its full intensity. She said, "I think I'm afraid of the person that I will find out I am. Angry." I interpreted her fear that I would back away from a full expression of her anger. She tearfully acknowledged this fantasy and began to confront her early responses when both parents engaged in extraordinary efforts to avoid her aggression.

We explored Dora's need to view me as one who prohibits, and she began to examine fantasies of violent retaliation. Following this piece of analytic work, Dora became much freer in direct expression of both her anger and her feelings of longing in her interactions with me.

When she spoke of feeling conflict over presenting herself as "tough" or "wimpy," I told Dora that both stances are ways of keeping others at a distance. Dora said, "I really like that idea. If you turn into what you think the other person wants so they will like you, you aren't really close, because, at least part of the time, you feel mad at them, and if you are tough as nails, you aren't really close either." Following this, within the context of the transference, Dora was able to explore her fears of intimacy on a deeper level than previously.

When Dora argued regularly with her father over possible vocational alternatives and he threatened to disown her if she chose an occupation that was not "ladylike" and "in keeping with family tradition," I said that the struggle with Dad seemed to be more important than the actual content of their discussion. Dora conceded that she really liked the fight, and she recognized both her "feminine" side and her impulses to represent herself as "very tough," thus enraging her father. As we began to examine Dora's presenting herself as an object of pity in peer and family relations, I interpreted her trying to get her parents to show love by demonstrating pity for her and her fear of the anger she experienced in response to her parents when they did not. These interventions provided developmental assistance in addition to offering an interpretation of her defenses. Following my interpretations, Dora smiled and said that her whole body relaxed when I said that. She then recalled numerous examples of her fear of her anger and her early misperceptions of links between pity and love.

When this material emerged within the transference, I interpreted Dora's wish for me to feel pity for her, and she acknowledged that she feels frustrated when I don't respond in that way. When I commented on the contradictory elements, she said, "I guess it's that struggle again. Getting so excited about the fight with an authority person that I forget the issues." As this was reworked in the transference from a variety of perspectives, she began to talk about experiencing love that is distinct from pity. For the first time in years, Dora accepted her parents' invitation to join them on a trip to visit the extended family in Buenos Aires.

Dora expressed anxiety over feeling close to me, and I said that while she wants to trust me, she worries about what she describes as feeling "too close." She said that when she was younger she felt she had to keep some feelings and thoughts to herself that she imagined most girls shared with their mothers. At first she viewed this as based entirely upon her mother's lack of affective availability. My interpretations within the transference led to Dora's recognition that perhaps her own acute sense of shame about her body was a significant factor in her keeping some thoughts private.

Dora imagined fighting with me over which school to attend next, yet she recognized this conflict as one that was taking place in her own thoughts. With an expression of surprise and excitement, she said that she was thinking of a new concept from her course in elementary psychology. "It's a defense," she exclaimed. "The way it works is that if I give a thought to you, and I don't own it, then I don't really 'go for it.' I sort of drag around, feeling forced, and feeling not as capable as I know that I really am!"

When Dora's associations to her feelings of envy, episodically projected onto the object, were related to my professional work, I told her that she may worry that I will be envious if she reaches the top of her field. She felt that was accurate because in psychiatry you "can never really get to the top of the medical field—although," she added, "people don't realize that sometimes your whole life changes because of your work with your analyst."

Dora linked her fantasies of physical defectiveness to her pattern of holding back her feelings in intimate relations with a man. As she explored her fantasies, I raised the possibility that this "holding back" might be connected to other types of holding back—such as repeatedly engaging with boyfriends whose difficulties present overwhelming problems or considering vocational plans that did not permit her to use her gifts. Dora offered confirmatory material at once. By then her identificatory wish in professional choice was firmly replaced by a career in which she could pursue her genuine interests. Dora presented her new career plans to her parents and became aware that as soon as her mother displayed interest in or curiosity about her ideas, her own interest waned.

I interpreted this material as an expression of her fear of closeness with her mother, and she exclaimed that sounded exactly right. "It's sort of like I'll lose my brain, my sense of myself, if I don't keep some things separate from Mom," she said ruefully. "I know it's a fantasy, because I've been feeling very good about my brain. Sometimes I feel that I am smarter than both of my parents. Now I can reason in a deeper way, and I used to be afraid to think, but now I am not!" she asserted.

Dora re-examined her anxiety about feeling too dependent upon Mom, whom she feared emulating, by finding a man on whom to depend completely. She recalled a series of distressing exchanges in which she felt that her father belittled her mother by denigrating her professional achievements. She said that she realized once more that she feared climbing to the top of her field because it might alienate her father, who "deep down" believes women to be inferior. She attributed her father's notions to "cultural background." Then she experienced a fleeting feeling of "glory" when her father "put down Mom." She added, "Maybe if I were successful my Dad would admire me terribly.

Scary. Like Dad and I might spend lots of time together, talking about work." "Oh boy," Dora exclaimed with a smile, "is this what my psychology professor means by Oedipus complex?"

Dora spoke of fear of my disapproval of her sexual thoughts, and I interpreted her conflict over expressing herself freely. She referred to a (then) recent vacation at Club Med, where she overheard a discussion of masturbation. She responded by feeling "stunned and ashamed" because she did not share the comfort of other people of her age in discussing this subject. From earliest childhood, she had thought of genital touching as "repulsive." When I commented on her concern over extremes in behavior, she said she imagined that if she really liked masturbating, it might take up too much of her time. At once she expressed fears of my criticism of her sexual fantasies. I said it was difficult to think of me as an adult who was not critical, but also that her worry about whether she could trust me served to protect her from the discomfort of talking about things she perceived as embarrassing.

When she spoke of her self-defeating posture, she recalled that her parents forced her to comply, her friends forced her to do things for them, and she sometimes thought that I forced her to continue in treatment. I related those feelings to her masturbatory fantasies. Surprised, she acknowledged that ideas of powerful, dominant men and submissive women suffuse her personal interactions. Exploring this material during the succeeding months, particularly in the context of the transference, Dora expressed a wish for a more consensual relationship with a man.

When Dora examined her intense feelings of wanting direction from me, yet her certainty about her own decisions, she was puzzled. She examined, in various contexts, her inclination to seek, and adopt, the opinions of others, even when she felt confident in her own position. In her associations to a dream, prompted by transference material in which she yearned for me to give her direction, she recalled a sequence of events at about age five, when she was severely reprimanded by her father for urinating behind a tree, a position that appeared to her very private. Her father became enraged over this "unladylike behavior" and spanked her. Continuing to believe that she had broken no rules because the behavior would have been acceptable for her brothers, she recalled deciding, over a period of weeks or months, to perpetually seek the opinions of others "to find the right way." "Taking the opinions of other people also got me away from the crazy feeling of having very different strong feelings at the same time." At age four, Dora felt that the experience of two conflicting intense feelings indicated "craziness," like some of the adults and older children in her family. "But," she continued, "before I started taking other people's opinions I was an independent little kid, and everybody talked about how mature and independent I was; very different from my mother and older sisters. Maybe I didn't really lose all that, but it was in a kind of deep sleep. Maybe I can get that part of me back to work again!" she said with delighted excitement.

Dora dated a man whose parents were from Chile and whose warmth and admiration she enjoyed. She said that she used to feel it was necessary to work to have people like her and now she just accepts it. She enjoyed her sexual relations with him more than with any man previously. She was pleased to have established a congenial circle of close women friends.

When a boyfriend raised the possibility of marriage, Dora smiled and said, "I don't plan to marry until I have finished graduate school. After all, how can a woman my age make a decision that will affect her whole life? I still have a lot to learn."

DISCUSSION

My work with Dora involved both the analysis of conflicts within the transference and work with developmental issues. In addition to the interpretation of conflict within the context of transference and the use of reconstruction, specific developmental needs emerged that required particular attention from the viewpoint of technique. Relatively early in our work, it became clear that Dora sought approval from the "other" to an extraordinary degree, frequently with such intensity that she neglected her own wishes (sometimes to the point of being unaware of them). And most of her relationships were based on mutually intense need-fulfillment, characterized by Dora's serving as "rescuer" for a number of her friends. Dora was terrified of engaging in a relationship of mutual partnership, because she feared that her "faults" would "drive the other person away."

To address these developmental issues, I worked slowly and carefully to help Dora identify and delineate her affects and examine them in the context of our relationship. We linked her experiences (intense object hunger, for example) to what she had perceived as early maternal absence. In addition, I permitted idealization to continue (without the usual interpretation) for much longer than usual, even that typically required for an adolescent (Chused, 1987). It was my impression that the requisite reparative work called for a level of identification and internalization that was somewhat more extended than that typically required in the analysis of an adolescent who is deeply engaged in struggling with neurotic conflict. Dora identified with my mode of affect regulation and responses to her intense anxiety—exploring, considering, waiting patiently. This permitted her some opportunity to examine the intensity and urgency of her responses.

With respect to our extended work in displacement and externalization, Dora's keen interest in modern literature helped her become familiar with her sadism. This exploration bore profound likeness to working in the playroom with a child. That is, we explored the many possible feelings and experiences of fictional characters—murderers, victims, and bystanders. As this material was analyzed, Dora became more comfortable with her fantasy life, with tolerating conflict, with her affective expressions, and with differentiating herself from the idealized object.

Maturational shifts included a level of object constancy that did not appear to be present previously, a capacity to acknowledge her strengths and weaknesses as distinct from the object, an ability to engage in intimate relationships without fear of destroying the other or of being abandoned, and a substantial ability to manage affect modulation. Some of the shifts were notable in Dora's responses to interruptions in our work. During the early phase, Dora did not acknowledge feelings in response to my absences but instead externalized her feelings, conflicts, and compromise formations. Later in treatment, she was bereft at interruptions in treatment, in a panic, wondering what she would do in my absence "if something happened." During those vacations, she telephoned me on several occasions. Finally, she accepted interruptions with ease, able to analyze her affective responses, conflicts, and compromise formations.

My confidence in Dora's ability to work at resolving these difficulties may have been a factor in her willingness to enter an extended (and intensive) treatment situation. Dora was a worker—always thoughtful and interested in exploring, despite her fears of the risks that this might require. In the transference, it took some time before Dora was able to see me as different from her parents; ultimately she was able to analyze her wish to see us as identical. Early in our work together, it seemed to me that the therapeutic alliance was shaped in part by Dora's need to take time away from school, her long-anticipated pathway, and, in a sense, from development. Dora's many responses to her mother's episodic absences during her early years of life had to be engaged in a meaningful therapeutic struggle. It is possible that the moratorium Dora chose from school was her way of wrestling with some of those feelings and responses.

An early therapeutic issue was Dora's recognition that she needed to discover her preferred mode to develop as an independent person, without the caretaker that, as a midadolescent, she felt that she had needed urgently. Part of our work consisted in dealing with Dora's persistent invitation to me to be a "better" mother, and we examined both the invitation and the disappointment that followed my declining to engage with her in this manner.

Early in treatment, Dora expressed the fear that closeness with her mother would lead to her acquiring some traits of her mother's that she did not particularly admire; then she would risk, from her adolescent viewpoint, both social isolation and disrespect of her father. Difficulties at the level of identification, internalization, and object constancy provided an encumbrance to Dora's separation-individuation phase and substantively influenced both the shaping of the Oedipus complex and the second separation-individuation of adolescence. Various developmental issues, such as the struggle between intimacy and independence, which Dora viewed as mutually exclusive phenomena, appeared rooted in her very early experience and presented obstacles to her engaging in expectable adolescent growth, with its attendant emergence of new structures.

The transference was examined from a range of perspectives. I was the mother of early childhood whom she idealized but from whom she anticipated episodically acute disappointments. Alternately, I was the father of early childhood who periodically also assumed maternal functions, a fact that burdened her oedipal constellation. This was particularly prominent when she feared competing with me, as father, who might then deny her maternal care that she believed was otherwise unavailable. When I represented the mother of the negative oedipal stage, Dora longed for intimacy, yet feared retaliation from my "boyfriend or husband." Later, she experienced me as a "mean witch," threatening her relationship with a boyfriend whom she considered "far better" than the male colleague with whom she saw me in a public situation. She also examined, in substantial detail, her fear of competing successfully with me, linked in her fantasies to killing her mother. Additionally, I was a developmental object that Dora required for her continuing development, idealized during a significant piece of Dora's adolescence. When Dora was able to attain the distance to examine her relationship with Roberto, her first boyfriend, she explored her own derogated self-image.

As a result of this work, Dora could crystallize the kind of emotional foundation she needed in order to begin to approach the normative adolescent issues, with which she had previously been unable to engage. I always felt profound respect for Dora's needs for self-determination, experimentation, and action in the extrafamilial and extraanalytic worlds, as we continued to analyze the conflicts that interfered with her negotiation of adolescent struggles. Dora's multiple needs, in this sense, were a constant challenge.

In summary, my work with Dora involved working with oedipal conflict, engaged competitive, libidinal, and murderous wishes in the transference, and confronted substantial developmental issues as well. These included, but were not limited to, problems of object constancy and separation-individuation reworked at adolescence and gave us the opportunity to observe the emergence of organizations of middle and late adolescence, as well as of early adulthood. Some of the issues we addressed in treatment could not have been approached until Dora was developmentally prepared to engage them. At the conclusion of treatment, Dora was able to think before acting, had access to, and was increasingly tolerant of, a wider range of affects than previously, enjoyed increasingly satisfactory intimate relations with boyfriends, and had established a group of friends and a best girlfriend. Consolidation of identity in general and sexual identity in particular had demonstrated substantial progress.

BIBLIOGRAPHY

CHUSED, J. (1987). Idealization of the analyst by the young adult. *J. Amer. Psychoanal. Assn.* 35:839–859.

The Psychoanalytic Treatment of a Child with Deviational Development

ALAN B. ZIENTS, M.D.

This paper presents the analysis of Peter, a five-year-old boy with compromised ego functions including difficulties in maintaining stable internalized object representations. Despite these serious problems, which are often seen as contraindicating analysis, a predominantly traditional psychoanalytic position emphasizing dynamic interpretations was utilized. Detailed clinical material is presented to demonstrate the effectiveness of this approach in facilitating therapeutic changes in Peter.

PETER, A FIVE-YEAR-OLD BOY, WAS REFERRED TO ME WITH A DIAGNOSIS of gender identity disorder and organizational deficits. He presented not only with unresolved intrapsychic conflicts but also with constitutional (equipmental) deficits and developmental problems that were evident quite early in his life. My approach to his treatment relied primarily on psychoanalytic technique rather than milieu management, parental guidance, or psychopharmacology. His treatment required

Training analyst and supervisor in child and adolescent analysis at New York University Psychoanalytic Institute, New York Psychoanalytic Institute, and Columbia Psychoanalytic Institute; associate clinical professor of psychiatry at New York University College of Medicine.

Many of the ideas discussed in this paper emerged in a discussion group entitled "Coordinating Developmental and Psychoanalytical Goals in Child and Adolescent Analysis," sponsored by the Psychoanalytic Research and Development Fund, Inc. I especially want to thank Samuel Abrams, Albert Solnit, and Peter Neubauer for their careful review of the manuscript.

The Psychoanalytic Study of the Child 54, ed. Albert J. Solnit, Peter B. Neubauer, Samuel Abrams, and A. Scott Dowling (Yale University Press, copyright © 1999 by Albert J. Solnit, Peter B. Neubauer, Samuel Abrams, and A. Scott Dowling).

an approach that not only facilitated the reactivation of old conflicts but also assisted him with his impaired functioning by providing with actual life events in the interaction with the analyst that served as a platform on which positive developmental predispositions could be organized and actualized. This paper emphasizes some aspects of conducting an analysis when important ego functions are compromised, demonstrating the need to coordinate the induced process of psychoanalysis with the natural process of development.

Peter lacked the capacity to form and maintain stable mental representations of either himself or others over time. My impression was that this difficulty was closely related to his overwhelming problems with modulating his anger appropriately. He was also limited in his ability to move from imitation to internalization. Furthermore, he had difficulty in the synthesis and amalgamation of new psychological data.

From the point of view of defenses, Peter's tendency to use extreme denial and isolation of both affect and content posed a serious obstacle to the establishment of a therapeutic process based on understanding. The ease and rapidity of his regression as well as his determined preoccupation with his own internal world severely limited his capacity to engage issues. Partly as a consequence of these impediments, Peter showed little motivation for change, seeing treatment as an intrusion while insisting that he be left alone. To Peter, growing older usually meant having to cope with new, unwanted, and probably overwhelming responsibilities.

My technical approach emphasized interpretations and clarifications. While interpretations are more commonly thought of as assisting in the analysis of conflicts, in particular through the analysis of transference and resistance, my articulation of his preconscious fantasy life also provided a narrative scaffolding around which Peter could actually, for the first time, organize his experiences. This actualizing of experience through narration and interaction in the hour facilitated internalization and the pulling together of ego structure. In addition, my emphasis on understanding Peter through interpretations and on continually clarifying and summarizing his communications offered him a stable, reliable, and consistent relationship. This was especially valuable for Peter, whose capacity for stable object representation was so shaky. He slowly responded to my efforts to understand and assist him. Over time, he came to imitate my approach and eventually made it his own. I would suggest that a traditional psychoanalytic technical approach may secondarily provide the best "real" relationship for patients such as Peter. At various times, according to need, Peter used me as a valued teacher, close friend and ally, or surrogate parent.

History

Peter was referred to me for treatment by an analyst who had diagnosed him as having primarily a gender identity disorder. This analyst told Peter's parents that the only hope of resolving his bisexual conflicts was through an analysis.

The milieu was not uneventful. Two years prior to Peter's birth, his mother had delivered her first child, Ronald, who lived for only six days because of a congenital abnormality that could not be surgically corrected. Despite Ronald's brief life, he remained a living presence in the house. He was frequently referred to by the parents as Peter's older brother. Peter's mother became severely depressed and preoccupied after Ronald's death. Despite constant bickering and strife and the considerable risk that any additional pregnancy also would be problematic because of what had happened with Ronald, the parents decided to have a second child. Mother become pregnant with Peter. Although the pregnancy was uneventful, Peter did inhale amniotic fluid at birth; as a result, both Peter and his mother remained in the hospital for ten days after his delivery.

Mother described Peter as a studious, compliant youngster with artistic tendencies. He sucked his thumb continuously from soon after birth. Mother tried to breastfeed him but, feeling insecure and fearful that he was not getting sufficient nourishment, she quickly switched him to a bottle. At six weeks Peter developed severe colic, which lasted for approximately two months. Mother appeared disappointed when she talked about how easily he would always go to strangers. She stayed home with Peter for ten months before taking a job at a local factory. During Peter's first eighteen months, his mother would spend long hours lying on the couch, feeling depressed and lethargic, watching television with Peter resting against her naked breast.

Peter walked two weeks after his first birthday. He always had a blanket that he clung to at bedtime. Mother indicated that the only time the usually docile Peter would get agitated and scream was when father would return home from work and would verbally attack his wife, sometimes loudly denigrating her. Mother felt constantly belittled by her husband but continued to seek and require his approval. During this period of marital discord, she pulled Peter closer and closer to her. He would frequently sleep in her bed with her at night.

When Peter was twenty-seven months old, his brother Robert was born. This child had serious physical handicaps, possibly related to an unspecified intrauterine accident. Robert has had repeated major surgical procedures to ameliorate his physical deformities. He has normal intelligence. An extremely aggressive and demanding child, Robert has consumed much of the family's resources, both financial and emotional. Both parents confessed that they felt that Robert had received much more of their attention than Peter, who was superficially so cooperative and undemanding. A few months after Robert's birth, Peter refused to go to sleep and would wake up repeatedly throughout the night. His parents were puzzled by this behavior and didn't understand what had prompted it.

Shortly after his second birthday, Peter began to talk about how he wanted to be like his mother and about how frightened he was of his father. His interest in wearing women's clothing was first observed at about twenty months and has been constant since that time. He experimented with his mother's make-up, particularly her lipstick. When this was forbidden, he used a chapstick.

Peter's entrance into preschool at age three was recalled as uneventful, although it was at about this time that his parents separated. His teachers described him as cooperative but isolated and without friends. Both at school and at home, he preferred to entertain himself, drawing pictures or playing at solitary make-believe games.

At four years of age, Peter had recurrent dreams in which his mother was dying and somebody was going to kidnap him. During this period he was fascinated by his mother's large breasts and constantly tried to stroke or hit them. He frequently expressed the wish to be a girl like his mother. In addition, Peter seemed scattered, forgetful, and often oblivious to obvious social clues. While he was superficially compliant, he stubbornly refused to yield to parental direction and seemed impervious to external input. While father was possibly cruel and rejecting of mother, he was usually kind and maternal toward Peter.

Peter's mother was thirty-nine at the time of his referral the following year. A large, masculine-appearing woman, she showed little understanding of her children or their special needs. Peter's birth so soon after Ronald's death, compounded by the devastating marital difficulties and Robert's handicaps, left her preoccupied, depressed, and only minimally available to Peter. Peter's father responded to the losses by dedicating his energy to his successful new law firm. He discharged his paternal responsibilities by making sure that Peter had all the help he needed rather than by spending much time with him.

Mother had finished only two years of college before her marriage and had held several jobs of short duration. She had difficulty focusing and taking direction. She became bored easily and, like Peter, preferred to have no responsibilities. She often appeared to drift off into fantasy. Her impulsiveness and unreliability presented a problem during Peter's analysis. She would frequently "forget" to bring him to the one appointment a week she had agreed to drive him to. (His father, who had the responsibility for getting Peter to his other sessions, was more reliable.) Sometimes she was an enthusiastic supporter of the analysis; at other times, she would suddenly raise questions as to whether a particular appointment should be the last one for Peter.

Mother's own childhood had been extremely difficult. Her father was inconsistent, chronically depressed, and frequently lost his temper over seemingly trivial matters. Her mother was self-preoccupied and not very attentive to mothering.

Mother had a waiflike quality and a lack of responsiveness to environmental cues. She had been in supportive psychotherapy since the marital separation but had no comprehension of the extent of her son's difficulties, tending at times to minimize his problems or expressing the opinion that the outcome was preordained and unmodifiable anyway.

During the second year of Peter's analysis, his parents divorced. Mother remarried a man twelve years her junior. Shortly after their separation, Peter's father had met a slightly older woman, a former pediatric nurse, with three children of her own. (He told me that his highest priority in selecting a new wife was to find a woman who was capable of handling his two difficult sons and who would agree to dedicate all her time to mothering.) The couple was married after a three-year courtship. Peter was sent to live with his father's new family; his mother had visitation rights two or three weekends a month.

Peter's new stepmother, a highly organized woman, was a strict disciplinarian who expected the children to live up to their potential. She had difficulties with Peter's passivity, intransigence, and constant underachievement.

COURSE OF TREATMENT

In my first appointment with Peter, he separated hesitantly from his mother. After entering my office, he immediately talked about how much he preferred girls' things to boys'. He thought girls' clothes were prettier than boys' clothes. He told me that his father was angry at him because of Peter's wish to be a girl. During this first hour, he assiduously avoided anything with male connotations. The only play materials he used were female puppets, whose hair he gently stroked and whose clothes he rearranged. He appeared timid, tentative, and self-absorbed. Physically, Peter was a handsome, almost pretty boy with subtly effeminate mannerisms.

Although Peter did not initially impress me as being very intelligent, that impression probably derived from his obliviousness to much of what was going on around him and his lack of responsiveness to my inquiries. I would frequently have to repeat a statement or a question in order to elicit any response from him. He seemed to lack curiosity and engagement.

During our first appointments, Peter spent most of his time drawing countless pictures. With encouragement, he would narrate his drawings, describing in minute detail stories such as Cinderella or the Little Mermaid. In one version of the Little Mermaid, a male "merman," bigger in size than the world, had the power to turn a little mermaid into a girl. I noted that someone with such power could possibly do anything he liked to a person's body. Peter responded by drawing numerous variations of the possible transformations of a mermaid's body. Initially creative, these drawings became repetitious and prototypic of how he manifested his resistance to treatment. During many hours Peter would become regressed; he would speak in baby-talk, crawl around the office, and imitate his crippled younger brother. Often he seemed to ignore my interventions and to be oblivious to my presence.

Peter's case raised many diagnostic questions in my mind. How much of his difficulty was related to dynamic inhibition as opposed to incapacity or constitutional deficits? Did his total self-absorption augur poorly for his engagement and active participation in the treatment? How could treatment be effective when he showed so little of the motivation to move forward and mature typically observed in boys his age?

The backward pull seemed greater than any positive developmental momentum. He wanted to be left alone and to have no interference with his wish to do things as he had always done them. I was concerned not only by the absence of any obvious motivation for treatment but also by his complacency about his various difficulties at home, at school, and with his peers.

At the same time, there was the suggestion of some oedipal-phase development. Peter's wish to be a girl could be conventionally constructed as a defense against his intense castration anxiety, especially given his brother's damaged body and his mother's overpowering and intrusive early presence.

Whatever the sources, it seemed to me that Peter's life was on a disastrous course, given his gender difficulties, organizational deficits, insensitivity to environmental cues, and blanket refusal to cooperate with his stepmother's instructions. To compound these difficulties, he spent his weekends with his mother, who provided an environment that was the antithesis of his stepmother's home. Mother encouraged regression, making no demands, and overstimulated Peter with exces- sive nudity and physical contact. I was hopeful that his strong identifi- cation with his mother would be responsive to our therapeutic inter- action and not unmodifiable.

During the initial consultation, I got an occasional glimpse of Peter's sadness, longings, and perplexity about why the world reacted so ad- versely to him. He appeared "frozen" and terrified of growing older. I hoped that the early part of the treatment would clarify some of the ambiguities and provide access to more internal conflict than was evi- dent on the surface. I thought he could benefit from a consistent ther- apeutic interaction and the emergence of a stable transference. I also hoped that I would be able to engage Peter in such a way that he would recognize the difficulties in his adaptation and begin to believe that he had the capability of improving.

Despite many misgivings, I decided to proceed with the analysis. I was impressed by his father's determination to do everything possible for Peter. I hoped that the limitations that I regarded as related to deficits in Peter's equipment might turn out to be at least partially at- tributable to dynamic inhibition and his extreme castration fears. I was also curious about the effect the non-interpretive elements of the treat- ment would have on Peter. For example, would his relationship with me have a positive impact on his difficulty in maintaining stable rep- resentations? I hoped that the treatment would facilitate his stalled de- velopmental progression. In any case, I thought that no alternative treatment approach could offer Peter as much potential gain.

The first six months of Peter's analysis did little to clarify my ques- tions about how he would utilize the analytic situation. The hours were very repetitive. Peter was afraid that my primary goal was to make him want to be a boy and stop acting like a girl. He feared that I was his fa- ther's agent and devoted his energies to making sure that I did not un- derstand him. He dismissed my reassurances that my objective was to help him better understand who he wanted to be and what would make him happy. He desperately tried to maintain control over the hours. For example, he would enter the office and immediately pick up a toy telephone, "calling" me and asking me to come out and play ball with him. He would toss a plastic ball back and forth and then declare that he was too busy to play and had to rush to work. He called me on his "business" phone but would then keep me waiting because he had so many other calls. He then would dial one number after the other, in- dicating to me how he experienced his father: as inconsistent and un- available.

In other hours, he was preoccupied with female anatomy and the potential for anatomical change. He showed me through his drawings that women could be with breasts or without them and could have bodies of all sizes and shapes. His drawings of the genital area were ambiguous. He drew pictures of mermaids depicting them with legs so that they could walk on land but adapting them to water by replacing the legs with tails.

In endless discussion of Cinderella, he ignored my observations and would just draw one picture after another. Alternatively, he would fill the hour by pretending he was Cinderella, doing repetitive routine domestic chores such as vacuuming, washing dishes, and dusting. In one hour, Cinderella was preparing to attend the ball. The wicked stepmother was doing everything to sabotage her efforts to dress. In a manner atypical for Peter, he acknowledged my comparing the wicked stepmother in the fairy tale to his feelings about his own new stepmother. He then elaborated his fears about what changes might occur when his stepmother moved in with her children. This encouraging response was in marked contrast to Peter's more typical blank stares in response to my efforts.

As our work continued, Peter became more organized, and the hours gained in thematic consistency. He acknowledged and enjoyed my attention. More and more he wanted to please me, as he did his father, by talking about issues he thought I wanted him to consider.

After the first two years of treatment, Peter, then aged seven and a half, was less tentative and more related and available during his analytic hours. A typical hour from the end of the second year illustrates some of these changes. During this hour, three weeks after summer vacation, Peter initially drew a picture of fairies about which he wanted to tell me a story. I noted that he had often told me that he draws pictures and creates elaborate stories about them because he doesn't want to talk about other more upsetting things. Much to my surprise, he responded by telling me to shut up. He was furious. He stuffed tissues in his ears and told me that he could not hear anything I was saying. I said that he had had it with all my unwanted and upsetting comments. He said that was true and crawled under the couch, informing me that there was nothing to talk about. I told him I was puzzled about what had caused such a violent reaction. He said, "Okay, I will tell you. Matthew, at school, is so mean to me. He is always teasing and saying, here comes Peter, and getting the other kids to laugh at me." I said, "You don't know what to do about it and talking about it just makes you feel worse." He replied, "Don't you understand, I have no problems. I have never had any problems. I hear everything you tell me even when I act like I don't. I do want my mommy and daddy to be back together again. I think I want to be a boy. I don't want to be a girl at all. I know that I draw pictures of girls all the time. It doesn't mean anything." Peter crawled back under the couch, covering his ears with tissues and telling me that he couldn't hear anything. I responded with a smile because his mood had clearly lightened and said, "Maybe by pretending you can't hear, you have to respond only to the things you want to talk about and can pretend not to hear what you don't want to talk about." He responded, "Well, maybe."

Then he took a piece of paper and requested that I ask him questions, something he had done in previous hours. I said I wasn't sure what questions he wanted me to ask. He said, "Ask about my feelings. That's what you are always interested in. I don't like feelings." I said that discussing feelings was upsetting and reminded him of all of the things he was unhappy about. He responded, "Yes, I just want to be left alone. Everyone picks on me. My stepsister picks on me. She tells me I am ugly and stupid. I hate her. I want to be left alone."

I suggested that maybe I seemed like his stepsister when I talked about his feelings and activities rather than just discussing his drawings and make-believe. He said, "That's right. I can do everything the other boys can do. They just don't think I can. What more does everyone want? Matthew is different. He can do more. He can climb up the jungle gym better than I can." Then he said, "Look at this," pulling up his trousers to show me his nonexistent leg muscles. He proudly stated, "I don't have arm muscles, but I do have leg muscles. Matthew's muscles are bigger and stronger." I said that maybe Matthew used his stronger muscles to force Peter to do things he didn't want to do. Peter agreed and added, "That's why I hate my stepsister. She pushes me around all the time too." He continued complaining until close to the end of the hour, when he lay down on the floor and began to crawl around. I observed that maybe we had talked about too many upsetting issues and that he was once again acting like his younger brother, who he felt had so few responsibilities. He exclaimed, "Robert poops in his pants. He's a little baby. Everybody does everything for him." I suggested that because Robert had so many problems with his body not as much was expected of him. Peter angrily agreed, indicating that this was unfair.

I told him that he wished I would perform an operation that would help him with all his problems, just as an operation had helped his brother with his physical problems. In response, Peter expressed his despair and his opinion that he just wasn't as capable as other boys. He did wish that something could be done to make him stronger and better able to compete with other boys. He was angry with me because I might be withholding an operation that would help him in the same way that his crippled brother, Robert, had been helped.

This hour was unusual in its coherence, relatedness, and rich content. It illustrates how my interpretative efforts also promoted a narrative structure about which Peter organized his otherwise ambiguous thoughts and feelings. More customarily, Peter filled the hours by emphasizing his helplessness and confusion, insisting that he didn't have what it takes to change. He tried to convince me that he was weak, inept, and incapable of functioning more independently. He insisted that he needed to be withdrawn and self-absorbed because he was not equipped to deal with the increasing demands and insults of the real world.

It was important for Peter that I acknowledge his limitations because my approval meant so much to him and he didn't want to disappoint me. My efforts to interpret his reluctance to venture forth and put himself on the line as a defensive compromise formation seemed unsuccessful. Although Peter typically did not respond to my interventions by bringing forth new material, my comments did help him organize his experiences. My perspective and method of observing and organizing his experiences provided a scaffolding on which he could organize his somewhat chaotic inner life and experiences, bolstering his fragile synthetic capacities. His ability to tell me how bad Matthew made him feel was a product of our previous work. Even at this point in his treatment, there was still little thematic continuity from hour to hour. Peter didn't seem to learn easily from experience, to carry forth earlier gains into later sessions.

In a dramatic hour a few months later, Peter insisted, with tears flowing down his cheeks, that he was no longer going to see me because coming to his appointments was his only problem. He was tired of everyone constantly talking to him about his problems. I said it seemed that to have problems meant that everything was wrong, and that if there were no problems everything was right. He agreed and asked me to be quiet. I agreed not to talk because I knew there were times when he was so upset that he felt no matter what I said he would just get more upset. He seemed relieved and a few moments later softly said, "I just don't know who I am. I have no idea who I am. I don't understand. I copy what other people do, and I think I will become like them and then the boys won't hate me any more. I want to be a regular person. I don't know what that is. I don't want everyone to tease me." I said that it hurts him so much to be teased that he would give anything to figure out how to stop it. He said, "That's right. I copy lots of people, but I don't really become them. I copy you most of all. That seems to help because then I do feel better and their words don't hurt me as much." Peter elaborated on his confusion about who he was and who he wanted to be. He told me that he preferred it when I asked him questions and talked more to him because then he felt better and knew what to talk about. He then explained that people thought he wanted to be a girl but that was not the truth. "I find myself acting like a girl. It's not something I decide I want to do." As the hour ended, Peter told me that he wanted to continue talking because he felt that I did understand what he was telling me and that I was helping him to know better who he was and who he wanted to be. He thought that I just wanted him to be a happier person.

Soon after this hour, Peter, now almost eight years old, became preoccupied with the life stories of various imaginary people. He drew detailed pictures of people at various points in their life cycle and would then tell me stories of their childhood, their adventures, their mishaps, their accomplishments, their children, their terminal illnesses and death. He was doing research on what a life is about and whether he could find a prototype he could emulate. Peter was uncertain whether life was a series of snapshots or whether there was something that provided continuity from moment to moment and year to year. This reflected another feature of his psychological organization: his identifications had no staying power; they were transitory. Even the potential for identifications within the therapeutic interaction lacked cohesiveness and durability.

Peter's research into how other people functioned began to focus on specific actors and actresses. For two to three weeks at a time, he would repeatedly watch the same movie, memorize all the lines of a particular performer, and then act out the role during the hour. Imitation was possible; internalization of the imitated functions was far more difficult. However, Peter's persistent efforts in this direction signaled his emerging determination to move forward in his development, to cast himself in some available mold. He was trying to find a path he could follow that would permit him to feel safe enough to grow up.

The following hour from the fourth year of his analysis, when Peter was nine years old, illustrates this phase of the analysis. Peter told me that he wanted to discuss and illustrate the story of "Indiana Jones and the Last Crusade," the movie he had been watching lately. He said, "I really like that movie. I saw it again with my mother last night. It's the third in the series of movies about Indiana Jones, the one where he searches for the Holy Grail." Peter became very animated and excitedly told me how one evil man tried to find the Holy Grail. The next thing you see is his head rolling down the floor. He told me that nobody seemed able to survive the search for the Holy Grail.

In an attempt to interpret his underlying anxiety about the threat to his body integrity at different levels of psychological organization, I observed how difficult and dangerous it was to try to get the Holy Grail and wondered why Indiana Jones would take such risks. Peter impatiently explained that Indiana Jones had no choice because if he got the Grail he could bring his father back to life. We talked about how miraculous it was that he could obtain the power to bring his father back from the dead after he had been shot and killed. No wonder he would courageously face such hardship and terror. Peter described how one man drank from a diamond-covered container, convinced that it had to be the Holy Grail, but then was immediately transformed into a monster and destroyed. He drew a detailed picture of this man, portraying him as a decaying corpse. I observed how rapidly he had changed from being strong and alive into someone who looked as if he had been dead for a long time. Peter nonchalantly informed me that this was just the way it happened. Excitedly, he said, "Indiana Jones was so smart. He decided to pick the plain dirt container to drink from it, and it was the right one. He saved his father." Proudly mimicking the successful hero, Peter showed me how Indiana Jones then poured a special fluid on the dead father's wounds, which healed magically. His father immediately returned to life.

Peter then added, "There was this woman, a Nazi, who was helping Indiana Jones. She grabbed the container from Indiana Jones and tried to steal it. She fell down a bottomless pit and supposedly was dead. Indiana Jones wanted to get the container back from her, but his father told him it would be too dangerous to try, and probably saved his son's life." I emphasized that first Indiana Jones had brought his father back to life and then the father saved him. Peter agreed that that was the way it seemed to work. He said it was not so bad that the woman had been killed because she was a Nazi anyway. I noted that he had said that she also was a friend of Indiana Jones. Peter looked at me and said, "Well, they slept together." He added with considerable animation, "She also slept with his father." I said, "That's really something. She slept with both the father and the son." He said, "Not 'something.' That's disgusting." He then explained that both Indiana Jones and his father were archaeologists. They worked close together and loved each other. The father was not that old. I again observed that the son was so dedicated to his father and took so much risk to restore his life and in return had his own life saved. Peter said they would have done anything to save each other. At the end of the hour, he talked about how strange it was that the Nazi woman had been with both the father and the son. What seemed most important in this story to Peter were not the obvious and intriguing oedipal themes but how the father and son looked out for each other and, most importantly, protected each other. Through repeatedly acting out the role of Indiana Jones, Peter developed a better understanding of how one person can assist and not destroy another person he cares for.

When I compared Indiana Jones' close collaboration with his father to our work together, Peter readily accepted the comparison. He then pointed out that I wasn't there to protect him from danger the way Indiana's father protected him. I noted that he was disappointed that I did not do that for him, and he agreed. This echoed Peter's earlier hope of being rescued by an omnipotent therapist or through some special surgical intervention. At the same time, Peter was beginning to recognize that I was helping him to understand himself and that as a result he could make the world a safer and better place for himself. He could learn how to get assistance when he needed it and also could see that his own actions affected other people. I thought this phase of the work boded well for enhancing his capacity for object-relatedness.

Peter continued in subsequent hours to portray himself as Indiana Jones, imitating Jones' courage, intelligence, and virtue. This made him feel more powerful and capable. He responded positively to my comments that when he was Indiana Jones he felt better able to face the day. These hours also had significance in that they represented one of the few times that Peter portrayed himself as an intelligent and effective man. He thought it would be wonderful to be Indiana Jones because of his strength, wisdom, and seeming invulnerability, but he also recognized that in his play he was using his idea of Indiana Jones to muster his own courage and capacities. Development was moving forward as he became more organized around his new sense of a more together self.

The thematic organization of these hours was in marked contrast to earlier material that had been more fragmented, less related, and lacking in richness. It illustrates Peter's finding coherence from an outside source and the difficulty of making that coherence his own. The forward move reflected Peter's greater stability and increased capacity for affect tolerance. In the transference, Peter viewed me as invulnerable despite his earlier denial that I protected him from danger both within the hour and in the rest of his life. Peter responded enthusiastically when I communicated an empathic recognition of his problems or discussed the details of his various roles. Although he seemed unresponsive to interpretations of his conflicts and inhibitions, the unfolding and consolidation of the therapeutic relationship suggested that they were having an impact other than accessing hitherto unrecognized conflicts.

During a subsequent hour, Peter told me that I didn't understand his unwillingness to discuss home or school and that enacting movie roles was his life. I noted that that was a life that he could control, and so much happened in his daily life that he disliked and felt helpless to change. He cried and said that in the world of plays and movies he did not feel the terrible pain of his days at school and home. Peter constantly experimented with different movie roles, roles that provided thematic coherence while they were being enacted and relief from the pain of his everyday life.

As we continued to discuss his portrayal of these roles, his descriptions became richer. Through his imitations of various actors, Peter gradually found different ways of expressing feelings and interacting with other people. These roles provided a scaffolding upon which he constructed a more coherent view of himself in the world. Peter made significant strides in his capacity to understand affects and ideas in an increasingly discriminate manner. This was an additional response to my efforts to help him become more specific through identifying affects and pursuing a better understanding of what various ideas signified to him. It demonstrated that interpretations of conflicts can have different therapeutic effects. Traditionally, we know they help patients by providing a fresh encounter and perspective on unconscious conflicts. In Peter's case they also helped by offering narrative constructs to facilitate the emergence and growth of developmental organizations. Those new developmental organizations may then make it possible to use interpretations in the more conventional way.

Peter's capacity to utilize more of my interventions concerning unconscious conflicts was amply demonstrated in the subsequent period of the analysis. More organized negative oedipal material emerged. I would be excluded while he drew female models such as Cindy Crawford, who could get whatever they desired just on the basis of their physical beauty. Peter, now ten years old, again became oppositional with me, contending that his only problem was his father's insistence that he continue his treatment. Without me, his life would be problem-free. In many hours, he would pretend that he was a beautiful, promiscuous model who could get anything she wanted from me. He would act seductively toward me, wanting me to take care of him and to have sex with him. I would protect him, and he would agree to satisfy my every desire. He also revealed his fantasy that penises and vaginas are interchangeable. He claimed that he might have been born with a vagina that was changed to a penis. Peter thought that a vagina might be restored surgically. Another fantasy was that he could die and return in a totally new form.

While Peter showed only moderate improvement at school and home, the transference was more clearly demarcated. At times, I was the all enveloping and consuming early mother whose attention was directed elsewhere. More frequently, I was the admired powerful father whom he wanted to seduce and from whom he sought protection and the source of his power.

Although identification with the early mother, the traumatic influences in the early years of his life, and dispositional factors contributed to Peter's wish to be a girl as well as his belief that he was a girl, he saw the issue as simply his not having the resources and capacities other boys possessed. His body could not compete and his mind was different from that of other boys. As a boy, he couldn't compete with other boys. But if he was a beautiful girl, he would be taken care of and could pursue his most coveted interests, many of which he thought were more appropriate for a girl. Given Peter's difficulty in maintaining stable internal mental representations, being female, a long-standing wish, provided Peter with a more coherent picture of himself. I urged him to discuss freely both his wish to be a girl and his feelings that he was a girl, being careful to be neither critical nor encouraging.

During this period of the analysis, his mother's second marriage came to a stormy conclusion when she discovered that her husband was having an affair. In his characteristic manner, Peter minimized his stepfather's importance, but over time he admitted that he had liked him and that he missed him. His mother remained antagonistic to the treatment, continuing to bathe both her sons together and in many ways encouraging Peter's female proclivities. Her naturalistic approach to parenting included continuing to grant Peter free access to her body, especially her breasts.

Peter continued to have difficulties with his stepmother, who, despite her own disappointment and frustration with Peter, persevered in her attempt to provide structure for him and encouragement for his school participation. Although his school performance improved, he still was not fully available for his studies. Peter continued to prefer being left alone in his room but was willing with strong encouragement to arrange play dates. At his father's insistence, he reluctantly participated in a martial arts class.

Unfortunately, Peter's analysis was prematurely interrupted because of circumstances in my own life. Peter was superficially nonchalant about the upcoming termination but in response to it seemed to consolidate certain therapeutic gains. Although he was oppositional during termination, he was also more direct in his wish that I take care of him. He would mimic me and make fun of me but would also talk about how if he were I, he would be able to do so much more in the world. In his last hour, he expressed his sadness in the only mode that he could tolerate; he became an actor, pretending that he was sad and crying as he walked out the door.

DISCUSSION

Peter made significant advances during his six years of analysis. At termination, he insisted that he now wanted only to be a boy, not a girl, and that he enjoyed primarily boys' activities. His castration anxiety was considerably reduced, and he was more appropriately assertive. My impression was that he continued to be more ambivalent about his gender preference and identity than he was willing to reveal to himself or to me.

Perhaps Peter's major accomplishment was that he possessed a more coherent picture of himself. His internal self representations had greater stability and integration that permitted him to process new material in a manner that was not possible before. Peter was less preoccupied with his fantasy life and more available for school, family, and friends. He showed more enthusiasm for the benefits of growing up and less apprehension about the challenges ahead. The developmental push forward was substantially increased. Peter could more accurately assess his assets and liabilities and act accordingly.

To delineate the mechanisms of change or the mutative therapeutic factors for Peter is a daunting but necessary challenge. My technical approach emphasized neutrality and non-intervention into his day-to-day life; this was generally consistent with my method of analyzing less disturbed children. I resisted the temptation to advise, cajole, and direct Peter. I had the impression that my consistent interpretive approach enabled Peter gradually to come to hear what I was saying and to organize previously confusing thoughts, feelings, and fantasies so as to facilitate more stable internal representations. The actualization in the hour of certain experiences contributed to this increased stability and coherence and thus furthered development. It also helped to stabilize the relationship of one experience to another. Although my intentions were to clarify unconscious meanings, Peter often used what I said as a source of organization and coherence. As the analysis progressed, he also identified with my efforts to deal with upsetting affects in a calm, understanding manner, mimicking and eventually identifying with my tolerance for affects in the course of our exchanges. Peter seemed to feel that the more he could be like me, the less helpless he would feel.

Peter's experience in the hours helped him to understand more about himself as he applied it to what occurred in other settings. Peter responded positively to the consistency and predictability of my efforts; he knew that I would be patient and would try to deal with even his angriest moments through understanding.

Especially early in the treatment, Peter rejected my interpretations of his conflicts and inhibitions because they threatened his fragile internal representations. He was too impressionable and easily overwhelmed by new ways of thinking. He lacked motivation for learning and facilitating his own development. What might be seen as an inherent pull forward in development was not discernible when the treatment began. Even Peter's resistance to understanding his wish to be a girl was partially determined by how long he had thought of himself as a girl and how this view of himself anchored his shaky self representations.

Peter was responsive to my help in identifying and discriminating among his more diffuse feeling states. As his capacity to identify feelings and experiences increased, he felt more confident and more capable of accurately communicating in a manner that permitted meaningful give and take. The movie roles he enacted during the hour provided various trial identifications and experiences in relating. Roles such as Indiana Jones represented an intermediate structure that he utilized to integrate experience. These roles provided a temporary way-station prior to the establishment of more stable internal representations.

As Peter's sense of self became more integrated, he developed an increased capacity to be responsive to interpretations of repressed conflicts and transference. Peter required a more stable sense of self before he could identify and begin to resolve his intrapsychic conflicts.

Peter's transference varied in intensity and duration. For long periods of time when he was regressed and wanting to be left alone, I was the early mother, barely separate and discouraging of separation and autonomy. Sometimes I was the frightening father, critical and not understanding of his fragility. Toward the last years of the analysis, I was more consistently an idealized, omnipotent paternal figure who could protect him from injury and lend him my strengths. Much of this was expressed as negative oedipal longings. During the entire analysis, a positive oedipal transference characterized by competitiveness and rivalry never consolidated.

The relationship with me, the actualization of experiences within the hour, identification, naming of affects, the creation of narrative structures, the consistency and predictability of our time together— all these contributed to Peter's increasingly stable self representations. These byproducts of the analytic situation (Harley 1958) took center stage during much of my work with Peter. They were what he required for his stalled development to resume. What is more difficult to understand is the effect of my interpretations aimed at understanding his oedipal conflicts, castration anxiety, and aggressive inhibitions. Given the progression of the analysis and the emergence of a more formed negative oedipal transference, these interpretations may have been more effective than I considered them to be during much of the analysis. As Peter's internal representations stabilized, he was more capable of integrating both ongoing and past interpretive efforts. The same is true with regard to his development. Even the observed lack of motivation to move on and become more independent was in part a consequence of conflict and inhibition. As conflict was resolved, the constraints to development were freed. The reciprocal relationship between developmental and analytic needs are especially clear in Peter's treatment, as is the difficulty in dealing technically with both in the course of the work.

I hope that Peter will return to treatment at some point. Although his progress was considerable, I feel that a more thoroughgoing examination and resolution of his antecedent childhood conflicts would probably prove very fruitful.

BIBLIOGRAPHY

COATES, S., FRIEDMAN, R. C., & WOLFE, S. (1991). The etiology of a boyhood gender identity disorder: A model for integrating temperament, development and psychodynamics. *Psychoanalytic Dialogues, 1*(#4):481–523.

FREUD, A. (1965). *Normality and pathology in childhood.* New York: Int. Univ. Press.

HARLEY, M. (1986). Child analysis, 1947–1984: A retrospective. *Psych. Study of the Child,* 41, pp. 129–155.

HARTMANN, H. (1929). *Ego psychology and the mechanisms of adaptation.* New York: Int. Univ. Press, 1958.

McDEVITT, J. (1995). A childhood gender identity disorder: Analysis, pre-oedipal determinants and therapy in adolescence. *Psych. Study of the Child,* 50:79–105.

RITVO, S. (1978). The psychoanalytic process in childhood. *Psych. Study of the Child,* 33:295–305.

Coordinating the Developmental and Psychoanalytic Processes: Three Case Reports

Discussion

SAMUEL ABRAMS, PETER B. NEUBAUER, AND ALBERT J. SOLNIT

EACH OF THE FOREGOING CASE PRESENTATIONS AND THE TREATMENTS they describe was prepared, presented, and written up for consideration and discussion by the Study Group described in the Introduction. These clinical presentations uniquely put forth how each of the child analysts involved treated his or her analysand and how each responded to the theoretical and clinical questions raised by the Study Group.

Theoretical and clinical questions were referred to in an earlier contribution (Abrams and Solnit, 1998) and briefly reviewed in the Introduction to these case histories (Abrams, Neubauer, and Solnit, 1999). Here we (S. Abrams, P. B. Neubauer, and A. J. Solnit) briefly summarize and clarify many of these questions and issues, as a way of pointing to future discussions and study.

Development spans an anticipated sequence of hierarchically ordered phase organizations, periods when certain dilemmas are confronted in the course of human growth. Intrapsychic issues of all kinds erupt early, and psychoanalysts are especially attentive to the nuclear infantile intrapsychic conflicts that leave their residue in unrecognized structures and unconscious fantasies. In latency, a different dilemma is confronted. Development pulls the growing child toward ego growth and extrafamilial contacts. The shift toward these facets can sometimes be so intense that it pulls the child away from the intrafamilial, with its constellations of intrapsychic conflicts. Later, during adolescence, the growing child confronts a struggle between the lure of the past and the needs of the future. This developmentally induced dilemma creates an additional focus for analytic work.

Attending to the complexities introduced by developmental forces requires a transactional field in which the analyst may be used as a "new" object to assist in the patient's developmental progression. Generally, in latency, patients use analysts as new extrafamilial objects; and in addition to being used for transferences and for necessary new experiences, analysts are always "real" individuals, readily available for identifications, for example. Identifying with the affect tolerance or the psychological-mindedness of analysts is useful in both analytic and developmental-processes settings.

How were developmental forces and components of the child's deviant and neurotic make-up taken into account by each of these three psychoanalysts as they evaluated and treated each of the three children? We find it useful to ask how child analysts coordinate their therapeutic technical approach with the developmental assistance they provide in their treatment of neurotic children, children whose primary condition is one of developmental deficit or deviance, as well as children who have a mix of neurotic and developmental difficulties. Analogously, how are the various phases of development taken into account?

The case illustrations demonstrate how three analysts engaged the fundamental therapeutic dilemma of balancing the need to solve the issues evoked by intrapsychic conflicts with the requirements for facilitating developmental pulls. The problem was compounded in two of the three cases because they were diagnosed as having ego deviations that impaired their capacities for forming unconscious fantasies and their derivatives. These deviations also affected emergent new phases. But in spite of the fact that two children were diagnosed with serious disturbances, it appears that all three benefited from their treatment by their respective child analysts. It is likely that what is learned from these cases can be usefully applied to more normative circumstances.

Overlapping questions and issues emerge:

(1) How were developmental forces and the components of each child's deviant or neurotic make-up managed technically by these three psychoanalysts as they established the treatment setting to best serve their patients?

(2) How do different normative developmental stages influence the kinds of therapeutic strategies available to the child analyst? Does ado-

lescence require its own particular strategy, different from that used in latency?

(3) Differences in diagnostic categories affect therapeutic strategies. How do child analysts go about determining the child's psychological capacities and limitations in order to plan how to proceed within the therapeutic relationship?

(4) What methods of appraisal are available that allow child analysts to decide when to promote the transferential features to resolve the neurotic underpinning and when to promote the "new" object potential within the therapeutic encounter to facilitate developmental progression? This question contains two basic assumptions: (a) that transference ("old" object) is significantly—albeit not exclusively—the "motor" for analytic treatment, and (b) that the analyst as "new" object with whom the child can identity is often the "motor" to promote the resumption of development. In brief, what are the prevailing features of development and diagnostic categories that determine the emphasis within the therapeutic interaction?

(5) This leads to the specific technical tool of interpretation. (a) Under what circumstances can interpretations interrupt the developmentally promoting experience of the therapeutic relationship as contrasted with serving to promote insight? This question has a long history—interpretations that aim to induce regressions during latency, for example, are known to hinder that developmental period. (b) Under what circumstances can interpretation aimed at promoting insight turn out to serve developmental goals instead or as well? (c) In which cases do interpretations intended to gain access to unconscious fantasies or narratives *create* narratives instead? (d) Are there useful distinctions between narrative-reducing interpretations (customary in analytic work) and narrative-promoting ones?

The clinical data highlight these issues while suggesting further pathways for research. The selection of these case reports was not intended to provide examples of each developmental phase, to feature diverse diagnostic categories, or to force into view gender differences or various developmental vicissitudes or deviations. These examples were selected to enlarge our general awareness of integrating analytic and developmental issues while broadening the analytic landscape. There has always been a question about how child analysts can function effectively within a context influenced by variations and deviations in development. This study brings a sharper focus to the issues we have specified and approaches a more systematic view of how theory and technique in child analysis can be responsive to developmental considerations.

BIBLIOGRAPHY

ABRAMS, S. & SOLNIT, A. J. (1998). Coordinating developmental and psychoanalytic processes: Conceptualizing technique. *JAPA* 46, 85–103.

THEORY

Constant Mental Change and Unknowability in Psychoanalysis

LEON BALTER, M.D.

Conflict and compromise formation are central aspects of mental life. They dispose to constant mental change. Limitations of knowability in psychoanalysis are inextricably connected with constant mental change— the latter sometimes diminishing unknowability and sometimes exacerbating it. This paper explores three kinds of unknowability in psychoanalysis and their relation to constant mental change. That relation clarifies to some degree the implications of certain controversial proposals for change in psychoanalytic theory, method, and technique.

THIS PAPER WILL DEMONSTRATE THAT THREE KINDS OF UNKNOWABILITY in psychoanalysis have a substantive relation to the mind's active, reactive, and auto-mutative nature. This constant and inexorable change in mental life reflects the basic mental property of conflict resolution through compromise formation, as adumbrated by the principle of multiple function. Unknowability of the first kind pertains to inherently unobservable unconscious mental processes and how they are inferred. Unknowability of the second kind pertains to practically unobservable extra-analytic determinants of psychic functioning in the psychoanalytic situation. Unknowability of the third kind pertains to practically unanalyzable effects of the analyst's own technical and investigative interventions in the analytic work itself. Standard aspects of psychoanalytic method and of the psychoanalytic situation address

Training and supervising analyst, The New York Psychoanalytic Institute.

Presented in earlier form and under another title at the annual meetings of The American Psychoanalytic Association, Los Angeles, May 4, 1996.

The Psychoanalytic Study of the Child 54, ed. Albert J. Solnit, Peter B. Neubauer, Samuel Abrams, and A. Scott Dowling (Yale University Press, copyright © 1999 by Albert J. Solnit, Peter B. Neubauer, Samuel Abrams, and A. Scott Dowling).

these three kinds of unknowability. Indeed, that is the reason they have become standard.

This discussion may contribute to the clarification of issues intrinsic to the current diversity in psychoanalytic theory, technique, and method. Crucial to the extreme pluralism that characterizes psychoanalysis today are diverse views concerning what is proper psychoanalytic knowledge and its limitations, what is actually knowable, and what is not. This paper constitutes an examination of this fundamental problem in psychoanalytic method.

CONSTANT CHANGE IN MENTAL LIFE

For the sake of conceptual clarity, it should be stated at the outset that the centrality of conflict and compromise formation was one of the most immediate implications drawn from the structural model of the mind conceptualized by Freud in *The Ego and the Id* (1923) and *Inhibitions, Symptoms and Anxiety* (1926). Waelder's formulation of the principle of multiple function in 1930 was the first important step in the direction of recognizing conflict and compromise formation as universal aspects of all observable mental phenomena. Even so, the centrality of conflict and compromise formation, so evident in Freud's monographs, was only implicit in Waelder's conceptualization. It became progressively more explicit in the psychoanalytic literature following the publication of Waelder's paper, reaching its acme of expression in *The Mind in Conflict* (1982). The following discussion of psychic change will be mostly in terms of conflict and compromise formation. Waelder, to some degree, discussed these matters in his early paper.

Brenner's consolidating synthesis defined *conflict* as follows:

> Under certain circumstances, [infantile] drive derivatives pressing for gratification arouse anxiety and depressive affect. Both of these are unpleasurable, sometimes intensely so. This is what accounts for the fact that the ego, which develops as the executant of the drives, as the agency for the gratification of drive derivatives, can on occasion oppose them. Such an opposition between ego and drive derivative is the essence of psychic conflict (pp. 53–54).

And also:

> [C]onflict occurs whenever gratification of a drive derivative [from childhood] is associated with a sufficiently intense unpleasurable affect. I should add here that superego demands and prohibitions which arouse anxiety and depressive affect of sufficient intensity will also occasion conflict (p. 55).

In a more general statement about conflict, Brenner (1982) wrote:

> Its components are several. They include [childhood] drive deriva-
> tives, anxiety and depressive affect, defense, and various manifesta-
> tions of superego functioning. These components interact in ways gov-
> erned by the pleasure-unpleasure principle. The consequences of
> conflict are compromise formations (p. 7).

While conflict produces compromise formations, it is the latter that
are the actual data of psychoanalytic observation.

> It is compromise formation one observes when one studies psychic
> functioning. Compromise formations are the data of observation
> when one applies the psychoanalytic method and observes and/or in-
> fers a patient's wishes, fantasies, moods, plans, dreams, and symptoms.
> Each of these is a compromise formation, as are, indeed, the entire
> range of psychic phenomena subsumed under the heading of mater-
> ial for analysis (p. 109).

Put succinctly, while conflict is a basic property of mental life, it is not
directly observable. The compromise formation, the resultant of conflict, is the basic unit of psychoanalytic *observation*. The conflict is the
basic unit of psychoanalytic *inference*.

Of greatest importance for the investigation of constant psychic
change is the fact that every compromise formation entails a dynamic
equilibrium among its various components of conflict. As Brenner
(1982) stated:

> [A] dynamic interaction among the components of psychic conflict
> underlies much or all of the subjectively conscious and objectively ob-
> servable phenomena of adult psychic life and behavior (p. 214).

> Conflict is always dynamic, always mobile. A successful defense does
> not fetter and immobilize a drive derivative [from childhood]. It does
> not render ineffective the psychic striving to be warded off. The mea-
> sure of the success or failure of a defense is the degree of diminution
> of anxiety and/or depressive affect it produces, not the fate of the [in-
> fantile] drive derivative that aroused those unpleasurable affects in the
> first place. The ego's function is to oppose id derivatives to the extent
> necessary to eliminate or to mitigate unpleasure. In their role as exe-
> cutants of the drives and, later, of the superego, ego functions will grant
> to both the fullest expression compatible with a tolerable degree of un-
> pleasure. When anxiety and/or depressive affect become too intensely
> unpleasurable, defense is heightened to mitigate them. When there is
> less intense unpleasure, more satisfaction is achieved (pp. 115–116).

Thus, the dynamic interaction among the components of conflict in
any compromise will cause each component to be both maximally ex-

pressed and minimally constrained. However, the obverse is also true: no component will be fully expressed, and every component will be expressed to greater or lesser extent in the compromise. The inherent limitation on the expression of each component ensures that its fulfillment must be partial. This is the paramount meaning of the term "compromise"—that is, each component is *compromised* regarding its complete fulfillment (see Waelder, 1936 [1930], p. 49).

Another corollary of this view is that any quantitative change in any one component of conflict will cause quantitative change in all the other components. The altered equilibrium will necessarily be in the direction of maintaining the compromise among the constituent components of conflict. That is, the re-equilibrating process must take place according to the pleasure-unpleasure principle, continuing to maximize infantile drive gratification but also continuing to minimize affective unpleasure. However, quantitative change may occur in one or several of the components of conflict such that infantile drive gratification is intolerably too little and/or affective unpleasure is intolerably too great. The compromise will then come undone, the original conflict will be re-evoked, and the result will be the formation of a qualitatively different compromise, which will be a derivative of the previous one, now taking into account the altered component(s) of conflict. The transformation of one compromise into a qualitatively different derivative one is the basic unit of psychic change.

The foregoing discussion points to the fact that both conflict and compromise formation are intrapsychic in nature. They are purely mental entities. The quantitative changes that occur in the components of conflict are due to the vicissitudes of mental life. However, this does not mean that the extrapsychic environment—material, interpersonal, and social—is always irrelevant. Clearly, it is not. Indeed, Brenner (1982) pointed out that a great many compromise formations are greatly affected by the environment. The environment may allow, or disallow, the various components of conflict the *means* for fulfillment of their respective tendencies:

> The environment influences compromise formations because of the opportunities it offers for the satisfaction of drive derivatives and the impediments it places in the way of their satisfaction; because of the fear or misery it brings, or even hints at, and the reassurances it offers against fear and the ways in which it assuages misery; because of the ways in which it reinforces defense as well as the ways in which it undermines it; and because of the opportunities it affords for supporting or for subverting morality in all its many aspects (Brenner, 1982, p. 225).

This is, in effect, a restatement of Hartmann's (1939) view of adaptation. It allows a more precise description of the process in that the specific environmental factors are brought into functional relation with the specific components of conflict in specific compromises. Compromise formations can then be classified according to whether they are influenced by the immediate environment and, if so, which element in the environment correlates with which component of the conflict. This view also provides much more precise insight into why certain environmental elements are actively sought and even actively constituted and why some are actively avoided and even destroyed.

The preceding discussion provides a general outline for understanding mental change. Quantitative changes in the drives biologically over the course of life and, intercurrently, through stimulation and frustration will have selective effects on specific components of conflict in specific compromises. Because anything the ego does may be used in the service of defense (Brenner, 1982, p. 75), quantitative changes in ego functioning will have selective effects on specific components of conflict in specific compromises. Quantitative changes in superego functioning, from endogenous sources (e.g., narcissistic gratification) or exogenous sources (e.g., group or social participation), will have selective effects on specific components of conflict in specific compromises. And quantitative changes in the environment will have selective effects on specific components of conflict in specific compromises. All these changes will cause shifts in the dynamic equilibrium of the affected compromises. If the shifts are great enough so that drive frustration and/or unpleasant affects are beyond toleration, qualitative change in the effected compromises will take place. Such change will range between gradual and abrupt, evanescent and stable, circumscribed and ramifying in its effects on other compromise formations, pathological (i.e., painful and/or dysfunctional) and healthy. The vicissitudes of everyday life provide a virtually endless and infinitely variable set of endogenous and environmental circumstances, which prompt and promote psychic conflict and therefore psychic change. The mind has, in its own functioning, a constant impetus to change itself. It is both active and reactive in this regard. This automutative nature of mind is based upon the omnipresence of mental conflict. *Constant psychic change, driven by psychic conflict, is a fundamental fact of psychic life.* This fact has great importance for the psychoanalytic enterprise.

The environmental circumstance of greatest interest to the psychoanalyst is the psychoanalytic situation. It is absolutely unlike any other situation. It is non-spontaneous, non-naturalistic, and artificially constructed so as to accomplish certain psychoanalytic goals. Of greatest importance among them is the elucidation of the components of conflict in certain crucially important compromises that automatically develop in the properly configured psychoanalytic situation. These are transference and resistance. They are conceptually distinguishable from each other, but operationally they are inextricably intertwined. The psychoanalytic work that elucidates their components of conflict (i.e., interpretation) leads to a certain kind of psychic change. Painful and/or dysfunctional compromises undergo qualitative transformation into ones characterized by greater tolerance of infantile drive derivatives and/or diminished anxiety or depressive affect. It is not clear whether this occurs in one or many ways (Fenichel, 1941, pp. 110–116). But the original pathogenic conflict persists; it is the resulting compromise formation that undergoes change in a salutary direction.

Now, every psychoanalyst every day observes the mind's constant conflict-driven changeability and considers it in his therapeutic approaches to each patient. Even so, constant psychic change is generally taken for granted as a crucial fixture of mental life, and its full implications have not been seriously explored. The recent work of Paul Gray (1990) on the analysis of resistance has turned attention to the inexorable flux of mental life as it pertains to psychoanalytic therapy. An example of this emphasis in Gray's work is the following statement:

> In listening to the patient, I focus on the flow of material with an ear for evidence, at the manifest surface level, of some identifiable expression of an instinctual drive derivative. This might appear from the patient's words alone—what is actually being said—or it might be evident from one or more of the many sounds or nuances of affect accompanying the words. I have in mind particularly affects deriving characteristically from libidinal or aggressive sources . . . As long as the drive derivative that has drawn my attention continues unabated, I tend to restrain interventions. I wait for this particular instinctually associated trend to continue into the patient's awareness as far as the patient's ego can tolerate it. Once there is evidence that the patient has encountered a conflict over this trend, for which the ego initiates a form of resistance, my interest is in assessing if and how best I might be able to call the patient's attention to the event—the sequence—which has just taken place (pp. 1085–1087).

At the same time that Gray was pursuing this line of technical development in the United States, Betty Joseph (1985) was pursuing a comparable line of development in London.

> My stress throughout this contribution has been on the transference as a relationship in which something is all the time going on (p. 452).

> [M]ovement and change is an essential aspect of transference . . . ; the
> level at which a patient is functioning at any given moment and the na-
> ture of his anxieties can best be gauged by trying to be aware of how
> the transference is actively being used; . . . shifts that become visible in
> the transference are an essential part of what should eventually lead to
> real psychic change (pp. 447–448).

And on the level of general psychoanalytic theory, Michael G. Moran
(1991) correlated the "fluidic nature of the mind" to its "interacting
with itself, or intra-acting" (p. 213). This may be seen in his description
of systems that have the "fluidic" quality that characterizes the mind:

> Mathematical approaches to modeling have for a number of years ex-
> amined systems that work on themselves over time, that "flow." . . .
> Many systems that are so modeled work on themselves, or "flow": the
> old "output" becomes the new "input." . . . Such fluidic systems char-
> acterized by this kind of feedback are prone to exhibit "chaotic" be-
> havior over time: behavior that is *apparently* random, disorganized, and
> without order (p. 211).

While Gray, Joseph, and Moran all emphasized the constant auto-
mutative aspect of mental life, they barely (if at all) approached its relation to essential unknowability in psychoanalysis. It is to this relation
that we now turn.

Unknowability of the First Kind: Unconscious Mental Processes

The most important problem of unknowability in psychoanalysis concerns the inference of inherently unobservable unconscious mental
processes through the use of inwardly directed attention—that is, introspection (see Freud, 1940, pp. 144, 196). It is in this process that the
auto-mutative nature of mental life manifests itself most immediately.
The perceptions of mental contents made conscious by attention hy-
percathexis are constantly fluctuating, sporadic, and ephemeral. Nevertheless, they are the primary data from which corresponding and
complementary unconscious mental processes are inferred. This inferential process is very much a matter of rote in psychoanalysis. However, the crucial roles of constant mental change and unknowability in
the inferential process do not appear to be so well understood. The following discussion may clarify these issues.

First of all, *unconscious* mental life is understandable only in terms of
what is apprehended in *conscious* mental life. But since conscious mental processes are essentially different from unconscious ones, the result

is a fundamental problem of unknowability regarding unconscious mental life. Freud (1940, p. 158), addressed this problem operationally, stating that psychoanalysis, like all other natural sciences, has to infer processes that cannot be observed directly through the human sensory apparatuses. But these other sciences can "follow [the] mutual relations and interdependencies" of the unknowable, unobservable processes "unbroken over long stretches," which greatly facilitates their inference. Psychoanalysis, by contrast, cannot follow *its* unknowable—i.e., unconscious—processes "unbroken over long stretches," for the observation of the complementary *conscious* phenomena is broken and discontinuous. This is where constant change in mental life enters as a problem peculiar to psychoanalysis, a problem that exacerbates the more general scientific one of inferring essentially unknowable (*because* unobservable) unconscious mental activities.

Freud in 1917 (p. 143) referred to this issue when he termed the perception of the contents of consciousness "incomplete and untrustworthy" for the understanding of unconscious mental life. Much later, in 1933, he referred to this issue when he stated that the criterion of being conscious is itself "untrustworthy" in the endeavors of psychoanalysis. And still later, in 1940, Freud stated: "[C]onsciousness is in general a highly fugitive state. What is conscious is conscious only for a moment. . . . The whole position is made clear in connection with the conscious perception of our thought-processes: these . . . may persist for some time, but they may just as well pass in a flash" (p. 159). The conscious mental life perceived by introspection in the psychoanalytic endeavor pertains principally to conscious "perceptions, feelings, thought-processes and volitions" (p. 157). Of these objects of direct internal observation, Freud stated: "It is generally agreed . . . that these conscious processes do not form unbroken sequences which are complete in themselves" (p. 157).

And further, in Freud's (1925a) remarkable paper "A note upon 'the mystic writing pad'," in which he elaborated upon his notions of consciousness and perception, he was especially concerned about their highly fluctuating and ephemeral nature, "the flickering-up and passing-away of consciousness in the process of perception" (p. 231). He then expanded on

> the method by which the perceptual apparatus of our mind functions. . . . My theory [is] that cathectic innervations are sent out and withdrawn in rapid impulses from within into the completely pervious system *Pcpt.-Cs.* So long as that system is cathected in this manner, it receives perceptions (which are accompanied by consciousness) and passes the excitation on to the unconscious mnemic systems; but as

soon as the cathexis is withdrawn, consciousness is extinguished and the functioning of the system comes to a standstill. It is as though the unconscious [ego (Freud, 1925b, p. 238)] stretches out feelers, through the medium of the system *Pcpt.-Cs.*, towards the external world and hastily withdraws them as soon as they have sampled the excitations coming from it. Thus the interruptions [are] attributed by my hypothesis to the discontinuity in the current of innervation; and the actual breaking of contact . . . by the periodic non-excitability of the perceptual system (p. 231).

In these passages, Freud was principally concerned with the *unconscious* ego in its engagement with the consciously perceived external— that is, extra-psychic—world. But his formulation applies equally to the unconscious ego's reflexive, introspective engagement with that most analytically pertinent sphere, the awareness of one's own thoughts and feelings (Freud, 1993, p. 75). Thus, the unconscious ego's function of conscious internal perception, while generally quite active, is also incomplete and discontinuous. Freud was in effect stating that unconscious ego activities determine the ego's functions of attention, consciousness, and perception and that these ego functions operate in a broken and discontinuous manner when the mind perceives its own conscious contents in the analytic situation.

However, Freud did not explain just how and why the "interruptions" and "periodic non-excitability of the perceptual system" occur. Insight into this problem derives from the work of Jacob A. Arlow, Martin H. Stein, and Ernst Kris.

Arlow (1961, pp. 374–375) extended Freud's notion of the unconscious ego "stretching out feelers towards the external world," of its sending out small amounts of cathexis into the perceptual system." Of greatest importance here, he showed that the ego function of consciousness operates characteristically according to the pleasure-unpleasure principle—particularly in the search for conscious pleasurable perceptions. Arlow's elaboration itself drew upon certain other basic propositions about consciousness. He referred to "an additional mental operation, a certain kind of cathectic investment." This is the mobilization and directing of the cathexis of attention by the psychic sense organ, the system *Cs*. The cathexis of attention is indivisible and limited in quantity. The ego unconsciously directs attention cathexis to perceived sensory data, causing these data to become conscious. The result is what Arlow termed "the awareness of perceiving." According to Arlow, the cathexis of attention is discontinuous—and therefore so is conscious perception. He emphasized that the pressure for instinctual discharge embodied in unconscious fantasies motivates this discontinuous directing of attention cathexis to scan sensory data in a discriminating manner. The play of attention will then not only be indivisible, limited in quantity, broken, and discontinuous in its duration; it will also be selective in its object. It will tend toward those perceived sensory data that seem useful as sources of pleasure, as vehicles for instinctual discharge. However, it should be noted that Arlow did not explain just why attention is characteristically discontinuous.

Martin H. Stein (1965) helped to clarify this issue. In his discussion of states of consciousness, he emphasized the factor that is often in opposition to pleasure-seeking—namely, defense. While Arlow pointed to the pressure for instinctual discharge as motivating the mobilization of attention *toward* preconscious perceptions (thus making them conscious), Stein pointed to defense as motivating the *withdrawal* of attention cathexis from conscious perceptions (thus rendering them, again, descriptively unconscious). He pointedly asserted that the withdrawal of attention cathexis is truly defensive; it entails a countercathexis. Stein was describing a species of denial or disavowal and was particularly concerned with painful memories. But this would pertain to any and all internal perceptions that evoke painful affects and therefore conflict—and so *a fortiore* to internal perceptions that are most characteristic and prevalent in the psychoanalytic situation. Stein stated: "It becomes desirable then to push the memory [or any other internally perceived mental content] away from the fore-front or *fovea* of attention, to ignore it. (In economic terms, we postulate the development of a countercathexis)" (p. 72). Accordingly, both the pleasure-seeking extension of attention cathexis to internal perceptions and its defensive withdrawal from them occur according to the pleasure-unpleasure principle and in the context of conflict. Here, then, is the beginning of an explanation for the discontinuity of conscious internal perception in the psychoanalytic situation.

Stein further demonstrated that the withdrawal of attention cathexis from conscious perception results, secondarily, in the seeking of gratification through fantasy activity. He showed this through the extreme case of traumatic situations. But he could then argue that this withdrawal of consciousness from perception and the shift to gratification through fantasy is an exaggeration of a normally occurring phenomenon. That shift entails a radical change in the state of mind, or "ego state," for the orientation to reality that is so characteristic of perception is abandoned in favor of the orientation to pleasure in fantasy. Seen in another way, the dynamic configuration of mental forces undergoes great change. It was Ernst Kris who elucidated this fact.

Kris (1950) explored quite productively the ego state of conscious fantasizing, or daydreaming, in his classical paper "On preconscious mental processes." His argument there was that the defensive turning toward gratification in fantasy which Stein described results in an intensification of the fantasies involved, along with a realignment of defensive forces. "[Turning to fantasy] is characterized by the facility with which id impulses, or their closer derivatives, are received. One might say that countercathectic energies to some extent are withdrawn, and added to the speed, force, or intensity with which the preconscious [fantasy] thoughts are formed" (p. 313). Thus, not only are conscious and unconscious fantasies intensified, but two sets of countercathectic forces undergo change: those denying the painful internal percept are mobilized, those inhibiting the drives are weakened. Accordingly, in the complex process Stein described, there is an alteration of instinctual and defensive configurations to achieve a new intrapsychic balance, a new ego state—or, using the basic terms of this investigation, there is a transformation, prompted by conflict, of one compromise formation into another.

Arlow's, Stein's, and Kris's insights, taken together, affirm that the discontinuous fluctuations of conscious perception are a very special case of the transformations of compromise formations driven by perceptual mental conflict, usually taking place in extremely small time spans. As Arlow indicated, in the compromise formation oriented toward internal perception, the instinctual impulses inherent in conscious and unconscious fantasy will often cause attention to be directed outwardly—but, especially in analysis, also inwardly—in pursuit of conscious pleasurable perceptions. But those perceptions may or may not provoke anxiety or depressive affect. To the degree that they do, and thus provoke conflict, the internal perception itself provokes its own transformation into another—now fantasy-oriented—compromise formation. For the dangers or calamities evoked or perceived will cause the defensive withdrawal of attention cathexis, as Stein described. Through that transformation, conscious perception will undergo extinction, and conscious fantasy will become the locus of pleasure. But also, in the new compromise formation, the orientation of pleasure in fantasy will result, as Kris asserted, in the strengthening of conscious or unconscious wishful fantasies. The resultant drive frustration will motivate the disruption of the fantasy-oriented compromise and its transformation back into the perception-oriented one—that is, toward the pursuit of pleasure in the perceptual sphere. And so the cycle of mobilization and the withdrawal of attention to perception—the discontinuity of the perceptual process, driven by pleasure-seeking and conflict—will play itself out again and again.

It is important to emphasize here that the pleasure-unpleasure principle holds total sway in the shift from internal perception to gratification in fantasy and back again. These cyclical processes most often take place easily and rapidly. They occur most naturally in situations of social isolation, of which the psychoanalytic situation is an approximation. Also, all the time this cyclical oscillation between these two extremely unstable compromise formations continues undisturbed and unmodified, the mind (specifically, the ego) constantly changes its orientation or motivational set regarding completely internal, intrapsychic, interests. The external world, the environment, is literally of no concern. This is the mind "interacting with itself or intraacting" (Moran, 1991).

In the analytic situation, introspective perceptions of conscious mental life relatively devoid of drive frustration and/or unpleasant affects will affect the cycle in a characteristic manner. The near-absence of active conflict in internal perception will cause a relative fixity of attention to non-fantastical thoughts and feelings and thus a temporary cessation of the cycle. This results in reflection, unwavering absorption in conscious mental activity. On the other hand, internal perceptions associated with intense active conflict will have the opposite effect; that is, defensive withdrawal from the internal perceptual sphere will supervene, to the enhancement and intensification of fantasy life. If that defensive removal to fantasy is sustained, the result is reverie and also a temporary pause in the cycle. Most often, however, conscious internal perception in analysis operates somewhere between the two relatively fixed extremes of reflection and reverie—that is, between no active conflict at all and sustained intense conflict. The moment-to-moment vicissitudes of the cycle will be affected by how much conflict the conscious internal perceptions evoke. And there can be no consistency or regularity in the content, timing, or meaning of the internal perceptions. Accordingly, the contingent resultant between instinctual pressure and painful affects in conscious internal perception will never be constant, regular, or consistent.[1] The cyclical process of extending and withdrawing attention cathexis, while it always occurs in the analytic situation, will thus mostly occur unpredictably, irregularly, and erratically.

It is, then, little wonder that introspective attention and conscious internal perception, being oriented mostly according to the pleasure-unpleasure principle and subject to the constantly changing forces of unconscious conflict, should operate in a variable and discontinuous

1. See Gill, 1963, pp. 156–157, for the many and various conflictual factors and circumstances—quantitative and qualitative—that go into "the likelihood that a mental content will attract attention cathexis." These factors and circumstances would apply to the special case on internal perception in the analytic situation.

manner. This is the auto-mutative nature of the mind, driven by conflict, operating in the special case of attention, consciousness, and internal perception. And this is the reason that conscious perceptions of mental life in psychoanalytic method are so "incomplete and untrustworthy," filled with gaps and breaks in continuity.

Freud (1940) elaborated upon this problem of the direct unknowability of the unconscious in relation to absolute dependence upon "fugitive," "incomplete and untrustworthy" conscious perceptions of thoughts and feelings. He stated the problem's radical nature, which distinguishes psychoanalysis from all other natural sciences: "Every science is based on observations and experiences arrived at through the medium of our psychic apparatus. But since *our* science has as its subject that apparatus itself, the analogy ends here" (p. 159). All other sciences use the mind and all its perceptual and intellectual faculties to infer essentially unobservable processes in the extrapsychic world. But only psychoanalysis uses the mind to study the mind—that is, to study itself. And that mind—in its auto-investigative mode—is characterized by "fugitive," "incomplete and untrustworthy" conscious internal perceptions.

Therein lies the problem. Using a scientific strategy so characteristic of him, Freud turned the principal methodological difficulty—the discontinuities and irregularities of *conscious* internal perceptions—into the very foundation for the scientifically valid inference and construction of *unconscious* mental life.[2] While absolute knowability of the unconscious is inherently impossible, in this way one may nevertheless achieve relative certainty about it. He stated:

> We make our observations through the medium of the same perceptual apparatus [that we are investigating], precisely with the help of the breaks in the sequence of [conscious] "psychical" events: we fill in what is omitted by making plausible inferences and translating it into conscious material. In this way we construct, as it were, a sequence of conscious events complementary to the unconscious psychical process. The relative certainty of our psychical science is based on the binding force of these inferences. Anyone who enters deeply into our work will find that our technique holds its ground against any criticism" (Freud, 1940, p. 159).

And again:

> Our procedure in psychoanalysis is quite similar [to those used in all the other natural sciences]. We have discovered technical methods of filling up the gaps in the phenomena of our consciousness, and we

2. Freud also turned two other intractable difficulties in psychoanalysis—transference (Freud, 1916–1917, p. 444) and sadomasochism (Freud, 1933, p. 104)—into the bases of later radical changes in theory, method, and technique.

make use of those methods just as a physicist makes use of experiment. In this manner we infer a number of processes which are in themselves "unknowable" and interpolate them in those that are conscious to us. And if, for instance, we say: "At this point an unconscious memory intervened," what that means is: "At this point something occurred of which we are totally unable to form a conception, but which, if it had entered our consciousness, could only have been described in such and such a way" (pp. 196–197).

Now, what Freud called "our technique," "our procedure," the "technical methods of filling up the gaps in the phenomena of our consciousness," and the "artificial aids [which] increase the efficiency of our sense organs to the furtherest possible extent" (1940, p. 196)—what Freud was referring to is the psychoanalytic method developed specifically to infer unconscious processes. That method entails a combination of the patient's free association and the analyst's evenly suspended attention. These two complementary modes of observation were termed "the analyzing instrument" by Otto Isakower (Balter, Lothane, and Spencer, 1980). To counter the usual, ubiquitous, and naturally occurring fleeting quality of conscious internal perceptions, this method emphasizes the unnatural, non-habitual, uncritical application of attention toward the objects of observation on the part of both analytic participants. But because of the difference in their functions in the analytic endeavor, the two parties differ in the alternation of attention. The patient oscillates his attention inwardly and outwardly—that is, between uncritically perceiving his conscious thoughts and feelings and uncritically reporting his perceptions to the analyst. Of course, this is the essence of free association. In complementary fashion, the analyst oscillates his attention outwardly and inwardly—that is, between listening uncritically to the patient's reports and perceiving uncritically his own conscious thoughts and feelings. This is the essence of evenly suspended attention (Balter, Lothane, and Spencer, 1980). Thus, both free association and evenly suspended attention entail directing attention toward and away from the internal perceptual sphere in each analytic participant.

This relatively regular and regimented oscillation of attention takes the irregular and broken play of attention and perception to some important degree out from under the dominance of the pleasure-unpleasure principle. The very context of doing psychoanalytic work—that is, collaboration between the two participants in the service of the rigorously defined pragmatic goal of inference-making—sets up a rational and reality-oriented overarching motivational set in both. It places the extension and withdrawal of attention to internal perceptions more under the dominance of the reality principle. Attention and conscious internal perception become more regulated, controlled, and useful within the activity of the analyzing instrument. Operationally, this occurs through the communicational circuit between the two analytic participants. Each must articulate to the other his internal perceptions *mutatis mutandis* in rational and syntactically adequate language—that is, through expressions that are organized mostly according to the secondary process (Balter, Lothane, and Spencer, 1980). The relatively simple extension and withdrawal of attention to internal perception become enmeshed in a more complex movement of attention that must also include concern with language and verbalization.

It is here, through the concern with the other participant in the communicational transactions, that the transference and countertransference, with their associated unconscious conflicts, are inextricably coupled to the crucial analytic work itself—dedicated to the inference of unconscious mental life and embodied in free association and evenly suspended attention. Because of this, in the very context of inferring unconscious mental processes, the discontinuities in the patient's internal perceptions are transmuted into resistances—that is, compromise formations that are analyzable as the result of unconscious conflict—over the transference itself (Freud, 1916–1917, pp. 286–302).

To be sure, even with the functioning of the analyzing instrument, the gaps and discontinuities of internal perception persist. For the pleasure-unpleasure principle can be "tamed" only partially and relatively. The ego function of attention will, of necessity, still adhere to its "fugitive," "incomplete and untrustworthy" nature much of the time. But even so, the discontinuities of conscious perception in the operation of the analyzing instrument will now be harnessed to provide crucial data for the inference of the essentially unknowable unconscious mental processes. That harnessing consists in the analysis of conflict, which causes the very discontinuities of conscious perception to occur.

This formulation is, in essence, equivalent to that described by Gray (1990) in his discussion of the analysis of resistance. Gray isolated and highlighted precisely that aspect of constant mental change which is most pertinent to the analysis of conflict: the fact that these discontinuities in conscious internal perception are the direct consequence of current, ongoing mental conflict. They thus provide an immediate and direct indicator of the presence of such conflict and, even further, evidence as to the content and meaning of the conflict. This is because introspective attention is automatically directed toward mental contents that apprise the analyst of the current instinctual pressure, and the withdrawal of the patient's attention from those contents reveals the meaning of the associated anxiety or depressive affect. Psychoanalytic method thus induces unconscious conflict to cause discontinuous conscious mental change in attention and internal perception. Unconscious conflict accordingly reveals itself through its conscious effects in a very controlled and well-defined context. This greatly facilitates the investigation of unconscious conflict and allows valid inferences about it. Seen another way, the psychoanalytic method is designed to produce, first and foremost, data pertaining to unconscious conflict. Data pertaining to other aspects of mental life, conscious and unconscious, are less available and less indicatory.

Further, the uncritical nature of the deliberate and voluntary deployment of introspective attention particularly enhances the tasks of inferring unconscious mental processes. For, as Arlow pointed out, the ego selectively fixes upon those perceptions that promise to be of use for drive gratification. If critical judgment is temporarily suspended, the ego will have greater freedom to exercise its selectivity regarding the internal perceptual sphere. Attention will then be maximally attracted to precisely those thoughts and feelings that most closely correspond to the ascendant instinctually oriented unconscious fantasies. At the other pole of conflict—that of defense—the uncritical nature of directing introspective attention will allow for the maximum play of attention away from pain-evoking (pre)conscious mental contents (Balter, Lothane and Spencer, 1980, pp. 498–500). Thus, the suspension of criticism magnifies discontinuity in the perception of conscious mental life. This makes the context of the conflict easier to discern. The analyst can then "fill in the gaps" of the concomitant discontinuity.

Another consequence of the suspension of critical judgment is moderate and controlled regression in the conscious mental life of each analytic participant, a regression that universally occurs with the deliberate abrogation of directive control over conscious mental life (Kris, 1950; Balter, Lothane, and Spencer, 1980). Accordingly, the conscious data thus perceived approximate in form and content the correlated unconscious mental processes in the patient and in the analyst. This regressive phenomenon greatly facilitates the scientific activity of inferring and constructing the associated unconscious mental processes (see Fenichel, 1941, p. 32).

Thus, free association and evenly suspended attention—both of which entail the suspension of critical judgment—provide relevant observations of relatively regressed conscious mental contents in both analytic participants. And those contents are fundamentally related to current conflict in the patient. This allows the analyst to create a broad array of hypotheses about the patient's unconscious mental life. He may then broach empirically grounded suppositions (i.e., interpretations) to the patient, who may then respond in a confirming or disconfirming manner (Freud, 1937). The progressive refinement of these hypotheses about the patient's unconscious mental processes is an ongoing collaborative activity between patient and analyst. Arlow (1969) described very well the way in which the analyst, in the joint enterprise with the patient, approximates asymptotically a relatively certain understanding of the patient's unconscious mental life. This is actually a further refinement of the oscillation of attention and perception which is "tamed" to some degree through the analyzing instrument. In it, the analyst's proffered hypotheses about the patient's unconscious mental life enter the patient's oscillating attention as *external* perceptions related directly to the patient's *introspective* perceptions. And the same process is echoed back to the analyst through the patient's responses. Arlow's discussion referred more to "the patient's past" but in effect the method refers to the inference of his unconscious mental life.

> The joint search by patient and analyst for the picture of the patient's past is a reciprocal process. In a sense, we dream along with our patients, supplying at first data from our own store of images in order to objectify the patient's memory into some sort of picture. We then furnish this picture to the analysand, who responds with further memories, associations, and fantasies; that is, we stimulate him to respond with a picture of his own. In this way the analyst's reconstruction comes to be composed more and more out of the materials presented by the patient until we finally get a picture that is trustworthy and in all essentials complete (p. 49).

Arlow showed that, even though the analyst's conscious mental contents are used, the resulting inference leads to the understanding of the patient's unconscious mental contents. That understanding then becomes the basis for the interpretation of transference and resistance. This is why psychoanalytic investigation (i.e., method) is a sine qua non of psychoanalytic therapy (i.e., technique).

The crucial position of this method in the foundation and development of psychoanalysis cannot be overestimated. The most essential insights of psychoanalysis derive directly from the inference of the patient's unconscious mental life through free association and evenly suspended attention. Those insights extend much further than the very existence of unconscious mental life and its intrinsic connection to unconscious conflict—monumental as these insights are. Because they stem from a common method and theory, they form a relatively self-consistent, internally coherent set of propositions. Hartmann (1939), who understood the mutual ramifications of theory and method, made an extremely perspicacious observation about psychoanalysis in this regard:

> The distinctive characteristic of a psychoanalytic investigation is not its subject matter but the scientific methodology and the structure of the concepts it uses. All psychological investigations share some of their objectives with psychoanalysis. . . . Recent developments in psychoanalysis have not changed its salient characteristics, namely its biological orientation, its genetic, dynamic, economic, and topographic points of view, and the explanatory nature of its concepts. Thus, when psychoanalysis and nonanalytic psychology study the same subject matter, they will, of necessity, arrive at different descriptive and relational propositions. . . .
> [P]sychoanalysis . . . is . . . a cohesive organization of propositions, and any attempt to isolate parts of it not only destroys its over-all unity, but also changes and invalidates its parts (pp. 4–6).

The unique and characteristic insights of psychoanalysis include: the predominantly infantile and instinctual nature of unconscious mental life; the omnipresent influence of unconscious mental life on conscious mental life; transference, analytic and extra-analytic; the meaning of dreams and slips; infantile sexuality and psychosexual development, including the Oedipus complex; the genesis of neurotic symptoms and perversions in the Oedipus complex; the oedipal origin of a universal unconscious moral agency (the superego); the existence of narcissistic object relations. These and other insights are interrelated and constitute a relatively coherent—but open-ended—view of the mind and its development. They can best be validated and confirmed through the unique psychoanalytic method of inferring unconscious mental processes—free association and evenly suspended attention—the very method that fostered their genesis in the first place.

And so, observational methods concerning mental life that eschew free association and evenly suspended attention will tend to provide little or no information concerning unconscious mental processes. They will produce strategic unknowability about that crucial part of mental life. Such methods will highlight other aspects of mental life, predominantly in the conscious sphere. The necessity to postulate unconscious conflict, instinctual drives and their development and defensive operations—or even unconscious mental life at all—will not be evident, and other psychological theories of explanation and corresponding therapeutic techniques must evolve. This is, in fact, what happened after Kohut, in 1959, announced that empathy and introspection were *the* essential observational method of psychoanalysis. His subsequent publications (e.g., Kohut, 1971, 1977, 1984) deviated further and further from the uniquely psychoanalytic insights noted above, from established psychoanalytic theory, and from the central technique of resistance analysis. Kohut's innovative approach was consciously, deliberately, and consistently attuned to observational method, and this clarified the causal correlation between his methodological revision and subsequent changes in his theory, technique, and view of mental life (see Spencer and Balter, 1990; Balter and Spencer, 1991).

However, there are psychoanalytic "schools" that neither renounce the essential methodological position of free association and evenly suspended attention nor concentrate on it. The contemporary Kleinians of London (Schafer, 1994) informally neglect the analyzing instrument in favor of another methodological pair: the patient's projective identification and the analyst's analysis of the countertransference. It is not clear from their publications or more personal communications whether this pair actually accomplishes free association and evenly suspended attention, for the analyst's openness and attention to the patient's projective identification may supply the same sorts of data free association does. The same may be said for the analyst's analysis of the countertransference and evenly suspended attention. The difference between the two pairs may be a matter of emphasis, not of qualitatively different methods. However, a comment by Schafer (1994) suggests that the contemporary Kleinians are *not* concerned with any operational equivalent of free association to guide them to a "relative certainty" concerning "unknowable" unconscious mental life in their work. Schafer stated: "[T]here is no well-developed theoretical provision for what standard Freudians call the observing ego and the ego's synthesizing function—that is, the analyst's structurally and functionally stable and intact collaborator and dialogical partner in the [analytic] process" (p. 427). Thus, it is not self-evident whether, or to what extent, this "school" of psychoanalysis effectively relies on standard psychoanalytic method to ascertain unconscious mental processes. It may be that these psychoanalysts collectively have no coherent and consistent approach to the inference of unconscious mental life. (There may well be very wide variation among them in this regard.)

Fortunately, they publish extremely lucid accounts of their clinical work. What is most striking is the very active use of their own subjectivity and intuition, which seem to be highly developed and used to great effect in the analysis of resistance. Because they rely so much on themselves and their keen clinical sensitivity, they do not wait for many of the patients' free associations and do not suspend their own attention very much. Rather, their main concern is to interpret quickly and accurately. Their inferences of patients' inner lives may well be correct, but the alacrity of their interventions does not allow for extensive observations by analyst or patient. There is an absence of (in Gray's [1990] words), "the particular form of attention to which I give priority." There is little of the rich array of possible hypotheses about unconscious mental life that the analyzing instrument provides for the analyst. And there is little description of the approximating "reciprocal process" that Arlow described.

Thus, the predominant use of projective identification and countertransference analysis in the writings of the contemporary Kleinians necessitates that the analyst's understanding of the patient rests more on his idiosyncratic intuitive talent than on inferences derived from a standard, generally employed method. The contemporary Kleinian method cannot be taught but only demonstrated. The accuracy or validity of the data presented therefore cannot be appraised by other psychoanalysts. Generalization from its observations is very difficult and, in fact, these analysts do not claim much generality for their clinical inferences. Their theorizing is therefore sparse; and the more general the theory, the sparser it is (Schafer, 1994, pp. 426, 428). It is to be expected, then, that the progressive development of psychoanalytic theory and technique will not come from such a method.

UNKNOWABILITY OF THE SECOND KIND: EXTRA-ANALYTIC DETERMINANTS OF ANALYTIC DATA

Unknowability of the second kind concerns the influences brought to bear upon the patient's mental life *inside* the psychoanalytic situation by events and circumstances *outside* it. Quite simply, the analyst cannot directly observe relevant events, circumstances, and relationships that have often intense and far-reaching effects on the patient's mental life during the analysis. These determinants are extra-analytic owing to displacements in time or space—that is, they may be antecedent to the analysis itself or contemporaneous with it but take place in another geographical locus. As with knowability of the first kind, the auto-mutative nature of mental life intensifies this problem of unknowability. However, where constant change in mental life provided the essential psychoanalytic method for addressing unknowability of the first kind, it only partly contributes to the solution of unknowability of the second kind. Consequently, other means must be employed to make the necessary observations and inferences.

Considering first extra-analytic influences that are contemporaneous with the analysis, every analyst every day experiences phenomena within the analysis that have a tendency to change their functions and meanings to integrate events that have occurred contemporaneously outside the analytic situation. This occurs because the conflicts and compromise formations related to the analyst and the analytic work do not remain operative only in the analysis. As noted above, the analytic work itself exacerbates conflict about the transference. The patient carries acute transference conflict and the resulting compromises to situations outside the analysis. The auto-mutative aspect of mental life, driven by conflict, facilitates the transformation of compromise formations referable to the transference. Events and conditions outside the analysis may then provide the means and material for derivative compromises to form, compromises that do not manifestly refer to the transference at all. (This process of transformation is frequently subsumed under the rubric of "acting out.") Accordingly, the compromises based in the analysis are replaced by new ones manifestly referable to circumstances outside the analysis. This sort of psychic change is driven by intensified conflict pertaining to the analysis itself and takes place principally according to the logic of the primary process.

Thus, the auto-mutative nature of mental life constantly presents the psychoanalyst with new psychic configurations in the analytic material derived from ones that were previously understood to pertain to the transference but are now correlated with events and circumstances that are unknowable because practicably unobservable. Further, the primary-process logic of the transformations is not necessarily obvious, reasonable, or realistic. This is why Betty Joseph (1985) stressed "transference as a relationship in which something is all the time going on" and also noted that "movement and change is an essential aspect of the transference." She accordingly emphasized "trying to be aware of how the transference is actively being used."

Psychoanalysts are exquisitely sensitive to this tenacious difficulty. Much analytic effort is directed toward undoing it, by exposing the continuity within the change, demonstrating that the newer compromise is actually an unconsciously derived version of the older one. Only in this way can the original compromise formations, manifestly pertaining to the transference, be kept operative in the observational field of the treatment and thus available for continued psychoanalytic investigation. (See Fenichel, 1941, pp. 98–99, for a concise discussion of this matter.)

Thus, the essential activity of keeping the transference available for analysis is now addressed to the extra-analytic derivatives of the transference. Certain standard properties of the psychoanalytic situation provide time and opportunity to undo these effects of the mind's unceasing auto-mutative nature as it pertains to contemporaneous influences outside the analysis. Those properties are, most notably, the relatively high frequency of analytic sessions and their relatively long duration. These fixed elements of the psychoanalytic situation in effect help the two analytic participants apply to the extra-analytic circumstances the same sort of investigatory concerns that are applied to the intra-analytic circumstance. They thus make possible persistent interpretative work on the analyst's part to transform the derived compromises back into the original ones referable to the transference conflict itself. This aspect of analytic work keeps psychic phenomena that are pertinent to the analysis from undergoing too much alteration according to the logic of the primary process. Transference phenomena thus remain available for analysis and may ultimately undergo modification somewhat more according to the secondary-process logic of causal self-understanding—that is, insight.

The so-called Monday crust noted by Freud (1913) is a clinical consequence of the incessant, spontaneous auto-mutative aspects of mental life which change transference manifestations into other phenomena pertaining to contemporaneous circumstances outside the analysis. During any temporary cessation of analytic work, the tendency to form derivative compromises based on current experiences outside the analysis goes unchecked. That is the inner meaning of Freud's discussion of the matter:

> I work with my patients every day except on Sundays and public holidays—that is, as a rule, six days a week. For slight cases or the continuation of a treatment which is already well advanced, three days a week will be enough. Any restrictions of time beyond this bring no advantage either to the doctor or the patient; and at the beginning of an analysis they are quite out of the question. Even short interruptions have a slightly obscuring effect on the work. We used to speak jokingly of the "Monday crust" when we began work again after the rest on Sunday. When the hours of work are less frequent, there is a risk of not being able to keep pace with the patient's real life and of the treatment losing contact with the present and being forced into by-paths (p. 127).

In effect, Freud was referring to the mind's tendency to incorporate the practicably unobservable events of the patient's life outside the analysis into the compromise formations most useful for analytic investigation. Time, opportunity, and effort are necessary "to keep pace" with those events and transformations. Or, as Freud (1913) put it: "a necessary proportion must be observed between time, work and success" (p. 129). Frequent and lengthy sessions thus become necessary to avoid the possibility of "the treatment losing contact with the present and being forced into by-paths"—that is, into unknowability. Even so, frequent and lengthy sessions do not guarantee that contemporaneous extra-analytic determinants will be inferred well enough to restore effectively previous compromises to the observation field but only make that desirable result more probable. Frequent and lengthy sessions achieve a "relative certainty" about the dynamic effects of contemporary events and circumstances outside the analysis. They provide the opportunity for free association and evenly suspended attention— i.e., the analysis of the derivative compromises back to their original forms.

Freud also pointed out that the frequency of sessions addresses an essentially practical matter: the need to gather information to make inferences about the patient's current extra-analytic life. According to Freud, when little is known of the patient, highly frequent sessions are necessary. When much is known, three sessions per week are adequate. Freud did not indicate why he decided upon that number of sessions, but clearly the criterion used was whether the frequency of sessions allows the analyst "to keep pace with the patient's real life"; in terms of the present discussion, it was whether the frequency of sessions allows the analyst to keep the analytically based mental phenomena from losing their analyzable relation to the transference itself.

This pragmatic consideration is an individual matter, peculiar to each patient and analyst and changeable according to the phase of the analysis and the vicissitudes of the patient's life. This consideration makes it difficult, if not impossible, to specify the number of sessions per week that are necessary for adequate psychoanalytic work to occur. This problem becomes important for defining standard criteria for psychoanalytic treatment. "Standards" by definition can be useful or valid only when applied to a statistical average, but lose their utility and validity when applied to individual instances. Current controversies about the standard frequency of sessions pivot around this problem— a problem for which there may not be any adequate solution.[3] If, however, the problem is taken by fiat out of the practical clinical sphere and placed into the realm of standard "rules and regulations," error must

---

3. It is obvious that the same considerations which pertain to the *frequency* of analytic sessions also pertain to their *duration*. (Reference need not be made here to the notorious, legendary, and probably apocryphal five-minute Parisian session.)

necessarily occur through the incongruity between clinical indication and regulatory standardization. For practical clinical reasons, the inevitable error must be in the direction of higher frequency of sessions.

In shifting the discussion from the inference and neutralization of *contemporaneous* determinants outside the analysis to the inference of *pre-analysis* determinants, it should be noted that the difference between these two versions of unknowability of the second kind is essentially a matter of emphasis. Contemporary events and circumstances outside the analysis are located not only outside the analytic situation in space but also before their analysis in time. Conversely, the pre-analysis determinants of compromise formations in the analysis in time are positioned outside the analysis in space as well. Accordingly, relatively frequent and long sessions are required simply to glean sufficient historical information and to subject it to the essential psychoanalytic process of inferring their unconscious meanings and functions (see Blum, 1994, p. 155).

It is well know that the compromise formations that originated before the initiation of treatment may become transformed by the very fact that the patient is in a psychoanalytic treatment. The original pre-analysis compromise formations will then take on meanings and functions which refer directly to the transference. Freud (1916–17) noted that the ceaseless auto-mutative quality of mental life causes the analysand to transform the original meanings and determinants of neurotic symptoms into others that are referable to the analysis and to the analyst. Indeed, this transformation of the psychoneurosis into the transference neurosis[4] is the principal vehicle of both the psychoanalytic investigation and the psychoanalytic cure. Freud stated:

> We must not forget that the patient's illness . . . is still growing and developing like a living organism. The beginning of the treatment does not put an end to this development; when, however, the treatment has obtained mastery over the patient, what happens is that the whole of his illness's new production is concentrated upon a single point—his relation to the doctor. Thus the transference may be compared to the cambium layer in a tree between the wood and the bark, from which the new formation of tissue and the increase in the girth of the trunk derive. When the transference has risen to this significance, work upon the patient's memories retreats far into the background. Thereafter it

---

4. The term "transference neurosis" is used here in its most generic context. It means here *any* psychopathological compromise formation in the patient that refers to the analyst and the analysis. It would thus include: transference psychosis, transference perversion, transference depression, transference anxiety, transference psychopathy, transference conversion reaction, transference psychosomatic reaction, etc.

is not incorrect to say that we are no longer concerned with the patient's earlier illness but with a newly created and transformed neurosis which has taken the former's place. All the patient's symptoms have abandoned their original meaning and have taken on a new sense which lies in a relation to the transference; or only such symptoms have persisted as are capable of undergoing such a transformation. But the mastering of this new, artificial neurosis coincides with getting rid of the illness which was originally brought to the treatment—with the accomplishment of our therapeutic task (p. 144).

Now, despite the methodological and therapeutic advantages of this sort of transformation, there is nevertheless a price to pay in unknowability. This is clear from Freud's statements that the meanings and constituents of conflict of the original symptomatic compromise formations may be lost to analytic investigation. Inevitably, there will be a lack of correspondence between the original psychoneurosis and its derivative substitute, the transference neurosis:

> We can draw no direct conclusion from the distribution of the libido during and resulting from the treatment as to how it was distributed during the illness. Suppose we succeeded in bringing a case to a favorable conclusion by setting up and then resolving a strong father-transference to the doctor. It would not be correct to conclude that the patient had suffered previously from a similar unconscious attachment of his libido to his father. His father-transference was merely the battlefield on which we gained control of his libido; the patient's libido was directed to it from other positions. A battlefield need not necessarily coincide with one of the enemy's key fortresses. The defense of a hostile capital need not take place just in front of its gates (Freud, 1916–17, pp. 455–456).

However, Freud then pointed out that it may be possible for psychoanalysts to reconstruct "in our thoughts" what must have been the determinants of the original psychoneurosis. "Not until after the transference has once more been resolved can we reconstruct *in our thoughts* the distribution of libido which had prevailed during the illness" (p. 456). It must be added that the reconstruction "in our thoughts" of the pathogenesis of the original psychoneurosis does not have the advantage of the patient's confirmation or disconfirmation. Without the patient's participation, the degree of unknowability about the determinants of the original neurotic illness must be substantial.

Current psychoanalytic thinking in this matter is even more skeptical than Freud. Arlow's (1969) discussion of the effects of unconscious fantasy upon conscious perception militated against the notion that childhood experiences—especially pathogenic ones—can ever be analyzed sufficiently to infer the objective historical circumstances. All that can be inferred—using the standard psychoanalytic method of free association and evenly suspended attention—is the idiosyncratic mixture of perception and childhood fantasy, which cannot be distinguished fully from each other. This is the influence of current environment on current conflict and compromise formation, but now taking place in early childhood—that is, yet another instance of the mind's auto-mutative nature leading to unknowability. Further, Freud's own concept of *nachträglichkeit* (deferred effect) calls into question whether previous experiences can ever be analytically disentangled from subsequent retrospective distortion. This is yet another example of unknowability due to constant mental change. Even further, there is now real questioning as to whether Freud's basic assumption of unaltered mnemic registration of perceptions is correct at all. In other words, the effects of constant mental change are now generally assumed to reach into the very depths of the mnemic systems of the mind (see Blum, 1994, p. 138).

Thus, some degree of unknowability regarding the determinants of the patient's illness must be considered inevitable, and the effects of constant mental change are central to it. However, as with the other kinds of unknowability, this does not rule out "relative certainty" if the investigative tools available to the analyst are used to good effect. In the present instance, the main tool (besides the accumulation of historical data) is the analysis of the transference neurosis. Ultimately the procedure for analyzing the transference neurosis is the analyzing instrument—free association and evenly suspended attention. Their efficacy is necessarily limited, but their power is still great.

There is a current controversy in psychoanalysis regarding the analyst's need to infer the determinants of the patient's extra-analytic life, past and present. Some analysts believe that the analyst's *only* concern should be with the psychoanalytic situation itself and the analytic interaction between the two participants. This view maintains that all phenomena of the psychoanalytic situation refer to and must be interpreted as being co-constructed by the two analytic participants. Accordingly, the patient's past and present extra-analytic life either is of no importance or is of derivative concern. This position adheres to the postmodern tendency called "social constructivism." (See Hoffman 1983, 1991, 1992.)

There are probably many reasons for this very rigid monism. However, surely the most important is the frequent clinical observation that immediately current transference interpretations are the only, or the principal, mutative ones. This view was most cogently presented by

James Strachey in 1934. But even Strachey showed that extra-analytic transference interpretations could be, and very frequently are, preparatory for the mutative ones that pertain to the person of the analyst himself. This is a very neat example of "keeping pace with the patient's real life" and transforming phenomena referable to extra-analytic situations back into those referable to the analysis itself. Further, Strachey was quite clear that the transference must be interpreted in accordance with the patient's childhood development—that is, in terms of the patient's pre-analysis circumstances.

Thus, the view that immediate transference interpretations are the only mutative ones does not necessarily militate against investigation, inference, and interpretation of the patient's extra-analytic life, current or previous. However, the view that the *only* relevant subjects of analysis are the interactions of analyst and patient in the analytic situation runs the risk, stipulated by Freud, "of the treatment losing contact with the present and being forced into by-paths." Ignoring the other twenty-three hours of the patient's everyday life and the patient's past must lead to skewed concepts of the patient's unconscious mental life. Kimberly Leary's (1994) critique of this postmodern position spells out the consequences very well.

> [P]atient and analyst in essential respects are wedded to a constantly unfolding present. Given this, meaning can only be in the present tense, a moment in time, and nothing more. . . .
>
> The focus on the present moment obscures the fact that people behave differently at different times and can remember this. Social constructivist accounts of psychoanalysis are ahistorical: without memory, there is no history. Narrative reconceptualizations nod to historical reasons but these are then reinterpreted as present-day tellings. In key respects, postmodernism purges the analytic situation of the need to grapple with history, with things that once were and had an effect. . . .
>
> . . . The emphasis on the present and the unfolding moment diverts attention from that which *endures* in persons, in social transactions, and in the world in which they occur (p. 457).

This is a particularly nice example of how a basic change on a general theoretical level (postmodernism; the co-construction of psychic phenomena) leads directly to a change in method (the analysis of only the immediate transference). However, as noted above, investigative method is an essential ingredient of therapeutic technique in psychoanalysis. Accordingly, the associated technical change will lead to essential changes in method—that is, changes in just what data become knowable and unknowable. Hartmann and Kris, in 1945, saw the methodological danger consequent to such a change of technique. They stated: "[O]ne frequently is tempted to believe that those who advocate changes in technique . . . are not aware of the consequences such changes will have upon the set of data to which they will be able to obtain access" (p. 12). It is clear that ignoring the mind's incessant tendency to change will lead precisely "into by-paths"—that is, into errors and unknowability. Observations made from that very narrow perspective and the theories and therapeutic techniques thus derived must be held suspect.

UNKNOWABILITY OF THE THIRD KIND: THE EFFECTS OF THE ANALYST'S INTERVENTIONS

For some time psychoanalysts have recognized that the analyst's therapeutic and investigative interventions in themselves will affect the very object of the treatment and will introduce unknowability into the psychoanalytic endeavor. Robert Galatzer-Levy (1980, p. 79) was perhaps the first in the psychoanalytic literature to pose the problem of this kind of unknowability. He noted the analogy with the Heisenberg uncertainty principle. The following discussion will elaborate upon the inherent relationship between inexorable change in mental life and unknowability of this third kind.

As with unknowability of the second kind, there is the danger that the transference phenomenon's relation to its origins in conflict may be rendered difficult or even impossible to apprehend by too rapid and/or too extreme mental change—but here the danger is due to the interactions between the two participants in the psychoanalytic situation itself. The psychoanalytic situation is, accordingly, configured to minimize the speed and degree of the transformations of compromise formations that occur predominantly according to primary-process logic. Conversely, the configuration of the psychoanalytic situation attempts to maximize transformative effects which are more related to the secondary-process logic of causal self-understanding and must occur more gradually. The responsibility to keep the primary process mutability minimal must devolve principally upon the analyst. In this context, consideration of the constant change in mental life driven by conflict helps to explain another standard aspect of the psychoanalytic situation—the analyst's neutrality.

Neutrality has been defined in various ways: by Anna Freud's (1936, p. 28) "equidistance" formulation and by Warren Poland's (1984) formulation of the analyst's abstaining from personally invested influence over the patient. The definition suggested here is: the condition in the psychoanalytic situation intended to minimize the primary-process transformation in conflict and compromise formation where it pertains to the analyst's attitude and behavior. (But see Hoffer, 1985, esp. pp. 771–772, for a scholarly discussion of the term.)

Within the psychoanalytic situation, the neutrality of the analyst will minimize the distorting influence of the environment (which principally includes the analyst himself) on the patient's compromise formations. These will then refer maximally to the patient's own intrapsychic dynamisms of conflict and compromise and will provide a maximum of information about their principally unconscious determinants. This is the basis of the analyst's "behavioral minimalism" (Renik, 1995, p. 474)—an oft-criticized, much satirized, but enduring aspect of the analytic situation. It is, after all, simply the effort to keep the variables of an experimental situation (see Freud, 1940) to the fewest and the most constant possible. (See Fenichel, 1941, p. 72, for a discussion of this matter.) Seen this way, the analyst's neutrality is the methodological counterpart of Ockham's razor. This is particularly important for the inference of unconscious determinants of the patient's compromise formations in the form of transference and resistance. These determinants must remain over time not only as few as possible but also as stable, discernible, and available as possible for psychoanalytic investigation.

There is, then, a profound correlation between neutrality as a methodological approach in psychoanalysis and the essential procedure of any psychoanalytic investigation—that is, the inference of unconscious mental life through free association and evenly suspended attention. Theodore Shapiro (1984) stated this point very boldly: "The crucial aim of analysis remains the uncovering of the unconscious. As I understand it, that is the *sine qua non* of the science. If it is not the aim of analysis, then neutrality is no longer necessary and we can dispense with it" (p. 280). Alex Hoffer (1985), in an extremely important paper, echoed and elaborated this point:

> Neutrality, in a general sense, is the optimal position from which the analyst gathers his data from the analytic field using the free association method. While free association ([and] the analyst's evenly hovering attention) is the *process* by which the analyst observes the analytic field, neutrality is the *position* from which the analyst observes (pp. 774–775; italics added).

> [N]eutral exploration and explication of unconscious, unrecognized, and conscious conflict, compromise, and resolution are the foundation of the analytic approach and process. Neutrality, along with the patient's free associations and the analyst's evenly hovering attention, are the building blocks of that foundation (p. 777).

Renik (1995) reiterated this point in a paper particularly concerned with one crucial aspect of neutrality, the analyst's anonymity. However,

his remark would apply to neutrality in general: "Analytic anonymity is
. . . a strategy designed to maximize conscious scrutiny of a patient's
previously unconscious mental life" (p. 475).

As is generally recognized, *neutrality cannot be absolute.* The analyst's
anonymity must be only partial because obvious, subtle, and sublimi-
nal cues about him are presented to the patient constantly as a matter of course. Some of these cues will necessarily have instinctual and /
or moral dimensions. But, most radically, the analyst's own abstinence—his lack of personal influence on the patient—cannot be absolute. Any action or communication by one person to another necessarily entails a demand, implicit or explicit. Neither conscientious
phraseology nor egalitarian behavior can obviate this aspect of human relatedness—inside or outside the psychoanalytic situation. The
analyst, in his interactions with the patient, implicitly or explicitly
states: "*I want you* to tell me . . . " or "*I want you* to understand that . . . "
And, in the practical arrangements of the psychoanalytic situation—
relating to fees, schedule of appointments, the physical integrity of
the analyst and his consulting room, etc.—the analyst implicitly or
explicitly states to the patient: "*I want you to do* (this and / or / not that)
for me."

Thus, in the joint pursuit of the unconscious determinants of the patient's compromise formations and of their components of conflict,
the communicative and pragmatic rapport between analyst and patient must necessarily abridge the analyst's neutrality. Further, the
auto-mutative nature of the mind and the conflict-exacerbating nature
of psychoanalytic work ensure that these abridgments will affect the
patient's compromise formations in the analytic situation in ways that
must themselves be analyzed so that the patient's transference and resistance remain relatively discernible and analyzable. This sort of analysis does, indeed, provide extremely valuable information about the patient's inner life, but that very act of analyzing necessarily produces
further material to analyze. And the analysis of that further material
leads to still further material, and so on. Accordingly, by the very nature of the psychoanalytic investigative process, there must always be a
practicably unanalyzed residuum—constituting unknowability—concerning the non-neutral communication and interaction with the patient by the analyst himself.

This inevitable unknowability has practical importance to a *relative*
degree. That is to say: while unknowability exists, "relative certainty"
may often still be achieved. And, in fact, in many instances the inerad-
icable incompleteness of psychoanalytic investigation may be ignored—
for all practical analytic purposes. In other instances, it may not. Brenner

(1996), addressing methodological problems closely related to those presented here, took up this particular issue quite directly.

> The problem of the influence of observation on data arises in every field of scientific inquiry. . . . The question is not whether the observer influences the data. Of course the observer does. Always. The question is whether the observer's influence is a significant one for the purpose of the observations made and the generalizations one hopes to be able to draw from them. I believe that in a properly conducted analysis or, if one prefers, in a proper analytic situation the effect of the observer on the data is not so great as to render the data unreliable for the purpose to which one hopes to put them—i.e., as a basis for understanding the nature and origin of the patient's conflicts and, by extension, as a basis for conveying that understanding to a patient (pp. 28–29).

Brenner thus acknowledged inherent unknowability in the psychoanalytic situation, but he shifted the problem away from its inevitable presence to its degree. He correlated "a proper analytic situation" with a degree of the analyst's distortion of the analytic data that is still acceptable for psychoanalytic utility. Clearly, in any given instance, it is a matter of practical judgment how much of such unknowability—and what subject matter is unknown—renders a psychoanalytic investigation invalid.

Further, any modification of psychoanalytic theory that hypothesizes mental life as essentially, or principally, determined by interpersonal relationships must concentrate on the analyst's very active engagement with the patient in an effort to modify the patient's mental life in a salutary direction. There will necessarily be little concern about the analyst's distorting effect upon the patient's analytically pertinent compromise formations. This is the position set out by Stephen Mitchell in *Relational Concepts in Psychoanalysis* (1988) and *Hope and Dread in Psychoanalysis* (1993). The essential methodological goal of obtaining as much evidence as possible of the unconscious conflict pertinent to the patient's compromise formations must necessarily be discarded. The methodological centrality of the analyst's neutrality and of free association and evenly suspended attention will not only be impossible to implement, but must be considered as actually anti-therapeutic. Therefore, there will be no evidence of the unconscious determination of the patient's conscious mental life in the analytic situation, nor will there be indications of unconscious pathogenic factors in the patient's troubles. Correspondingly, this modified conception of mind and of therapy will not see as essential the patient's insight into himself, his unconscious conflicts and his repressed childhood past. Indeed, the basic theoretical hypotheses of a dynamic unconscious and of psychic determinism will appear not only as therapeutically irrelevant but also as without heuristic and scientific value. And, in fact, Mitchell has rejected virtually all the unique insights of psychoanalysis noted above. Necessarily, he has developed other—essentially, non-analytic—mutually compatible and mutually confirming theories of mind, pathogenesis, therapy, and method.

Robert Michels (1996), in his review of Mitchell's 1993 book, made this same point, showing the essential interconnection of changes in theory, technique, and method.

> Mitchell believes that the analyst's subjectivity and ideas, together with the patient's experience and understanding, co-determine the analytic process. . . .
>
> Mitchell is not concerned with the development of ego-psychology or the analysis of defenses; he is interested in far more basic concerns. "Psychoanalysis is a process involving, most fundamentally, the hopes and dreads of its two participants" (page 9). "[The] issue of the analyst's personal influence is one of the key features of the analytic process" (page 15). . . . "The hope inspired by psychoanalysis in our time is grounded in personal meaning, not rational consensus" (page 21). "The goal of psychoanalysis . . . is . . . the establishment of a richer, more authentic sense of identity" (page 24). There has been a shift in theorising about what the patient needs from insight to relationship, parallel to the shift from rationality to the search for an authentic personal experience" (page 39).
>
> . . .
>
> For Mitchell, psychoanalysis is not an empiric science: it does not provide us with a map of what the mind really is. In his words, "there has been a fundamental redefinition in our understanding of what psychoanalytic theorising is, from a representation and reflection of the underlying structure of the patient's mind to a construction, an interpretation of the patient's experience" (page 67). But which construction? How does Mitchell know whether a given construction is psychoanalytic? What makes one interpretation "psychoanalytic" while another is not? Or, does it make any difference if it makes the patient feel more "authentic"? (pp. 618–620).

It is clear form Michels's comments that generalizations of a psychoanalytic nature—that is, based upon the inference of unconscious mental processes—cannot come from such an approach. Indeed, there can be no advancement of psychoanalysis as a coherent discipline at all.

Not surprisingly, Michels made the same point regarding psychoanalysis as a therapeutic procedure. He quoted Mitchell: "'the analyst knows a collection of ways of thinking about how the mind works. . . .

[P]sychoanalytic knowledge is not anchored in enduring truths or proofs, but rather in its use value for making sense of a life, deepening relationships with others, and expanding and enriching the texture of experience' (pages 64–65). Many religions would lay claims to this domain as well, and Mitchell does not make clear how, or even whether, he would differentiate them from psychoanalysis" (p. 619). Michels went on to observe that the sort of therapy Mitchell was advocating is appropriate if the goal is "a richer, more authentic sense of identity," but not for the alleviation of neurotic suffering. Michels was, in effect, stating that Mitchell's technical innovation could not properly be termed "psychoanalytic" at all. Here, again, a change in basic theory leads to basic changes in method and technique.

CONCLUSIONS

Unknowability in psychoanalysis has three sources: the patient's inherently unobservable unconscious mental processes, practicably unobservable extra-analytic influences on the analytic material, and the practically unanalyzable effects of the analyst's activities. They all derive from the mind's constant auto-mutative nature, driven by persistent intrapsychic conflict. These inherent limitations are addressed by standard aspects of psychoanalytic method: free association and evenly suspended attention, analysis of the transference neurosis, relatively long and frequent analytic sessions, and the analyst's neutrality. The latter two aspects of analytic method themselves facilitate the application of free association and evenly suspended attention. This pair of operations function to infer unconscious conflict. And are at the heart of certain current controversies in psychoanalysis. Whether the controversy entails de-emphasizing the analyzing instrument itself, curtailing the frequency or length of analytic sessions, concentrating solely on the patient-analyst interaction, or abrogating the analyst's neutrality, the controversial proposals all ultimately interfere with the procedure of inferring unconscious mental life, particularly conflict. This procedure is central to psychoanalytic theory, technique, and method and is vitally important in addressing inevitable unknowability in psychoanalysis. Accordingly, any removal of the unconscious and its inference from their crucial position will lead to an increase in unknowability and a weakening, or even eradication, of the psychoanalytic insights gleaned over the past century, as well as their disjunction from analytic work. Other theories and insights, other modes of therapy, and other observational methods *that are not psychoanalytic* must supervene.

Of course, this has always been the case with non-analytic theories of mind and investigative methods, whether they see conscious mental life as deriving from social circumstances or from neurological processes. Neither approach can recognize and integrate what has been discovered by psychoanalysis—namely, the influence of unconscious mental processes in the context of mental conflict. In order for social scientific or neuroscientific disciplines to incorporate the insights of psychoanalysis, they too must employ the uniquely psychoanalytic observational method. Without free association and evenly suspended attention their approaches must remain limited, skewed, and incomplete. Current proposals to modify traditional psychoanalytic method, theory, and technique pose the same danger within psychoanalysis itself.

Yet the history of psychoanalysis shows a robust continuity that follows the centrality of inferring unconscious mental life in the context of intrapsychic conflict. There have been many proposed changes in theory, technique, or method that deviated from this course—e.g., Freud's theory of the "actual neurosis," Jung's theory of the "collective unconscious," Adler's theory of the predominance of the "will to power," Freud's theory of neurosis as the "negative" of perversion, Reich's concretistic theory of "orgone" energy, Freud's theory of the "death instinct," Fenichel's and Reich's amalgamations of psychoanalysis and Marxism, Freud's theory of the "dissolution of the Oedipus complex," Jones's theory of "aphanisis," Greenacre's theory of the "biological economy of birth" and the "predisposition to anxiety," Erikson's "epigenetic" theory of human development, Ferenczi's and Rank's "active" therapy, Rank's theory of the predominance of the birth trauma and his associated technique of predetermined termination, Freud's technical injunction not to analyze "the unobjectionable part of the transference," Reich's technique of aggressive "penetration" of the patient's character "armor," Alexander's technical theory of the "corrective emotional experience," Felix Deutsch's technical strategy of "sector therapy," John Rosen's technique of "direct analysis." All these, and others too, fell away—because they had to. They either formed non-psychoanalytic theories, techniques, and methods or disappeared for lack of further development due to unknowability. Current proposals for revision appear destined to repeat this natural history. What will remain in psychoanalysis *as psychoanalysis* will be continued progress based on the inference of unconscious mental life through free association and evenly suspended attention.

BIBLIOGRAPHY

ARLOW, J. A. (1961). Ego psychology and the study of mythology. *J. Amer. Psychoanal. Assn.* 9:371–393.

――― (1969). Fantasy, memory, and reality testing. *Psychoanal. Q.* 38:28–51.

ARLOW, J. A. AND BRENNER, C. (1964). *Psychoanalytic Concepts and the Structural Theory.* New York: International Universities Press.

BALTER, L., LOTHANE, Z., AND SPENCER, J. H. (1980). On the analyzing instrument. *Psychoanal. Q.* 49:474–504.

BALTER, L. AND SPENCER, J. H. (1991). Observation and theory in psychoanalysis: The self psychology of Heinz Kohut. *Psychoanal. Q.* 60:361–395.

BLUM, H. P. (1994). *Reconstruction in Psychoanalysis: Childhood Revisited and Recreated.* New York: International Universities Press.

BRENNER, C. (1968). Archaic features of ego functioning. *Int. J. Psycho-Anal.* 49:426–429.

――― (1976). *Psychoanalytic Technique and Psychic Conflict.* New York: International Universities Press.

――― (1982). *The Mind in Conflict.* New York: International Universities Press.

――― (1996). The nature of knowledge and the limits of authority in psychoanalysis. *Psychoanal. Q.* 65:21–31.

FENICHEL, O. (1941). *Problems of Psychoanalytic Technique.* Trans. D. Brunswick. New York: *The Psychoanalytic Quarterly, Inc.*

FREUD, A. (1936). The ego and the mechanisms of defense. *Writings* 2:1–176.

FREUD, S. (1913). On beginning the treatment. (Further recommendations on the technique of psycho-analysis I). *Standard Edition* 12:123–144.

――― (1916–1917). Introductory lectures on psycho-analysis. *Standard Edition 15 and 16.*

――― (1917). A difficulty in the path of psycho-analysis. *Standard Edition* 17:137–144.

――― (1923). The ego and the id. *Standard Edition* 19:13–59.

――― (1925a). A note upon the "mystic writing-pad." *Standard Edition* 19:227–232.

――― (1925b). Negation. *Standard Edition* 19:235–239.

――― (1926). Inhibitions, symptoms and anxiety. *Standard Edition* 20:87–172.

――― (1933). New introductory lectures on psychoanalysis. *Standard Edition* 22:5–182.

――― (1937). Constructions in analysis. *Standard Edition* 23:257–269.

――― (1940). An outline of psycho-analysis. *Standard Edition* 23:144–207.

GALATZER-LEVY, R. (1980). Characterizing our ignorance. *Annual Psychoanal.* 8:77–82.

GILL, M. M. (1963). *Topography and Systems in Psychoanalytic Theory. Psychological Issues, Volume 10.* New York: International Universities Press.

GRAY, P. (1990). The nature of therapeutic action in psychoanalysis. *J. Amer. Psychoanal. Assn.* 38:1083–1098.

HARTMANN, H. (1939). *Ego Psychology and the Problem of Adaptation.* Trans. D. Rapaport. New York: International Universities Press, 1958.

HARTMANN, H. AND KRIS, E. (1945). The genetic approach in psychoanalysis. In: Hartmann, H., Kris, E., AND Lowenstein, R. *Papers on Psychoanalytic Psychology.* New York: International Universities Press, 1964.

HOFFER, A. (1985). Toward a definition of psychoanalytic neutrality. *J. Amer. Psychoanal. Assn.* 33:771–795.

HOFFMAN, I. (1983). The patient as interpreter of the analyst's experience. *Contemp. Psychoanal.* 19:389–422.

HOFFMAN, I. (1991). Discussion: Towards a social-constructivist view of the psychoanalytic situation. *Psychoanal. Dialogues* 1:74–105.

——— (1992). Some practical implications of a social-constructivist view of the psychoanalytic situation. *Psychoanal. Dialogues* 2:287–304.

JOSEPH, B. (1985). Transference: The total situation. *Int. J. Psycho-Anal.* 66:447–454.

KOHUT, H. (1959). Introspection, empathy, and psychoanalysis: An examination of the relationship between mode of observation and theory. *J. Amer. Psychoanal. Assn.* 7:459–483.

——— (1971). *The Analysis of the Self: A Systematic Approach to the Psychoanalytic Treatment of Narcissistic Personality Disorders.* New York: International Universities Press.

——— (1977). *The Restoration of the Self.* New York: International Universities Press.

——— (1984). *How Does Analysis Cure?* Ed. A. Goldberg with the collaboration of P. E. Stepansky. Chicago: University of Chicago Press.

KRIS, E. (1950). On preconscious mental processes. *Psychoanal. Q.* 19:540–560.

LEARY, K. (1994). Psychoanalytic "problems" and postmodern "solutions." *Psychoanal. Q.* 63:433–465.

MICHELS, R. (1996). Book review essay: Gill, Gray, Mitchell, and Reed on psychoanalytic technique. *Int. J. Psycho-Anal.* 77:615–623.

MITCHELL, S. (1988). *Relational Concepts in Psychoanalysis: An Integration.* Cambridge, Mass.: Harvard University Press.

——— (1993). *Hope and Dread in Psychoanalysis.* New York: Basic Books.

MORAN, M. G. (1991). Chaos theory and psychoanalysis: The fluidic nature of the mind. *Int. Rev. Psycho-Anal.* 18:211–221.

POLAND, W. (1984). On the analyst's neutrality. *J. Amer. Psychoanal. Assn.* 32:283–299.

RAPAPORT, D. AND GILL, M. (1959). The points of view and assumptions of metapsychology. *Int. J. Psycho-Anal.* 40:153–162.

RENIK, O. (1995). The ideal of the anonymous analyst and the problem of self-disclosure. *Psychoanal. Q.* 64:466–495.

SCHAFER, R. (1994). The contemporary Kleinians of London. *Psychoanal. Q.* 63:409–432.

SHAPIRO, T. (1984). On neutrality. *J. Amer. Psychoanal. Assn.* 32:269–299.

SPENCER, J. H. AND BALTER, L. (1990). Psychoanalytic observation. *J. Amer. Psychoanal. Assn.* 38:393–422.

STEIN, M. H. (1965). States of consciousness in the analytic situation: Including a note on·the traumatic dream. *Drives, Affects, Behavior II.* New York: International Universities Press, pp. 60–86.

STRACHEY, J. (1934). The therapeutic action of psychoanalysis. *Int. J. Psycho-Anal.* 15:127–159.

WAELDER, R. (1936 [1930]). The principle of multiple function: Observations on over-determination. *Psychoanal. Q.* 5:45–62.

Therapeutic Functions of the Real Relationship in Psychoanalysis

ARTHUR S. COUCH, Ph.D.

This paper attempts to give a comprehensive picture of the concept and therapeutic functions of the real relationship in clinical psychoanalysis. After introducing this theme, the author presents an extensive review of the literature, citing not only the major recent contributors to the concept but also many contributions from the past. A third part summarizes Freud's development of the analytic relationship and then quotes from Freud's patients' written accounts of their analyses in order to illustrate how Freud's actual analytic style contained many elements of a real relationship. The fourth part presents the author's own formulation of the therapeutic contributions of the real relationship to psychoanalysis and offers a clinical vignette as an illustration of its therapeutic role in the termination phase of an analysis.

INTRODUCTION

UNDERSTANDING THE THEORETICAL SIGNIFICANCE AND THERAPEUTIC functions of the "real relationship" in psychoanalysis has been the challenging goal of a long-recognized attempt to comprehend the full range of communications between patient and analyst, including the "non-orthodox" aspects. Such a concern frequently comes from a clin-

Training analyst at the British Psycho-Analytical Society.

This paper is an extensively revised version of a paper on "The Role of the Real Relationship in Analysis," given at a Scientific Meeting of the Boston Psychoanalytic Society on 10 January 1979.

The Psychoanalytic Study of the Child 54, ed. Albert J. Solnit, Peter B. Neubauer, Samuel Abrams, and A. Scott Dowling (Yale University Press, copyright © 1999 by Albert J. Solnit, Peter B. Neubauer, Samuel Abrams, and A. Scott Dowling).

ically derived awareness of the extent and importance of non-technical interchanges in the analytic situation.

The intuitive conviction held by most analysts, starting with Freud himself, that a genuine human relationship between analyst and patient is inherent in the analytic situation and is crucial for its functioning is so much taken for granted that it has almost no explicit place in our general theory of the therapeutic process. The human foundation of analysis is underplayed in our literature, partly because it seems to conflict with the explicit conceptual formulations and "rules" of the analytic process—that is, with the primacy of interpretations, and counter-transference reactions, and concerns for analytic neutrality, anonymity, acting out, unresponsiveness, and so forth.

I share with many analysts the view that the real human relationship is not in conflict with our basic analytic principles but, on the contrary, has always provided the essential foundation—the *Anlage*—for the full functioning of the analytic process.

The main purpose of this paper is to illustrate the positive contributions of the real relationship (the reality-oriented contact between patient and analyst) to the therapeutic process at the different phases of an analysis. I believe that the effective presence of a real relationship, both in its independent state and as interwoven into the fabric of the transference neurosis, creates the crucial conditions for the analytic process to enlarge the scope of the patient's ego. It does this through increasing the patient's awareness of the neurotic distortions in his self-perceptions and his perceptions of others, especially the analyst in the transference relationship instead of in the real relationship, which may be perceived quite correctly.

There are two aspects of the real relationship that must be carefully differentiated, although both are inherent in the concept: the nature of the *communication* between analyst and patient, and the nature of the *personality* of analyst and patient as real persons. Both aspects are part of the real relationship, which might best be described as the realistic communication between analyst and patient when they are functioning as their real selves, relatively free from transference or counter-transference influences. The real relationship is effectively present when both analyst and patient are talking to each other in reasonable ways as ordinary human beings.

Like most analysts in the classical tradition, I began clinical work with a primary focus on the issues of transference neurosis, resistance, character defenses, affects, reconstructions, unconscious derivatives in dreams and associations, and so forth. Thus, I initially gave only commonsensical and humane attention to the realistic aspects of communications with my patients about session arrangements and reality exigencies. But as I gained more experience as an analyst, I soon realized the need to bring the subtle, complex, and usually overlooked interactive presence of the real relationship in to my conceptual thinking about how the analytic process works. Believing that I was on the track of an original theme, I paused to review the literature and found that other experienced analysts had already recognized this issue and considered its implications for technique. But this process of rediscovery reinforced my conviction of the significance of the real relationship for psychoanalysis.

The issue of the role of the real relationship in analysis brings up some significant analytic controversies, such as the relative emphasis on ego vs. id analysis; the role of analytic anonymity and neutrality; whether an ego alliance should be a major part of analysis; whether all material should be reduced to unconscious references to the transference; or whether analysis should be insulated from reality as much as possible so as to promote transference and regression. Certain theoretical and clinical positions on these issues have influenced analysts to take very different positions on the role of the real relationship.

REVIEW OF THE LITERATURE

GREENSON'S FORMULATION

Much of what I have so far been discussing will be recognized as mainly derived from Greenson's classic presentations of the real relationship (1965, 1967, 1968, 1972, 1974). In Greenson's view, the full analytic relationship can be divided into three modes or levels: the transference (and countertransference) relationship, the therapeutic relationship or working alliance, and the real relationship. Here are some relevant passages from Greenson (1967) that illustrate his position:

> In adults, all relationships to people consist of a varying mixture of transference and reality. There is no transference reaction no matter how fantastic without a germ of truth, and there is no realistic relationship without some trace of a transference fantasy. All patients in psychoanalytic treatment have realistic and objective perceptions and reactions to their analyst alongside of their transference reactions and their working alliance. These three modes of relating to the analyst are interrelated. They influence one another, blend into each other, and can cover one another (p. 219).

> The term "real" in the phrase "real relationship" may mean realistic, reality-oriented, or undistorted as contrasted to the term "transfer-

ence," which connotes unrealistic, distorted, and inappropriate. The word real may also refer to genuine, authentic, true in contrast to artificial, synthetic, or assumed. At this point, I intend to use the term real to refer to the realistic and genuine relationship between analyst and patient (p. 217).

It is important to re-emphasize the organic *unity* of the analytic relationship itself, so that the differentiations Greenson makes among transference, therapeutic, and real relationships will be seen in a holistic perspective. As Greenson has noted, these relationships are always interwoven, and each always contains elements of the others. During certain phases of an analysis, one type of relationship may predominate, but the other components are silently present and latent in the background.

With this seminal contribution, Greenson established a significant new formulation of the nature of the psychoanalytic situation. His views express the vague uneasiness many experienced analysts feel about the sterile "orthodox" technique that had begun to dehumanize psychoanalysis. Greenson's position offered a new, humanistic standard to be set against the overtechnical rules about transference focus coming out of the post-Freudian schools of psychoanalysis.

LIPTON'S FORMULATION

Lipton's (1977) classic article on Freud's technique offered a significant critique of the rigid technical impersonality of the post-Freudian developments, which he termed "modern" technique. The many important points Lipton makes in this paper must be put in the context of his hypothesis that Freud excluded a substantial personal relationship with patients from his technique and that this "excluded" characteristic actually accounts for the decisive advantages of his technique over modern technique. This is a significant redefinition of the conception of the real relationship: namely, that as a "personal relationship" between patient and analyst, it is not part of technique but is a necessary part of analysis. Lipton explains, "I have chosen the adjective 'personal' to convey the idea that it is both outside technique and subject to individual variation" (p. 268). Here are some brief extracts from Lipton's (1977) paper that illustrate his position:

> In my opinion, the problem lies in the expansion of the [modern] concept of technique to incorporate matters which Freud did not consider technical but instead considered only as part of his non-technical personal relationship with [the patient] (p. 259).

What Freud called the unobjectionable element of the transference is now often referred to as the current, real, actual, or nontransference feelings of the patient (p. 261).

I think the essence of the difference between modern technique and Freud's is that the definition of technique has been expanded to incorporate aspects of the analyst's relation with the patient, which Freud excluded from technique (p. 262).

The criticisms of Freud's technique show that modern technique places great weight on minor matters [realistic interventions] rather than major ones. . . . Instead of occupying himself exclusively with comprehending the meaning of the patient's associations, the analyst presumably devotes some of his attention to excluding interventions which might become the subject of future associations. Then, to the extent to which such avoidance is prospective, it tends to move technique from collaboration to unilaterality (p. 262).

One of Lipton's main points concerns the influence of Eissler's (1953) paper defining the "parameters" of a modern "orthodox" analysis, which was, in fact, very different from the more natural and personal quality of Freud's technical style. Lipton writes:

With the pejorative connotation which the parameter acquired, it may be that it was from this paper that a sort of myth arose—that is, that the analyst uttered no words except interpretations. . . . [Also] [i]n formulating his basic model technique he [Eissler] explicitly excludes the personality of the analyst and the living conditions of the patient. . . . At any rate, it was in the period after this paper was published that the exclusion of the personality of the analyst and the expansion of technique to cover all utterances of the analyst gained acceptability (pp. 264–65).

In one respect, Lipton's view of the "personal relationship" differs from Greenson's conception of the "real relationship": while Greenson separates the real relationship from the therapeutic alliance, Lipton combines them: "Insofar as I understand the concept of an alliance with the patient, it is no more than the personal relationship which Freud established with his patients, based on the unobjectionable elements of the transference on the part of the patient and the recognition of the patient as an individual by the analyst, a relationship which Freud excluded from technique" (p. 265).

In a summary statement, Lipton presents his view that a technical style which includes a personal relationship has several clinical advantages over the modern technique, which tries to exclude it:

Paradoxically, modern technique can produce just what it may have been designed to avoid, a corrective emotional experience, by exposing the patient to a hypothetically ideally correct, ideally unobtrusive, ideally silent, encompassing technical instrumentality rather than the presence of the analyst as a person with whom the patient can establish a personal relationship. In addition, modern technique also incurs the danger of fostering iatrogenic narcissistic disorders by establishing an ambience in which the patient has little opportunity to establish an object relationship (p. 272).

VIEDERMAN'S FORMULATION

The significant article by Viederman (1991) on "The Real Person of the Analyst and His Role in the Process of Psychoanalytic Cure" sets forth a position complementary to Greenson's. The paper offers a very positive affirmation of the therapeutic value of the direct expression of the real person of the analyst at certain times in a session rather than hiding behind the "orthodox" façade of anonymity, neutrality, and abstinence. Viederman describes a number of clinical cases in which his naturalistic, "real person" interventions made important contributions to his patients' analytic progress. His very comprehensive presentation deserves careful reading by anyone interested in this complex topic. The following brief excerpts will give only a brief summary of Viederman's (1991) position:

> The influence of the real person of the analyst on "psychoanalytic cure" has, with few exceptions, been treated cautiously in the psychoanalytic literature. My intent . . . is to place the relationship at center stage as an aspect of the therapeutic process that leads to change, to examine the reluctance of analysts to acknowledge its role, and to explore the manner in which it manifests itself in the psychoanalytic process that leads to change. . . . By the "real" person of the analyst I refer not only to his outward traits, but also to his unique characteristics as a person and to his behavior in the analytic situation which goes beyond interpretation and clarification (p. 452).

> The affective presence of the analyst, namely his self-expression with feeling and conviction, when indicated, acts as a stimulus for an affective interchange and development of transference which has a different quality from transference evoked by an analyst who insists on absolute abstinence and interpretation as the only vehicle for communication with the patient (p. 454).

> To give theoretical status to the personal attributes and responses of the analyst understandably generates concern that the definition of the analytic process will be clouded and its scientific status compromised. . . . Psychoanalysts therefore have been hesitant to recognize the importance of personal influence lest it cloud the definition of

transference, countertransference, resistance, defense, interpretation
(p. 459).

Patients often remember moments in their analyses when the analyst
shows great feeling or deviates from a more usual abstinent approach. . . . These uncontrived moments have a special significance
for the patient because they reflect his awareness that he has had an influence on the analyst and that the analyst is involved in the relationship (p. 475).

My intent [in conclusion] has been to place the real person of the analyst at centre-stage as it relates to the curative process of psychoanalysis, and to focus on the analyst as a *presence* in the analytic situation.
Moreover, it is intended to encourage a freedom that has too often
been stifled by strict interpretation of the rules of psychoanalytic technique (p. 487).

The position Viederman expresses in this seminal paper is in line
with my own long-held views on the role of the real relationship
(Couch, 1979). While many others hold similar views and have similar human, non-rigid, analytic relationships with their patients, it is
rare for analysts to acknowledge this position as openly as Viederman
has.

It is noteworthy that Viederman's excellent paper does not differentiate between the two aspects of the real relationship that have been
previously conceptualized: realistic communication and the presence
of the real personality of the analyst in the analytic situation. This is
quite understandable, for the real relationship is a natural fusion of
these two aspects.

EARLIER LITERATURE

Since the 1930s many analysts have tried to point out the widespread
misunderstanding of the "neutrality" rule and have emphasized the
need for a natural and concerned human relationship in analysis. Thus
Ferenczi, Nunberg, W. Reich, Fenichel, Bibring, and Glover, among
others, wrote about technique in ways that conveyed a fuller picture of
the analyst at work. Ella Sharpe (1930), in her papers on technique,
very sensitively outlined the need for full humanity and personal integrity in the analyst: "Our own adjustment to reality should be proven
by our simplicity of purpose, honesty, and freedom from pose" (p. 19).
In a symposium on therapeutic results, Bibring (1937) expressed the
view that a real relationship is a precondition for the psychoanalytic
procedure.

Soon after 1940, more explicit references to the role of the real relationship could be found in the writings of Fenichel (1941), Menaker (1942), A. Freud (1954), Stone (1954, 1961), Winnicott (1955), Zetzel (1956), Nacht (1958), Loewald (1960), and Gitelson (1952, 1962). Greenson and Wexler (1969) conducted a comprehensive review of the relevant literature, so I will present only some highlights.

In 1942 Esther Menaker wrote about this topic in a surprisingly prescient way:

> It seems to us . . . important to distinguish between that part of the analytic experience which is relived *as* if "real" (not to question the genuineness of this experience) and that part which *is* real—that is, which constitutes a direct human relationship between patient and analyst, which has an existence independent of the transference, and which is the medium in which the transference reactions take place. In making the distinction between the real and the transference relationship in analysis, we must not become confused by the fact that both relationships have this in common: like all object relationships in the life of individuals they are characterized by the heritage of earlier relationships. . . . The real relationship, like the transference, repeats an earlier emotional pattern, but the impetus for this repetition comes not so much from the inner psychic life of the patient—as does the transference—as from the external situation of the analysis itself (pp. 172–174).

> In general, it is important that the real relationship between patient and analyst have some content and substance other than that created by the analytic situation itself. This is achieved if the analyst presents himself in a distinctly human role, unafraid to show his own personality and to function with friendly interest towards his patient, reserving his cooler objectivity for the material of the analysis. This functioning of the analyst as a real person, in the course of which he reveals something of his own ego, liberates the ego of the patient for freer functioning because the patient is able to relate himself to an image of the analyst which approximates his [the analyst's] personality rather than to one which places the analyst exclusively in the position of the authoritative, perfect parent (pp. 184–185).

Max Gitelson (1952), in his paper "The Emotional Position of the Analyst in the Psychoanalytic Situation," wrote as follows regarding the inevitability and necessity of self-revelation on the part of the analyst:

> One must conclude that the analyst as a mere screen does not exist in life. He cannot deny his personality nor its operation in the analytic situation as a significant factor. . . . In such a situation one can reveal as much of oneself as is needed to foster and support the patient's discovery of the reality of the actual interpersonal situation as contrasted with the transference-counter-transference situation. . . . An analysis

can come to an impasse because the analyst does not realize, or mis-understands, or avoids the issue of a patient's discovery of him as a per-son (pp. 7–8).

In 1954 Leo Stone made the first of his contributions toward a sepa-ration of the real relationship from forms of transference and coun-tertransference. During a discussion of his paper Anna Freud (1954) made the following remarks:

> I refer briefly to Dr. Stone's remarks concerning the "real personal re-lationship" between analyst and patient versus the "true transference reactions". To make such a distinction coincides with ideas which I have always held on this subject. . . . We see the patient enter into analy-sis with a reality attitude to the analyst; then the transference gains mo-mentum until it reaches its peak in the full-blown transference neuro-sis which has to be worked off analytically until the figure of the analyst emerges again, reduced to its true status. But—and this seems impor-tant to me—so far as the patient has a healthy part of his personality, his real relationship to the analyst is never wholly submerged. With due respect for the necessary strictest handling and interpretation of the transference, I feel still that we should leave room somewhere for the realization that analysts and patient are also two real people, of equal adult status, in a real personal relationship to each other. I wonder whether our—at times complete—neglect of this side of the matter is not responsible for some of the hostile reactions which we get from pa-tients and which we are apt to ascribe to "true transference" only. But these are technically subversive thoughts and ought to be handled with care (pp. 618–619).

Zetzel (1956, 1958, 1969, 1970) made a series of significant contri-butions to this issue by articulating the need for a separate conception of the relationship implied in Freud's (1937) statement: "As is well known, the analytic situation consists in our allying ourselves with the ego of the person under treatment" (p. 235). Zetzel (1956) termed this component of the analytic relationship the "therapeutic alliance" and felt it was closely related to the real doctor-patient relationship. In 1958 she wrote: "In terms of mature ego functions and reality testing, the ability of the patient to maintain a real relationship with the analyst as a separate individual—with both positive and negative attributes—ap-pears to be related to the capacity for a therapeutic alliance. In this con-nection it is recognized that the analyst's real personality and individ-ual characteristics inevitably influence the analytic situation" (p. 183). In this paper, Zetzel is saying that the presence of a real object rela-tionship is necessary for the "therapeutic alliance" to develop, and that these conditions are necessary for the analysis itself to proceed. In a 1969 article Zetzel developed this formulation:

> As the psychoanalytic method developed, the real personality of the physician became blurred, overshadowed or even lost as the sexualized transference neurosis took the center of the stage [p. 197]. The real doctor-patient relationship was still recognized by Freud as an indispensable feature of the analytic situation. . . . Though analytic work concentrated on interpretation of the transference neurosis, this would have been impossible without the clear separation of transference from reality, the mutual alliance towards a therapeutic goal, and the genuine object relationship which remained intact despite the expression by the patient of ambivalence, hostility and intense resistance (pp. 198–199).

In *The Psychoanalytic Situation* (1961), Stone outlined many implications of a neglect of the real relationships in an analysis. Here is one brief statement very pertinent to the theme of this paper: "There is, throughout the [analytic] process, the presence of the patient as an integrated adult personality, larger than the sum of his psychic parts or functional systems. Whereas purely technical or intellectual errors can, in most instances, be corrected, a failure in a critical junction to show the reasonable human response which any person inevitably expects from another on whom he deeply depends can invalidate years of patient and largely skillful work" (p. 55).

Stone (1981) makes the significant point that the "here-and-now" of the psychoanalytic situation contains not just transference material but also the manifestations of the real relationship, including "certain basic considerations of analytic technique, the recognition of the adult relationship between patient and analyst, and due respect for the sometimes critically important significance of the patient's extra-analytic activities and relationships as such" (p. 731).

In a paper on the multiple levels of the analytic relation, Paolino (1982) perceptively summarizes therapeutic functions: "The real relationship is just as important to the psychoanalytic process as the other aspects of the therapeutic relationship. If the real relationship is not actively recognized and utilized in the therapy sessions, then the patient is exposed to a relationship with the analyst that is interpersonally sterile and lacking the opportunity for the patient to develop a meaningful and therapeutic object relation" (p. 232).

Anna Freud made the following differentiation of transference from other aspects of the analytic relationship: "I have always learned to consider transference in the light of a distortion of the real relationship of the patient to the analyst, and, of course, that type and manner of distortion showed up the contributions from the past. If there were no real relationship, this idea of the distorting influences would make no sense" (quoted in Greenson and Wexler, 1969, p. 28).

Finally, I present some summarizing ideas from Greenson and Wexler (1969) to illustrate the kind of formulation I try to extend in later sections of this paper:

> To facilitate the full flowering and ultimate resolution of the patient's transference reactions, it is essential in all cases to recognize, acknowledge, clarify, differentiate, and even nurture the non-transference or relatively transference-free reactions between patient and analyst. The technique of "only analysing" or "only interpreting" transference phenomena may stifle the development and clarification of the transference neurosis and act as an obstacle to the maturation of the transference-free or "real" reactions of the patient (p. 27).

FREUD'S DEVELOPMENT OF THE ANALYTIC RELATIONSHIP

In the very earliest phase of psychoanalysis, Freud quite naturally grafted his new "talking cure" method of treatment onto the role of the physician. This age-old role has always served as a culturally sanctioned way of giving professional care to ill people. At the same time, it has provided enough leeway within that role for the doctor to express his humane, personal self to the patient. This humane aspect of the doctor's role has frequently been seen as secondary to the technical procedures for the care of the patient's illness. Freud overemphasized the technical, trying to bypass resistance and transference reactions in order to get to the curative tasks of uncovering the repressed traumatic memories. But Freud made use of his eventual discovery of these "errors" in formulating the major pillars of psychoanalytic technique: the analysis of transference and resistance.

As Freud took the crucial steps from hypnotism to suggestion to free association, he gradually developed a new kind of working relationship: therapeutic cooperation. The authoritative aspect of the physician's role turned into one of mutuality. In the aftermath of Dora's analysis, Freud (1905) became aware of the importance of transference, in terms of both the projections of earlier relationships and the resistances to analysis derived from it. Freud then, in a brilliant stroke, turned his perception of the power of transference into an awareness of the value of analyzing it as a major tool for acquiring insight into the patient's unconscious mind.

The point relevant to the theme of this paper is that the transference was at first unrecognized in its importance and was viewed mainly as an interference with the therapeutic work. There is a parallel in the way in which the real relationship has been overlooked, its presence seen as a kind of contamination or interference with the transference, and its therapeutic functions not clearly seen or recognized.

We will gain much understanding of how analysis works if we become more aware of the hidden functions of the real relationship, which is always present in the background of every analysis. Like the transference relationship, the real relationship should be seen as essential for the analytic process with important implications for technique.

CONTRAST OF FREUD'S TECHNIQUE AND HIS TECHNICAL "RULES"

Although there were undoubtedly many technical changes over the nearly fifty years of Freud's practice as an analyst, Freud always remained a very real human person in the analytic situation. Most importantly, he always made a sincere effort to engage his patients in a mutual effort to discover the deep psychological truths about themselves and their disturbances. This was the basic principle of his psychoanalytic technique, overriding any specific rules.

The quality of genuineness and naturalness is evident in all of Freud's published cases, as well as in the numerous reports by patients about their analyses with him (e.g., Grinker 1940, Wortis 1954, Doolittle 1956, Blanton 1971, H. Deutsch 1973, Lampl De Groot 1976, and Kardiner 1977). There are also summary descriptions of Freud's technique, by Ruitenbeek (1973), Sterba (1982), and Mogliano (1987). All these sources support the picture of Freud's natural, non-rigid analytic style.

For those early candidates who acquired their understanding of analytic technique from Freud himself and for the close circle of analysts around him, the human quality of the principles of analytic technique was conveyed directly by the way Freud described his clinical work. It was the later generations of analysts, far from his immediate circle in Vienna, who began to take too literally certain rules and metaphors in Freud's papers on technique (1911–1915) concerning: (1) the analyst as a mirror; (2) with the emotional detachment of a surgeon; and (3) imposing conditions of anonymity and abstinence. The result is that the learned model of "orthodox" technique is only a skeleton of the fully human analyst that Freud was personally and assumed others would become. This distortion of Freud's technique puts the rules ahead of the basic principles of psychoanalysis. The pitfall that awaits those who take Freud's written prescriptions too seriously is that the unprescribed but necessary human Anlage of the real relationship between patient and analyst will be overlooked as the equally fundamental basis of an effective analytic therapy.

As I have struggled with this large discrepancy between Freud's written advice on technique and the documented picture of how he actually worked, I have come to the conclusion that his technical rules of emotional detachment, anonymity, abstinence, and unresponsiveness apply *only* when the analyst is operating in the realm of interpretative work, where a nonjudgmental stance is imperative. When outside this special realm, the analyst, like the surgeon outside the operating room, can relate to his patients in quite normal and human ways, but always within the boundaries of the analytic situation. Unknown to me at the time, Lipton (1977) had previously come to the same conclusions about this issue:

> With his [Freud's] personal relationship with the patient excluded from technique, . . . his recommendation that the analyst be like a mirror, like a blank screen, and similar comparisons can be understood as purely technical recommendations. They were meant to emphasize the attitude of neutrality with which the analyst was to comprehend the patient's associations, an attitude which the patient understood and collaborated with. They were not meant to encompass the analyst's entire personality. The recommendation of neutrality is like that of aseptic technique for the surgeon. That necessity is confined to the operation itself and not, of course, to any other contacts with the patient which are necessary (p. 272).

Freud shares some of the blame for the widespread misunderstanding of classical technique in that he left out of his written formulations the way he constantly presented himself as a real person in the analytic situation. He expressed concern and warmth toward his patients and quite freely communicated his reactions to their significant life events. He was able to reveal his personal feelings about realistic issues while always maintaining the benign detachment necessary for the analytic process.

Unlike the strict conception of analysis as ideally "interpretations only," Freud certainly had many ordinary conversations with his patients, and he considered this a part of an analysis. Lipton (1977) commented on this issue directly:

> While the word "conversation" can be misunderstood, it is not one which Freud avoided. In one of his descriptions of analysis (Freud, 1904, p. 250), he wrote that the "session thus proceeds like a conversation between two people equally awake," and in his report on Lorenze [the Rat Man] he referred to "our conversation" (Freud,

1909, p. 185). . . . Unlike conversations in other situations, it [the conversation in analysis] is not carried out for its own sake but in the interest of the analysis. I have already alluded to one situation in which conversation becomes necessary, that is, in resolving conflicts over what will become the subject of analysis and what will not be. A second reason why conversations become necessary is for clarification, both of the patient's and the analyst's meaning (pp. 269–270).

REPORTS OF ANALYSES WITH FREUD

The essence of Freud's personal style can best be conveyed by a few excerpts from the reports of two American doctors analyzed by Freud in the 1920–1930 period. The first illustration comes from Dr. Smiley Blanton, whose diary notes of his analysis with Freud were published posthumously (Blanton, 1971).

September 1, 1929: [The first session with Freud] I handed the professor the letter which Dr. McCord had asked me to give Freud as soon as I saw him. "As I see your name mentioned," said Freud after motioning me to a seat, "I will read the letter." After reading the letter, Freud motioned me to the couch, while he too took the chair at the head. "You have written and spoken about analysis," he began inquiringly. I hastened to say that I had not. "But you have read about it?" "Oh, yes," I replied. "Well, how is it carried on?" I replied that the patient lies on the couch, with the analyst seated at the head, and freely speaks all that comes into his head. I mentioned that the patient should be completely relaxed. In point of fact, however, I was half sitting, half lying on the couch, rather tensely. "Well, then," said Freud, "why don't you relax." I stretched out in a more comfortable position. After I relaxed, Freud said: "You may wonder why I make so few comments, or help you so little." I then began to give Freud the thoughts that were in my mind. First, I discussed the chagrin I felt in being late. Then, I told him that I had always liked him and disliked Jung and Adler. When he asked me why, I said I did not quite know but simply felt that way. I then spoke of my feelings of insecurity. "About what?" asked Freud. "About my life in general," I answered, and then suggested that I [had] best give him a brief outline of my past life. Freud agreed, and so I drew a brief outline of my life. Occasionally Freud interrupted to question me about some of the points that came up. At all times he seemed in close touch with what I was giving him. There was none of that cold detachment which I had imagined was the attitude an analyst is supposed to take. As we went along, Freud's simple manner made me feel secure and easy. At the same time, there was a detachment which was not repelling but pleasant. I talked until I heard a clock strike four. I rose at once, stopping in the middle of my sentence. "I am sorry the hour was so short," said Freud as he accompanied me into the hall. He asked if I knew my way to the station, and I assured him that I did. Then I said, "May I ask how long you shall remain here?" "I leave on the 15th of September," Freud replied, "but I go to Berlin for a month." With a shrug, he added, "You can either accompany me, or you can wait until I return to Vienna." I assured him that I should accompany him. . . . I shook his hand and departed after confirming that our next session will be on Monday (pp. 19–20).

September 4, 1929: When I began to speak of my money matters, Freud remarked that this was my "anal side." I confessed that I was somewhat embarrassed in speaking of this because I was afraid it would influence him in his charges. "You must not let your critical side interfere with what comes to mind," he cautioned. I said something about how lucky I was to be with him, to which he replied, "Dr. Amsden wrote so well of you that I was glad to have you." Here I remarked that I had made many sacrifices to come over. "I know you have," said Freud, "and I hope you will be repaid for your sacrifices." The clock struck four, and I rose although again it was actually five minutes before the hour. "As you will," said Freud, spreading out his hands, and then adding, "This is very interesting. You must be patient. We will get to the deeper layers, and then I shall not be so silent, I shall give more of myself" (p. 28).

September 6, 1929: As I left, Freud remarked, "you see how much more interesting it is when you associate with your dreams." Again I was impressed by Freud's soft and easy manner. He does not push you. He does not make emphatic statements often. When he does, it is in a very undominating manner. I feel easy with him (p. 31).

September 9, 1929: On Saturday I had much resistance and did not get very far. "The way to treat resistance," said Freud, "is to let it grow until it defeats itself. Today has been absolutely sterile." But in order to encourage me, he said as I departed, "But I am sure you will be of much assistance in helping us to overcome it" (p. 32).

April 23, 1930: I spoke of my transference to Freud as not being negative. "There is just one thing, perhaps I should not mention it," Freud remarked, "but I will give it to you for what it is worth. Perhaps, you have not been entirely frank. It sometimes happens that a patient makes a mental reservation, which is easy to do, and then the analysis goes on happily and smoothly, with little or no negative transference" (pp. 57–58).

June 1930: I visited Freud a few minutes late on my last day. He gave me a letter of introduction to Dr. Ernest Jones, whom I expected to visit in London on my way back home. Freud asked me what my plans were, and I told him I had decided to work with Dr. Brill after I got back. "Do you think," I asked, "that after working with Dr. Brill for a year I will be ready to practice analysis?" "Yes," Freud replied, "I think you have the groundwork so you can go ahead" (p. 59).

A second illustration comes from a book by Dr. Abraham Kardiner (1977), whose analysis with Freud took place in the period 1921–1922.

> *First session:* [At the end of the first hour] Freud stopped me and said, "Did you prepare this hour?" I replied, "No! but why do you ask?" Freud answered, "Because it was a perfect presentation. I mean, it was, as we say in German, *"druckfertig."* I will see you tomorrow." He shook my hand, and I left elated, feeling impressed with the idea—I can really engage him (pp. 36–37).

> *A later session:* Freud had listened to my whole story [about a failed romantic relationship] without once breaking in to comment. Now, however, he spoke, "Your reaction to the breakup with Miss K. was unfortunately, as we say, in the cards. Her treatment of you was a repetition of your reaction to the death of your mother. It left you confirmed in your feeling of worthlessness, abandonment, and depression. However bad your reaction was, I can say this to you, and let this be a guide to your future—you may be down, but you will never be out" (p. 51).

> *In summary:* In our hours together, there were many personal interchanges. I was enormously fond of him. This was a very likeable and dear person. He was a charming man, full of wit and erudition. One could not tell from his behaviour in the office what a real giant he was, because he was unassuming and natural. I said to him many times . . . I can't reconcile the image I get of you in this room with the man who wrote all those great books. His reply to that was, "This is where familiarity breeds contempt" (p. 71).

Richard Sterba's book *Reminiscences of a Viennese Psychoanalyst* (1982) contains some pertinent comments:

> Some of Sigmund Freud's patients occasionally provided me with information on Freud's attitude as a therapist. John Dorsey told me that what impressed him most . . . was that he was completely natural. Philip Sarasin emphasized that he felt that Freud was continuously with him and that this supportive presence made it possible to go through all the emotional upheavals to which the analytic process exposes a patient. His remark fortified me in my conviction that the "blank screen" attitude of the analyst was not what Freud considered the optimal position (p. 122).

> Freud did not hesitate to transcend the so-called classical or orthodox behaviour of the analyst as it was prescribed by training institutes. He freely deviated from the straight and narrow path of "impersonality" and indulged in "parameters" that would have met with an outcry of indignation by the adherents to the strict and "sterile" attitude of the

analyst which is supposed to present the classical model of the analyst's behaviour (p. 123).

On the occasion of postwar visits to Vienna, I had lunch several times with the famous "Wolfman." He too emphasized how free and easygoing Freud was in the analytic situation and that Freud and he not infrequently talked about subjects other than his analytic material. It is certain that Freud did not suffer from the parameter phobia that became rampant among analysts in the fifties and sixties (p. 124).

These observations clearly reveal the discrepancies between the stereotype of the ideal "orthodox" analyst conveyed by the classical "rules" and the natural style of the originator of psychoanalysis. Freud was certainly far from being an aloof, purely interpreting, "mirror" analyst; instead he created a human and realistic atmosphere in which he subtly blended interpretative work with building a therapeutic alliance and a (personal) real relationship with his patients. I contend that Freud's clinical style is analytically sounder and more effective than the more rigid and impersonal technique of "modern" analysis.

CLINICAL ASPECTS OF THE REAL RELATIONSHIP

THE REAL RELATIONSHIP AND THE THERAPEUTIC BARRIER

As I pondered the lack of a theoretical place for the real relationship, I was surprised and impressed to come across a book by Sidney Tarachow (1963) in which he did formulate a theory of the therapeutic process that took the real relationship into account. In his view, the analytic situation is forged out of the real relationship by the analyst's act of imposing a "therapeutic barrier" to the inclination of both analyst and patient to respond to each other as real objects in their lives. He writes:

> Every patient regards his therapist as real, regards all the manifestations of the treatment situation as real, and strives to regard the therapist as a real object. The therapist, vis-à-vis the patient, strives to do exactly the same. He too wants to regard the patient as real and respond to the patient as a real object. Thus, both patient and therapist have a basic urge to mutual acting out.
>
> How is the therapeutic situation created out of this real relationship between the two parties involved? It is created by an act of the therapist. The therapist imposes a barrier to reality. We shall here term it the "therapeutic barrier." The imposition of this barrier creates a therapeutic task for both therapist and patient. The *real* situation is transformed into an *as if* situation demanding attention and comprehension (pp. 8–9).

The analytic form of this barrier sets the conditions of mutual deprivation through muting and restricting the full real relationship. This special act of withdrawal and detachment on the part of the analyst creates the unique situation in which a classical analysis can take place. The therapeutic barrier blocks an acting-out of wishes in overt activity, such as physical affection or aggression.

While I accept the main outlines of Tarachow's theory, I would add the qualification that while many aspects of a real relationship are blocked in an analysis, the core of the real relationship always remains in the background. For despite the restrictions imposed by the therapeutic barrier, much of a real relationship pertaining to genuine feelings and verbal communications remains open to expression within the confines of the analytic situation. This *limited* form of the real relationship is the foundation on which analysis can take place, but it should be emphasized again that it is the underlying basis of the analytic process, not a technical tool. It is the long-term maintenance of this barrier to a *full* real relationship that allows the transference neurosis to develop in an analysis, in contrast to the fragmentary transferences that appear regardless of the therapeutic technique.

RESOLUTION OF THE ANALYTIC DILEMMA

As Stone (1961) and Greenson (1967) have fully described, there is a fundamental dilemma facing the analyst as he attempts to create and maintain the conditions necessary for analysis. On the one hand, he must create an atmosphere of human concern and rapport so that a long-term commitment and working alliance can develop and be sustained. On the other hand, certain conditions of deprivation, frustration, and detachment must be imposed by the analytic situation so that the crucial aspects of the patient's unconscious past can emerge in a transference neurosis, without undue distortion or interference from the analyst's real personality and reality interventions. Achieving the appropriate balance between these antithetical conditions is the never-ending task of the analyst as he tries to promote the analytic process. Excessive unresponsiveness, impersonality, and rigid detachment can be as detrimental to the delicate fabric of an analysis as the opposite extreme of excessive impingement of the analyst's real personality and realistic gratifications or interventions.

Achieving the optimal balance is no easy task. The analyst's capacity to do so stems basically from his own analysis and technical training. The well-analyzed analyst should be able to allow an appropriate real relationship with his patient to exist without fearing that uncontrolled countertransference reactions will disturb the analytic situation.

Also related to the analytic dilemma is Nacht's (1962) point that in many fundamental respects what the analyst *is* has more importance than what the analyst says. Rephrased, the analyst's inherent ability to utilize his real self freely, with un-anxious confidence, allows him to find a natural resolution of the analytic dilemma suited to each individual patient. This ability to move naturally in and out of the real relationship comes from a confidence that realistic and commonsensical communications with the patient will not prevent the transference tendencies from emerging in full force from the unconscious (Couch, 1995).

The integration of the therapeutic function of the real relationship into clinical work depends on the analyst's acquisition of experience that convincingly supports the value of this perspective, on a lowering of the analyst's defensive distance from patients, and on his freedom from fear that such naturalness will lead to inappropriate acting-out in the analytic situation.

DIFFERENTIATION FROM TRANSFERENCE PHENOMENA

In order to place the concept of the real relationship in proper perspective, it is necessary to differentiate it from other types of clinical phenomena that bear a close resemblance to it.

As early as 1912, Freud approached this problem from his own viewpoint, distinguishing hostile and erotic transferences from friendly and affectionate transferences, which he accepted as the necessary underlying relationship of an analysis. Freud wrote: "If we remove the transference by making it conscious, we are detaching only these two components of the emotional act [hostile and erotic feelings] from the doctor; the other component [friendly feelings], which is admissible to consciousness and unobjectionable, persists and is the vehicle of success in psychoanalysis exactly as it is in other methods of treatment" (p. 105). This view supports Lipton's (1977) position that Freud placed the friendly personal relationship outside the realm of technique.

Starting with the simplest differentiation, the patient's *wish* for an idealized kind of real relationship—similar to the "Golden Fantasy" described by Smith (1977)—clearly belongs to the transference realm and is much more a product of the patient's past than a realistic reaction to the analyst as a real person. To gratify rather than interpret such transference wishes would constitute a fundamental error in analysis. In most cases, the underlying real relationship does not provide transference gratification. At times when it does provide such gratification, that aspect should be fully interpreted.

Such cases as adolescents, emotionally deprived personalities, and borderline patients sometimes overtly *demand* a real relationship. In these cases the transference wishes for support become completely egosyntonic and are carried to the point of actual verbalized demands that the analyst enter into their lives in a fully real way. In a previously reported adolescent case (Couch, 1977), the patient made the persistent demand that I enter into an equal, real, genuine friendship with her in which we would share information about our personal lives and sincerely care about each other's future. This demand was, of course, deeply related to her developmental problems, and as these were worked through in the analysis, she was able to accept a therapeutic relationship that helped her move into adulthood.

A more subtle form of *pressure* for a reciprocal real relationship manifests itself in the patient's constant transference wish that the analyst respond to him in a certain kind of desired role relationship derived from childhood. J. Sandler (1976a,b) has presented a comprehensive view of this widened scope of the transference and countertransference tendencies in analysis. The patient's transference wish to actualize the role relationship embedded in the past creates not only a distortion in his perception of the analyst but also a deep need and effort to force or seduce the analyst into responding in a certain realistic way. On the other side, the analyst can have a countertransference reaction of feeling pushed to take on that role—a role responsiveness. Thus, as Sandler formulates it, there is a driven tendency to actualize the role relationship embedded in the patient's transference. Furthermore, the analyst's awareness of this countertransference impulse to respond by taking on the role desired by the patient helps him to understand the early object relationships in the patient's life. While this is an important way to conceptualize the patient's drive and pressure for a certain kind of real relationship of the past, it is important to differentiate such phenomena in analysis from the genuine quality of the real relationship that exists in the present, independent of the transference.

This independent aspect of the real relationship is extremely difficult to define. It is certainly more than just unconsciously determined breakthroughs of acted-out transference or countertransference impulses or role pressures. Although such enactments may have the same form as real object relations, they bear only a surface resemblance to the authentic functioning of the real relationship. This is normally silent, in the background of the analysis, and most truly appears when it is not demanded nor expected, certainly not when one is put under pressure to respond in a wished-for way or to show expected feelings. The essence of the difference is well conveyed by these lines from *Merchant of Venice:* "The quality of mercy is not strained; it droppeth as the gentle rain from Heaven."

DIFFERENTIATION FROM COUNTERTRANSFERENCE

The concept of countertransference has been encumbered for many years by a diversity of definitions as well as differing conceptions of its role in the analytic process. These complexities must now be simplified so as to approach the present task of differentiating countertransference reactions from appropriate responses of the analyst to the patient as a real person—that is, in the real relationship as opposed to in the transference relationship.

Countertransference phenomena have usually been formulated along a dimension ranging from the analyst's unconscious reaction to the patient's transference (Freud's view), inappropriate emotional responses created in the analyst by the patient's transference material and role expectations, and all the feelings aroused in the analyst by the patient. The technical implications of these views fall in a continuum from Freudian to Kleinian: (1) countertransference reactions are interferences with the analyst's task and should only be the subject of corrective self-analysis; (2) countertransference responses can be utilized to understand the patient's developmental relationships; and (3) all the analyst's feelings are reactions to the patient's unconscious and thus are a direct guide for analytic interpretations of the current material.

The relevance of these different views to this discussion is how to differentiate a counter-transference reaction from an authentic emotional or realistic reaction to the patient's report of his real life experiences—that is, in the real relationship.

Many important contributions by analysts of the British School, such as Winnicott (1947), Heimann (1950), and Little (1951), have emphasized the clinical usefulness of the analyst's emotional responses, but the distinction between the real and the transference relationship has generally been overlooked. However, Pearl King (1977), in a relevant paper about affect in analysis, did acknowledge this concern by stating: "I do not . . . assume that every communication between patient and analyst relates directly to transference, and it becomes important to differentiate those feelings and moods which are related to the operation of the transference from those related to my reactions as a human being working with another human being" (p. 331).

This distinction is frequently overlooked by many "modern" analysts who are convinced that most of their reactions are complex unconscious responses to the patient's unconscious. A "classical" Freudian perspective could be briefly stated as follows: many of the analyst's reactions (feelings and thoughts) are quite ordinary responses to what the patient reports about his inner and outer life. Some of these responses may be useful for an empathic understanding of the patient's character and childhood experiences and thus can become the basis for eventual interpretations; other responses may be built into clarifications, confrontations, and explanatory comments; but many of the analyst's reactions are best seen and conveyed in a clinically appropriate form as genuine reactions to important aspects of the patient's life as a fellow human being. These natural interchanges are probably essential for creating an analytic atmosphere of real human engagement in which the full personality of the patient can emerge without constriction and can be fully analyzed. The absence of these natural responses by the analyst, especially when called for by actual tragedies, losses, failures, successes, disappointments, and other significant events in the patient's life, can be the cause of the most serious errors in an analysis—namely, the professionalized creation of an inhuman analytic situation, divorced from real life.

RELATION TO THE THERAPEUTIC ALLIANCE AND THE PHYSICIAN'S ROLE

The pioneer work in formulating the role and function of the ego alliance in psychoanalysis was by Zetzel (1956) in her description of the "therapeutic alliance," based on the ideas of an ego split in Sterba's (1934) paper on "The Fate of Ego in Analytic Theory." In her 1958 paper, Zetzel stated that the real relationship, which depends upon the capacity for object relations and reality testing, was the basis of classical analytic procedure: "If the analyst can actively convey his participation and partnership with the patient as a real person, development of a secure working relationship—the therapeutic alliance—will be encouraged. This participation is essential for the emergence of an analyzable transference neurosis" (p. 190).

While Zetzel fused the therapeutic alliance and the real object relationship, Greenson (1967) separated these components, claiming that the therapeutic alliance was a task-oriented relationship based on the assumed roles of analyst and patient doing therapeutic work whereas the real relationship was person-oriented and based on their natural and realistic relationship to each other as equal human beings.

A more complex differentiation remains to be made between the real relationship and the doctor-patient relationship which is also inherent in the analytic relationship. The centuries-old role of medical doctor in relating to an ill person has in it the subtle combination of physicianly concern, detachment during treatment, and a place for ordinary human contact. Zetzel (1966, 1969) has stated the widely held view that the doctor-patient relationship is the fundamental basis of *both* the real and the therapeutic relationship. This conceptual fusion arises when it is assumed that the physician's role is the bedrock of the analyst's real self when in interaction with patients, an attitude quite natural for medical analysts. It also reflects the accepted cultural norm of the diverse functions imbedded in the doctor's role, where the qualities of concern, competence, responsibility, and humanity are integrated parts of the doctor's self-conception. Furthermore, the doctor's role includes a taboo against full personal involvement with patients if that would unethically exploit the professional relationship; this is also a vital barrier in analysis. Therefore, a medical doctor's self-identity and role behavior is very close to his real self in the analytic situation, thus contributing to the conceptual fusion with the real relationship.

Stone (1961) and Greenson (1967) raise a relevant point in their similar views on the need for the analyst to maintain a physicianly attitude toward his patients. Concern, helpfulness, and integrity are natural parts of a doctor's self-conception and are therefore readily integrated into his role as medical analyst. For the more complex situation of the nonmedical analyst, the issue of the real relationship is actually put in clearer focus by the very fact that the physicianly attitude must still be present but derived from personal qualities. The physicianly attitude is integrated with the role of psychoanalyst and emerges in the real relationship with patients.

INTERWEAVING WITH TRANSFERENCE IMAGOES

One of the main therapeutic functions of the real relationship is to provide a human framework for the emergence of the unconscious structure of the patient's transference potentials. For the transference neurosis to develop fully, the real personality and behavior of the analyst must be interwoven with the skeletal imagoes of parental figures from the patient's past.

These transference imagoes and role expectations (Sandler, 1976) are like prototypal structures ready to be superimposed on all new relationships in the person's life, especially with the analyst who takes an analytic stance and conceals his personality and behavior. With absolute neutrality and mirror-like impersonality and unresponsiveness, the transference imagoes would appear like abstract projections in a human vacuum, put onto an analyst who is only a "cloth and wire" figure of a mother or father. While these transferences would be reflections of the past, they would lack the "life blood" connections to the real analyst. Much the same point has been made by Lipton (1977): "it is on those valid increments of knowledge about the analyst in current reality that the irrational elements of the transference find a foothold for expansion and elaboration. Without the actuality of the non-technical personal relationship, irrational elements of the transference remain imaginary or intellectual" (p. 271).

Of course, these disembodied transferences in the earliest phases of an analysis are useful for revealing the patient's unconscious dynamics, even if this information is not used for interpretations. More effective work can be done in later phases, when the patient's thoughts, feelings, fantasies, and expectations become more and more focused on the analyst and the analysis itself. Accompanying this evolution of the transference neurosis, the real relationship also develops more depth, scope, and particularity. As the real personality features of the individual analyst gradually emerge and are interwoven with transference elements the patient's skeletal transference patterns take on 'body' and more humanly intricate form. As Gitelson (1952) pointed out, it is an erroneous assumption that the patient continues to see the analyst as the neutral person presented by technique.

With the more human analyst emerging from the real relationship, the transference neurosis becomes the all-absorbing focus of the patient's feelings of love and hate, his wishes and fears, expectations and demands. These can now be attached to the ongoing nature of the analytic relationship itself and experienced as a new reality with this significant person whose characteristics and attitudes were partly correctly perceived and partly distorted by projections from the past. The gradual achievement of this realistic clarification about a previously misperceived "fantasy" analyst is a critical step in ego growth and part of the resolution of the transference neurosis. The success of this hard-won bit of reality helps the patient see his life more realistically.

The individualized interweaving of fantasy and reality makes the analysis of the transference neurosis a more genuine experience and helps bring alive the links between the patient's past and his current relationships. During the later phases of transference resolution and termination, the many interwoven elements are slowly untangled and worked through. If the process is successful, the patient can leave with sadness, but strengthened by the achievement of a more realistic perspective of his analytic experience, the real relationship, and his "real" analyst.

THE HIERARCHICAL PRINCIPLE OF THERAPEUTIC INTERVENTIONS

When one takes seriously the differentiation of the analytic relationship into its components of the real relationship, the therapeutic relationship, and the transference relationship, the analyst's awareness of where clinical material predominantly fits can be a guide to the appropriate kind of therapeutic intervention. To each component relationship, there is an appropriate level of response by the analyst.

When the patient becomes concerned about the analyst in ways that reflect deep-seated projections and fantasy distortions, the analyst should interpret these unconscious derivatives as coming out in the transference relationship. If the patient is blocked or highly defensive in talking about some unacceptable or painful thoughts, feelings, or characterlogical behavior, the analyst's interpretation should try to create an observing ego split (Sterba, 1934) for continuing mutual work for understanding the issue and thus maintain the therapeutic relationship. Finally, when the patient is reporting a very significant event in his life or brings up a realistic problem that impinges on the analysis, the analyst should first respond in a simple, human, and realistic way, in line with preservation of a real relationship. Paradoxically, with his acceptance of the realistic aspects of the issue, the real relationship again fades into the background, and the analyst can then attempt some interpretations of the possible unconscious factors intermixed with the reality issue.

A further extension of this differentiation of therapeutic interventions is a possible hierarchical ranking of priorities about such interventions. There are already some hierarchical principles in classical technique, such as the recommendations by Fenichel (1945) governing the order of analytic work: for example, defense before impulse, surface before depth, affect before content. Meyerson (1977) suggests a more complex priority: the need for the patient to understand the analyst's intentions before the analyst interprets repressed content. Some analysts advocate a focus on the patient's current anxiety, some on the transference, others on the here-and-now relationship.

On the basis of this differentiation of analytic relationships, a theory could be postulated for a hierarchical ranking of the attention paid to relationships in analysis. This hierarchical principle bears a similarity to the well-known conception of a hierarchy of basic human needs described by Maslow (1954). If a person is deprived of oxygen, the desperate need for air overwhelms all other considerations. Then, the need for water, food, and bodily warmth must be met before emotional needs can operate properly. If panic over security or grief over loss is severe, then the needs for love, sex, self-esteem, achievement, inner peace, and so forth take a secondary place. Only when the hierarchically more basic needs have been met can stable conditions be present for the more complex psychological needs and goals to become significant concerns in a person's life.

A similar formulation of hierarchical principles for analysis would be along these lines: as a first priority there should be stability in the real relationship before the more complex aspects of analysis can function effectively; if a serious disturbance occurs at the level of basic trust in the human relationship, the analysis itself is vulnerable to disruption. As the next priority, there should be a well-functioning therapeutic relationship, which needs to be maintained and repaired after occasional inevitable breakdowns; effective and sustained interpretative work cannot be done without a cooperative relationship. Finally, if the other levels are in good order, then the usual analytic conditions of neutrality and non-interference with free associations should be maintained, so that interpretative work on the transference and other unconscious dynamics can proceed. Many of these principles, even if not thought of in these explicit terms, are widely used and implicit in the careful timing, tact, and preparatory work of experienced analysts. This is just an attempt to conceptualize such clinical decisions.

Or course, in many analytic situations there are a circularity and intermingling of these differentiated analytic tasks, as when an urgently called-for transference interpretation serves to restore ego functioning and heal breakdowns in the therapeutic and real relationships. But despite such qualifications, the principle of hierarchical concerns can be a guide to a more balanced, natural, and humanistic analytic style.

RELATION TO THE WIDENING SCOPE OF ANALYSIS

As psychoanalysts extended the possibility of treatment to patients with serious ego disturbances, there were many differences of opinion as to whether analytic technique should be modified. Many analysts accepted the need for a shift toward an ego-oriented approach, others brought in more of the holding environment, while others thought that a purely analytic interpretative technique should be maintained. There is insufficient clinical evidence to resolve which is the most clinically effective approach.

However, in line with the first position of a modified approach, I support the view that the real relationship should take on a more central role in the therapy with such cases. Zetzel (1966) stated this point quite clearly: "In most therapy, . . . it is the reality of the relationship which remains in the forefront. It is the strengthening of the real object relationship which holds the potential for considerably increasing the patient's insights" (p. 153). Eissler (1951), in a paper on the psychoanalytic theory of schizophrenia, advocated changes in technique toward the realistic ego-level support needed to help such patients during periods of severe regression. Tarachow (1963), Semrad and Day (1959), and Wexler (1960) pointed out that with psychotic patients the traditional barrier to a real relationship with the analyst must be somewhat more relaxed than with neurotics since the first therapeutic task is ego-reconstruction.

With regard to the treatment of borderline and psychotic patients, Greenson and Wexler (1969) stated:

> In all likelihood it is even more important to sense, support, and develop the reality perceptions of this group of patients. This goes to the core of the symptom picture, and a failure to focus on reality perceptions or the "real" relationship in treatment would lead to a most serious breakdown in the working alliance. As a corollary, the exclusive focus on interpretation, whether of transference or resistance, seems to lead, in our experience at least, to increasing hostility and withdrawal or to an inert submission to ritual formulation (p. 35).

Lipton (1977, p. 272) goes so far as to suggest that the narcissistic disorders of patients can be exaggerated and not cured if the analyst adheres to an overly rigid technique of avoiding a real object relationship with patients.

In a contentious and unresolved issue such as the widening scope of analysis, it is worthwhile to point out that the concept of the real relationship has considerable relevance to analytic techniques with more disturbed patients.

RELATION TO THE RATIONAL FRAMEWORK OF ANALYSIS

Although psychoanalysis is widely regarded as a rather mysterious therapy aimed at uncovering the irrational depths of a person's mind, the main tradition of psychoanalysis is based on Freud's belief in the power of reason. Freud was seeking a scientific explanation of mental illness and gradually developed a rational method of discovering the nature of a patient's unconscious mind by using the principle of free association. In analysis, the patient and analyst together attempt to explore the meanings of the patient's material so as to give the patient insights into his unconscious and thus free him from these past determinants.

These basic assumptions of Freud have determined the procedures of psychoanalysis, and in many subtle ways a rational framework actually permeates the ambience of analytic sessions. Most patients know about or simply sense the premises of analysis and begin to talk about their problems and their past and present life, accepting that the analyst is listening attentively and trying to understand them. Only the most disturbed patients would follow their conception of the free-association rule and actually give disconnected word associations derived from their thought disorder. My point is that analytic sessions essentially have the form of rational conversations, even though at times the material is about dreams and fantasies as well as emotional outbursts and irrational thoughts.

In my view, the rational framework within which most analytic communication takes place has an underlying connection to the real relationship as that part of the analytic relationship which is based on the realistic communications between patient and analyst as real people. In his usual insightful way, Hans Loewald (1979) gave his own formulation of this complex phenomenon: "Thus there is a grid of rational adult mentation through which the analytic experience, and specifically the transference in all its primitive and more advanced variations, is sifted or screened. Analysis as a relatively continuous process, sustained over a protracted period of time, not constantly disrupted by irrational manifest behavior, requires the patient's capacity for this kind of rational mediation as a fairly reliable compass and overall guide" (p. 164).

This rational framework is perhaps more accurately described as the medium in which psychoanalysis takes place—an atmosphere of the process that is silently in the background in the same way as the real relationship.

CLINICAL MANIFESTATIONS OF THE REAL RELATIONSHIP

While it may sound convincing to describe the real relationship as the basic human relationship between patient and analyst, it is more difficult to convey concretely its clinical presence and manifestations in an analysis. Most of the time it is silently present in the background and shows itself occasionally only in those reality-oriented communications that are appropriately outside of technique.

The outer manifestations of the real relationship are much clearer at those times when the patient is not on the couch. They usually appear first in the initial face-to-face interview, where most analysts conduct a rather straightforward discussion of the patient's reason for seeking analysis, his current life situation, and various reality factors, such as fees and times of sessions, which are involved in a commitment to analysis. In these initial meetings there is a glimpse of transference potentials, but this first contact has lasting significance predominantly as the time when there is mutual assessment of each other as real persons, both forming judgments that are subject to all the usual errors of first impressions.

After the analysis begins, there are recurrent periods of off-the-couch behavior before and after every session as the patient enters and leaves the consulting room. Many very orthodox analysts try to minimize any communication in these brief encounters, but that pattern itself is a form of the real relationship. Other analysts, myself included, treat these brief encounters as a moment for a "normal" expression of the real relationship—a time for ordinary human contact and a bridge between the analytic situation and the outside world. The comments can be as short and simple as "hello," "goodbye," or "see you tomorrow." The point is that they express some sign of the real relationship. Freud seemed to have met this issue by shaking hands with patients as they entered and left his room. Sharp (1930) has put this issue very simply: "For anything that occurs while the patient is not lying on the analytical couch, we should be guided by the tact and courtesy we should extend to a formal guest. . . . The guide here is common sense. . . . The place for analysis is on the couch" (pp. 30–31). Sharp's advice, while simple, contains a good deal of wisdom, for the patient learns to perceive his analyst as a real person to some extent on the basis of these extraanalytic contacts. In my experience, these particular reality interactions reveal in brief flashes the degree of ego growth that has taken place and can be a penetrating indicator of changes in the patient's transference distortions and character defenses.

Once in the midst of the analysis, interpretations of the transference neurosis and all aspects of the patient's unconscious dynamics take center stage. But interpretations alone can be quite ineffective if used in isolation from other interventions to build a whole structure of understanding. These noninterpretative contributions, such as clarification, confrontation, and elaboration, are equally essential for analytic work and are the channels through which a degree of real communication takes place in a covert way, since they reveal the analyst's realistic thinking.

More directly expressive of the real relationship are those occasions when the analyst, after careful clinical considerations, answers the patient's questions about an important realistic issue, gives information about some circumstances that impinge on the analysis, or verifies a conclusion the patient has come to about his past or present life. Since mutual understanding is a clinical necessity, the analyst should ask for clarification of patients' communications that are unclear, acknowledge uncertainties or errors in interpretations, and proceed to make appropriate modifications. Such communications are in line with what Lipton (1977) called the "conversations" that should be part of analysis.

The most significant manifestations of the real relationships are revealed in those rare occasions when it is vital for the analyst to acknowledge real difficulties in a patient's life, to express genuine sympathy and concern about crucial or tragic events such as illness, an accident or death in the family, and also to express congratulations for successful achievements, marriage, the birth of a baby. An initial brief acknowledgment of the reality significance of such events is clinically more important than any interpretations or silent reaction by the analyst; in fact, a persistent lack of normal human responses at such times can easily destroy or sterilize an analysis.

Behind the overt manifestations of the real relationship are the genuine and appropriate feelings of the analyst and patient toward each other as real persons—that is, feelings that are relatively free of transference and countertransference coloration. In the early phases, the patient should feel some basic trust in his relatively unknown analyst as a reliable professional person; the analyst should feel this is a person he can comfortably work with and want to help. As the analysis proceeds, it is quite natural for the analyst to feel some sadness and concern over failures or tragic losses in the patient's life, some anger over the patient's cruelty to others, and some pleasure and satisfaction in the patient's successes and happiness. These are reactions that stem from and reflect the genuine human qualities of the real relationship, although the analyst must of course remain aware of the pitfalls of conveying too much of himself as a real person. Stone (1961) and Greenson (1967) have fully described the dangers and limitations of an analysis carried out under the opposite conditions of icy detachment and rigid unresponsiveness. If the analyst does not experience or express these human feelings, there is probably something fundamentally blocked in his countertransference that is disturbing the analytic relationship.

In some rare cases, hostile and distrustful feelings may develop on one or both sides of the real relationship. If these negative feelings remain strong and are seemingly irresolvable despite much analytic work, they make it unproductive to continue the analysis. The situation should be candidly acknowledged and a change of analysts arranged. The significant point here is that the real relationship is not always positive and therapeutically sustaining. A negative real relationship is probably a major factor in many prematurely terminated analyses.

On the patient's side there is the same range of genuine feelings about the real analyst and the real-life events of the analyst that become known to the patient. Although it is very difficult at times to untangle the transference elements from these reactions, it is important that the analyst recognize and accept the authentic component on a realistic level.

The most pervasive clinical manifestation of the real relationship appears in the subtle fusion with the therapeutic alliance. Greenson (1967) states this point very clearly: "The analyst's consistent attitude of acceptance and tolerance, his constant search for insight, his straightforwardness, therapeutic intent, and restraint serve as the nucleus upon which the patient builds a realistic object relationship" (p. 218).

To the extent that the analysis reaches a successful termination through a resolution of the transference neurosis, the real relationship emerges more clearly in the patient's communications in the ending phases. The transference distortions have diminished, insights have deepened, and the analyst's steady help through many tumultuous periods has been gratefully acknowledged. The many positive feelings about the analyst as a familiar real person begin to emerge more openly. In sessions, the real relationship becomes the central reality issue of the terminating analysis.

The character of this process may best be illustrated by some clinical material toward the end of a seven-year analysis of a young woman.

A CLINICAL VIGNETTE

At the start of a session, she told of seeing another girl walking near my house and feared that this girl would be her replacement when she leaves the analysis. I pointed out the constant return to her early childhood fear of losing her mother's full attention after the mother's remarriage. She then tried to untangle her feelings about me as her mother and me as a kind of real friend—someone she can talk to every day and whom she would like to keep as a friend when the analysis is over. I tried to help her understand how this effort to untangle her feelings about me was a necessary part of the ending.

In the next session, she started by saying for the first time that she now felt able to talk about ending and would like to try to sort things out. She felt that in the past year or so she had sensed a shift from seeing me as her parents to seeing me as an "analyst-cum-friend." She knew that if earlier in the analysis she had had to leave me while still seeing me as a parent, she would have felt deserted and would have become angry and depressed. However, if she can end when seeing me as an "analyst-cum-friend," she will feel differently—not deserted, but sad over the loss of such a good friend and counselor. She looked back at me to see my reaction. I said I agreed with her. Then she continued: "I may be going on too long by not ending until next April; perhaps I am pampering myself, for I no longer need you as I did earlier. But that is a good thing—a real change from feeling the deprived child to being the child that has had enough." I added that she wanted to be the satisfied child. She then went on to tell of feeling so differently in the past year compared to how she had felt for years: "I just see myself and you and life much more realistically." I agreed that she had made a lot of progress. She then recalled her early years in analysis and how depressed and fearful of life she had been. As she looks back, she more and more admires my great patience in the first two years, when I accepted her silences, her crying spells, and her blocks in talking openly about herself. She praised my patient approach, adding that she has told several patients she knows to stay with their analyses through the difficult periods in the first years. She ended the session by explaining why she chose April for the end—it will be her 31st birthday then. I commented that she would then feel old enough to go out alone in the world. She agreed and added that she was looking forward to having new freedom and more time for new activities.

In subsequent weeks she had many dreams that reflected her feeling of successful resolution of old problems. In one dream she is on a train that is going up a steep hill. Her associations were to her sense of potency about herself and her life. In another dream, she saves her mother from a terrorist bomb attack and later successfully captures the terrorists; she then tries to understand their motivations and gives them a psychiatric interview about the reasons for their behavior. Associations included a wish to become a child therapist. In a more complex dream she is with her mother, who brings in a man's penis on a biological tray; they sit down together and examine it with mutual interest; she feels closer to her mother for the first time in a dream. Her associations were to the old feelings of distance and alienation from her mother over frightening sexual matters that were to be kept separate from life. She now wishes she could share her new sexual freedom and her triumph over the frightening power of her hated stepfather. In working over these thoughts, she came to the conclusion that she might never be able to forgive her mother and stepfather—but she added that the analysis has rescued her from her old pattern of seeking revenge on others and from her old anxieties.

In a session a month later, she talked in a desultory way about yesterday's events, and then was silent for some time. Finally, she spoke of how this depressed mood came over her this morning, when she had a sinking feeling that this time next year she would have ended her analysis. Next session she reminisced about her old depression, linking it to some sadness because her 31st birthday is next month. She feels so much older now; then she added that I seemed to be looking younger than when she started. She supposed it was "because I never used to really look at you for years." I said I must have seemed inhuman to her. She agreed and started to cry: "I can't bear to think about the loss of you now. I don't think I can bear losing you as the one parent who did listen to me. But today I don't want to feel anything for you." I said that by this kind of blanking out she was trying to obliterate her love and attachment to me, so she can separate; this was the same thing she tried as a child. She responded: "Yes, it's the only way I could bear the pain—but I don't want to destroy my feelings for you when I leave." At the next session she acknowledged some vague feelings of anger at me, "as if you are pushing me out into the adult world before I am ready." I helped her go over again the clear link to the same feelings she had about her mother's pushing her away when she really needed her.

She left her umbrella behind one day, and the next time she spoke of how she feels more at home now in my waiting room and has even been able to pick up my mail from the hallway floor. She recalled how she felt herself a stranger in her stepfather's house, afraid she didn't belong there and afraid to show any angry feelings. Then she remembered the many times she had been very angry at me, and how she can now tell me when she's angry. She said one of the main changes she senses in herself is that she is no longer afraid all the time.

Just before the Easter break, she voiced her objection to my fixing vacation dates arbitrarily, instead of discussing them with her, as I had done about termination. Then she asked where I was going over Easter. I said I would tell her but suggested that we first explore the feelings behind the question. "Well, I feel I want to share something with you, and I suppose my old rage comes up whenever I feel left out." I noted her reference to rage. "Yes, I felt the rage just before I asked you where you were going—I think because I was afraid to ask." I said this was her problem in childhood, afraid to ask. "Yes, I felt in the dark all the time; I didn't know where my mother was when she was out, where my stepfather came from, or the new babies, or my period. My mother didn't tell me any of these things, and I was afraid to ask." We went over these thoughts for some time, and then she said: "Now I can see I had a strong need to know, and this is why I have been so pleased to be able to ask you things and gradually get more and more answers." At the end of the session I did tell her I was going to America for Easter.

For the next few sessions before the break, she engaged in a kind of mock display of anger at me for going without her consent. Once she turned around to look at me and said: "You are mean to go. I would really like to stop you." This honest expression of feelings led to some charged memories of how she had never been able to get her mother to do what she wanted.

In the last session before the break, she spoke for the first time of an awareness that she had "made a big fuss over the break before it happened" and that this had helped her to accept it. She added that knowing of my real plans had also helped her "because I can now think of you as a real person who is going away and whom I'll miss now and at the ending."

THERAPEUTIC FUNCTIONS OF THE REAL RELATIONSHIP

At this point I will summarize the therapeutic functions of the real relationship by briefly restating some key points made in earlier sections.

(1) *Initial Commitment.* In the first meetings, in which both analyst and patient acquire a sense of the other's personality, an early form of the real relationship provides the foundation for the initial commitment of both parties to the analytic endeavor. This is a crucial beginning phase before the "therapeutic barrier" is imposed. Thus the real relationship can be assessed in a clearer light to determine whether enough basic trust exists for the analysis to proceed.

(2) *Analytic Atmosphere.* As the analysis proper begins, the important real qualities of the analyst, such as integrity, warmth, sensitivity, soundness, gradually emerge more clearly from the background aspects of the real relationship and create an atmosphere in which the patient can begin to give expression to his thoughts and feelings.

(3) *Support of the Therapeutic Alliance.* The trustworthiness and competence shown by the analyst continually support the development and maintenance of the therapeutic alliance. On the patient's side, this depends on an awareness of analytic goals and the need for cooperation during the mutual work of exploring the unconscious past. This ego-level relationship is the task-oriented substitute for the real relationship as it fades into the background of an analysis, but the alliance is actually built on that foundation.

(4) *Full Emergence of the Transference Neurosis.* While fragmentary transferences will appear regardless of technique and atmosphere, a full-blown transference neurosis will more regularly develop if the real relationship has been sufficiently present and has created enough emotional significance to carry the weight of all the transferred childhood longings, fears, and fantasies. When the patient is in the midst of this crucial phase in analysis, the many real characteristics of the analyst serve as a focus for transference projections and displacements. These skeletal transference potentials are interwoven in remarkably intricate ways with what the analyst has said and *is* on a realistic level. Put simply, unless the analyst has become a real person to the patient, a full transference of deep feelings cannot take place in the analysis.

(5) *Resolution of the Transference Neurosis.* Hand in hand with the clinical process of interpreting the transference neurosis is the therapeutic function of the real relationship as the reality antithesis against which the infantile and neurotic projections, fantasies, and expectations are compared with the real person of the analyst as he has become known through the analytic experience. In many senses, the transference relationship is gradually given up for the limited but valuable real relationship that developed with the analyst.

(6) *Greater Acceptance of Reality.* The long-term therapeutic effect of gradually untangling the transference from the real relationship encourages the patient toward greater acceptance of the reality aspects of the world he lives in, as well as of himself and his past. This gain in ego functioning is further supported by an identification with the analyst's dedicated search for understanding and his integrity as a real person. The implicit analytic framework of rationality also contributes to the development of mature thinking in the patient's life.

(7) *Achievement of Greater Ego Synthesis.* As the analyst intersperses his interpretations of unconscious tendencies with realistic and therapeutic interventions in line with hierarchical concerns, the patient is helped to incorporate a similar balance of ego functioning within himself. This balanced perspective and the back-and-forth process of observation and communication in the shifting levels of the analytic relationship gradually lead to greater ego synthesis. As Freud (1937) wrote: "The analytic situation consists in our allying ourselves with the ego of the person under treatment, in order to subdue portions of his id which are uncontrolled, that is to say, to include them in the synthesis of his ego" (p. 238).

(8) *Working Through the Terminal Phase.* When the analysis approaches termination, the real relationship comes to the fore—this time serving as the major medium through which the meaning of the impend-

ing separation can be fully analyzed. As the patient works through the loss of transference objects that had been projected onto the idealized and denigrated "fantasy" analyst, the relationship to the "real" analyst takes up this loss for a while and provides a kind of compensation. But eventually, even the real analyst must be lost, at least as regards the intense relationship that had existed during the on-going analysis. When the patient reaches the stage in which he is sad about losing his real analyst, who has been his close companion through a difficult analytic journey, a proper termination to a successful analysis has been achieved.

CONCLUSION

To recapitulate briefly, the analytic relationship is created out of a matrix of the real relationship by imposing a special kind of task structure and a barrier to the real object relationship. Two other modes or ways of relating then emerge and grow to fill the interpersonal vacuum in the real relationship: namely, the transference relationship and the therapeutic alliance. However, a substantial part of the real relationship is left behind as a background Anlage and is always present and interwoven in the transference and therapeutic relationships of the on-going analysis.

The human qualities of this underlying real relationship are not to be viewed as a complicating residual in the analysis, to be suppressed and excluded through rigid detachment, anonymity, and unresponsiveness; if that were actually done, only a sterile and incomplete analysis would be possible. Instead, there should be a knowledgeable respect for the crucial role of the real relationship in the functioning of the psychoanalytic process during all phases, from the beginning through the growth and resolution of the transference neurosis to the mourning work of termination. By accepting the therapeutic need for the real relationship, the analyst can allow himself a natural and individual style that reflects his real self and can thereby create the human atmosphere vital for an effective analysis.

BIBLIOGRAPHY

ADLER, G. (1980). Transference, real relationship and alliance. *Int. J. Psychoanal.* 61:547–558.
BLANTON, S. (1971). *Diary of My Analysis with Sigmund Freud.* New York: Hawthorn.

BIBRING, E. (1937). Contributions to the symposium on the theory of the therapeutic results of psychoanalysis. *Int. J. Psychoanal.* 18:170–189.

COUCH, A. S. (1977). The demand for the real relationship. Paper read at the Hampstead Clinic, London, 1 June 1977.

—— (1979). The role of the real relationship in analysis. Paper read at the Boston Psychoanalytic Society, 10 January 1979.

—— (1995). Anna Freud's adult psychoanalytic technique: A defence of classical analysis. *Int. J. Psychoanal.* 76:153–171.

DEUTSCH, H. (1973). *Confrontations with Myself.* New York: W. W. Norton.

DOOLITTLE, H. (1956). *Tribute to Freud.* New York: Pantheon.

EISSLER, K. (1951). Remarks on the psychoanalysis of schizophrenia. *Int. J. Psychoanal.* 32:139–156.

—— (1953). The effect of the structure of the ego on psychoanalytic technique. *J. Amer. Psychoanal. Assoc.* 1:104–143.

FENICHEL, O. (1941). *Problem of Psychoanalytic Technique.* New York: The Psychoanalytic Quarterly.

—— (1945). *The Psychoanalytic Theory of the Neurosis.* New York: Norton.

FREUD, A. (1936). *The Ego and the Mechanisms of Defence.* London: Hogarth.

—— (1954). The widening scope of indications for psychoanalytic discussion. *J. Amer. Psychoanal. Assoc.* 2:607–620.

—— (1969). Communication quoted in: Greenson & Wexler 1969.

FREUD, S. (1905). Fragment of a case of hysteria. *S. E.* 7:7–122.

—— (1911–15). Papers on technique. *S. E.* 12:83–173.

—— (1912). The dynamics of transference. *S. E.* 12:99–108.

—— (1937). Analysis terminable and interminable. *S. E.* 23:211–253.

GITELSON, M. (1952). The emotional position of the analyst in the psychoanalytic situation. *Int. J. Psychoanal.* 33:1–10.

—— (1962). The curative factors in psychoanalysis: The first phase of psychoanalysis. *Int. J. Psychoanal.* 43:194–205.

GREENSON, R. (1965). The working alliance and the transference neurosis. *Psychoanal. Quart.* 34:155–181.

—— (1967). *The Technique and Practice of Psychoanalysis.* New York: Int. Univ. Press.

—— (1968). The "real" relationship between patient and psychoanalyst. In: *The Unconscious Today.* Kanzer, M. (Ed.). New York: Int. Univ. Press.

—— (1972). Beyond transference and interpretations. *Int. J. Psychoanal.* 53:213–217.

—— (1974). Loving, hating, and indifference towards the patient. *Int. Rev. Psychoanal.* 1:259–266.

GREENSON, R. & WEXLER, M. (1969). The non-transference relationship in the psychoanalytic situation. *Int. J. Psychoanal.* 50:27-39.

GRINKER, R. (1940). Reminiscences of a personal contact with Freud. *Amer. J. Ortho-Psychiatry* 10:850–854.

HEIMANN, P. (1950). On counter-transference. *Int. J. Psychoanal.* 31:81–84.

KARDINER, A. (1977). *My Analysis with Freud: Reminiscences.* New York: Harper.

KING, P. (1977). Affective responses of the analyst to the patient's communication. *Int. J. Psychoanal.* 59:329–334.

LAMPL-DE GROOT, J. (1976). Personal experience with psychoanalytic technique and theory during the last half-century. *Psychoanal. Study Child* 31: 283–296.

LIPTON, S. (1967). Later developments in Freud's technique (1920 to 1939). In: B. B. Wolman (ed.), *Psychoanalytic Techniques.* New York: Basic Books.

——— (1977). The advantages of Freud's technique as shown in his analysis of the Rat Man. *Int. J. Psychoanal.* 58:255–273.

LITTLE, M. (1951). Counter-transference and the patient's responses to it. *Int. J. Psychoanal.* 32:32–40.

LOEWALD, H. (1960). On the therapeutic action of psychoanalysis. *Int. J. Psychoanal.* 51:16-33.

——— (1979). Reflections on the psychoanalytic process and its potential. *Psychoanal. Study Child* 34:155–167.

MASLOW, A. (1954). *Motivation and Personality.* New York: Harper.

MENAKER, E. (1942). The masochistic factor in the psychoanalytic situation. *Psychoanal. Q.* 11:171–186.

MEYERSON, P. G. (1977). Therapeutic dilemmas relevant to the lifting of repression. *Int. J. Psychoanal.* 58:453–462.

MOGLIANO, X. (1987). A spell in Vienna—but was Freud a Freudian? *Int. Rev. Psychoanal.* 14:273–389.

NACHT, S. (1958). Variations in technique. *Int. J. Psychoanal.* 39:235–237.

——— (1962). The curative factors in psycho-analysis. *Int. J. Psychoanal.* 43: 206–211.

PAOLINO, T. J. (1982). The therapeutic relationship in psychoanalysis. *Contemp. Psychoanal.* 18:218–234.

RUITENBEEK, H. M. (Ed.) (1973). *Freud As We Knew Him.* Detroit: Wayne State Univ. Press.

SANDLER, J. (1976a). Actualization and object relationships. *J. Phila. Assoc. Psychoanal.* 3:3.

——— (1976b). Countertransference and role-responsiveness. *Int. Rev. Psychoanal.* 3:43–47.

SEMRAD, E. & DAY, M. (1959). Techniques and procedures used in the treatment and activity program for psychiatric patients. In: *Psychiatric Occupational Therapy.* Ed. W. L. West. Dubuque, Iowa: Boone.

SHARPE, E. (1930). The technique of psychoanalysis. In: *Collected Papers on Psychoanalysis.* New York: Hogarth Press.

SMITH, S. (1977). The golden fantasy: A regressive reaction to separation anxiety. *Int. J. Psychoanal.* 58:311–324.

STERBA, R. (1982). The fate of the ego in analytic therapy. *Int. J. Psychoanal.* 15:117–226.

STONE, L. (1954). The widening scope of indications for psychoanalysis. *J. Amer. Psychoanal. Assn.* 2:567–594.

——— (1961). *The Psychoanalytic Situation.* New York: Int. Univ. Press.

——— (1981). Some thoughts on the 'here and now' technique and process. *Psychoanal. Q.* 50:709–733.

TARACHOW, S. (1963). *An Introduction to Psychotherapy.* New York: Int. Univ. Press.

VIEDERMAN, M. (1991). The real person of the analyst and his role in the process of psychoanalytic cure. *Int. J. Psychoanal.* 39:451–489.

WEXLER, M. (1960). Hypotheses concerning ego deficiency in schizophrenia. In: *The Out-Patient Treatment of Schizophrenia.* New York: Grune & Stratton.

WINNICOTT, D. W. (1947). Hate in the counter-transference. In: *Collected Papers.* London: Tavistock Publications.

——— (1955). Metapsychological and clinical aspects of regression within the psycho-analytic set-up. In: *Collected Papers.* London: Tavistock Publications.

WORTIS, J. (1954). *Fragments of an Analysis with Freud.* New York: Simon & Schuster.

ZETZEL, E. R. (1956). Current concepts of transference. *Int. J. Psychoanal.* 37:369–376.

——— (1958). Therapeutic alliance in the analysis of hysteria. In: *The Capacity for Emotional Growth.* London: Hogarth Press. 1970.

——— (1966). The doctor-patient relationship in psychiatry. In: *The Capacity for Emotional Growth.* London: Hogarth Press. 1970.

——— (1969). The analytic situation and the analytic process. In: *The Capacity for Emotional Growth.* London: Hogarth Press. 1970.

Clocks, Engines, and Quarks— Love, Dreams, and Genes

What Makes Development Happen?

LINDA C. MAYES, M.D.

That psychological growth and maturation throughout the lifespan involve progressive linear processes is an implicit assumption of all models of development. Within psychoanalysis, a particular focus has been those processes that hinder forward development and manifest themselves as regressions or fixations or in character structure. However, the implicit assumption of progressive, linear development leaves unexplored the central question of what are the processes that govern developmental progressions. What makes psychological development happen in more or less predictable ways and yet allows for considerable individual variability? And are those developmental progressions inevitably forwardly progressive? Questions regarding what regulates and integrates development are relevant not only for understanding the normal building up of the internal world and of childhood psychopathology but also for those times of dramatic mental reorganization in adulthood surrounding events such as pregnancy and aging and for issues of psychological change during and after an analysis. Clinical material from

Arnold Gesell Associate Professor of Child Psychiatry, Pediatrics, and Psychology in the Yale Child Study Center.

Presented June 1, 1996, Western New England Psychoanalytic Society. Presented to the Vulnerable Child Discussion Group, Spring meeting of the American Psychoanalytic Association, San Diego, CA. May 15, 1997. This paper was a graduation essay for the Western New England Psychoanalytic Institute and was awarded the Heinz Hartmann Award from the New York Psychoanalytic Association, 1998.

analyses with a child and an adult and from interviews with four- to five-year-old children is used to explore individual fantasies of how development and change happens. The central role of internalization and object relations in regulating psychological development is emphasized.

IN 1862, EMILY DICKINSON WROTE, "COULD YOU TELL ME HOW TO GROW —or is it unconveyed—like Melody—or Witchcraft?" (Johnson, 1958). That sense of an unconveyed but received wisdom or expectation surrounds the question of how development happens and defines a problem pondered more or less explicitly by multiple generations and for any one individual throughout the lifespan. Fantasies of how development happens are replete with metaphors of inevitably timed events governed by internal clocks, instinctual urges driven by body-based engines, or unseen but powerful energies operating at a new atomic level. Often, developmental progressions are couched in terms of prophecies or dreams, growing because of the love of and wish to be like—or different from—one's parents, and fulfilling or defying one's genes. In fantasy, psychological development, like the biologic endowment it is so closely intertwined with, offers the prospect of unlimited change under the regulation of driven independence and, at the same time, a fated blueprint—out of our hands, forward, backwards, or sideways, but nonetheless an invisible preprogrammed process happening within us and simultaneously leaving us on the psychic sidelines to watch in mixed admiration and dismay.

What regulates, controls, and times development is a question of not only deep psychological meaning for any one adult or child but also for all theories of growth and change. At multiple levels of analyses ranging from cell migration and growth to the psychology of aging, the issue of the timing of development is a constant presence. To know that development happens is a different matter from knowing how it is regulated and timed, what are the implications of mistimed or failed events, and what is the room for error or normal variation in these timed processes. From its beginnings, psychoanalysis has been based on an epigenetic theory of development, that is, development as a staged, timed process with each stage building on the causal, antecedent one until reaching a kind of steady state in adulthood (Tyson & Tyson, 1990). Other psychoanalytic theories have emerged from that first foundation, taking as their basis the bedrock notion that later phases of development contain within them traces of earlier ones, but adding different emphases on environmental influences, utilizing notions of critical phases, and focusing on periods of development in adulthood. All psychoanalytic theories of development contain implicit assumptions about the question of what makes development happen that range from drives to adaptation, motivation, and object relations.

This paper will elaborate on three points: First, contemporary models of development offer additions to, and a fundamental paradigm shift from, the standard epigenetic approach that is the basis of much of a psychoanalytic developmental psychology. Current models of gene-environment interaction emphasize a dialectic between genetically timed events and biological substrate with environment and experience such that each influences the other, and the ensuing development is neither so linear or staged nor so intrinsically progressive and predictable. At any one developmental period, the complexity and number of interactions among genetic substrate, biology, and experience introduce elements of randomness into development that defy prediction or reproducibility. Also, in the context of these multi-level interactions, developmental progressions involve constant processes of loss, remodeling, and reorganization of functions so that behavioral and psychological properties may emerge that have few apparent antecedents in previous developmental periods.

Second, the fantasies of children and adults about how development happens capture some of the dilemmas inherent in the evolution of conceptual approaches to the same problem—the tensions between linear, progressive processes and interactive ones, between knowing and not knowing what will be, between holding on to all that has gone before and letting go so that other functions may emerge, and between development as a constantly additive, constructive process and one that involves loss, a certain amount of chance and destruction as well as transformation of function. In many ways, the fantasies of both children and adults about how development happens reflect traditional and persistent cultural notions of development as a staged, linear process with each successive stage building on the previous one, not a development that is interactive and only partially predictable. Third, these same fantasies particularly as they capture the mix of development as regular with some accidents versus random with a surprising regularity serve important object relations, defensive, and ego/super-ego functions. The fantasies allow each of us to at times deny the basic biology that governs our mental life, to live in fantasy outside of the body, and to deny our own responsibility in the regulation of developmental change and course.

Before turning to a brief overview of the evolution of theoretical approaches to the problem of how development is regulated, a few caveats provide some necessary boundaries for these three tasks. First is a caution regarding the limits of knowledge about the regulation of even the simplest developmental processes, for example, cell growth (Wolpert, 1994). These limitations become even more clear when we speak about psychological functions, e.g., affect regulation, that are never unitary and rarely emerge as single, easily distinguished events with a discrete timing. Thus, the integration regarding the regulation of psychological development offered in the next paragraphs will be in metaphorical terms subject to revision with more specific knowledge.

A related issue is a familiar caution about applying a language intended to describe development at one level of synthesis to psychological or mental constructs (Edelson, 1984). Surely the domain of discourse that applies to regulatory genes, neural maturation, or even perception is far different from that which applies to ego functions, mental representations, and internalized object worlds. The caution applies about reductionism in either direction—assuming that the genetic processes regulating physical growth are clear, simple, and unitary or that the metaphors for these same processes adequately capture the regulation of, for example, genderization or ego development.

Similarly, caution is in order regarding the use of the term development as if all aspects of physical, physiological, and psychological change fall under the same global rubric. Development is an extraordinarily complex term used in a variety of ways (Prechtl et al., 1981; Wolff, 1981), but it most often indicates a process of continuous change within the life history of the individual. These changes are usually assumed to occur in some, more or less, regular sequence and to be generally age related and largely irreversible, albeit with possible later compensatory revisions. Development is the superordinate construct to related processes including maturation, growth, adaptations, regressions, and even deterioration or decline.[1] Particularly in refer-

1. The concept of development inevitably evokes the harmonies of progressivism and is often used synonymously with maturation, change, and growth toward ever better capacities. Indeed, as several have suggested, development and evolution are hand and glove products of late nineteenth, early twentieth century optimism and the belief that within the developing child was the guaranteed hope of a better outcome for the next generation (Kessen, 1990). To define development solely as the process of progressive change or maturation from childhood to adulthood overlooks both the possibility that for any organism increasing functional complexity involves degradation as well as construction and intensifying chaos and uncertainty as the number of functional options increases; and that even senescence is a process involving remodeled capacities and relations among functions. Development might be more appropriately regarded as a process of continuous remodeling and restructuring governed by environmental demands and biologic imperatives. However, a notion of development as constructive progress is so built into our culture that it nearly obscures a critical effort to disentangle exactly what phenomenology a definition of development needs to explain.

ence to psychological functions, there tend to be separate theoretical positions regarding different functions—the development of a capacity for object relations, psychosexual, ego, or affective development (Tyson & Tyson, 1990). More likely than not, different regulatory systems apply to different functions—what works for cognition may not work so well for a capacity such as object relations.

Considering developmental regulatory processes also challenges us to define constantly what we call developmental functions. For example, the capacity for object relations is in and of itself a metaphorical construction and categorization. It is rather made up of many specific, more molecular capacities that come together to make differential social relatedness and attachments possible such as the capacity to recognize and remember faces and voices and to discriminate different affective states. These different capacities may be under the regulation of different timing functions and indeed their integration into a broader function such as the capacity for romantic love is in and of itself a timed reorganization. With these cautions in mind, the first task is to trace the evolution in the past century of approaches to the regulation of psychological development.

APPROACHES TO THE REGULATION OF PSYCHOLOGICAL DEVELOPMENT

Development, or the epigenetic notion that physiologic and psychological systems emerge and change in function as the child grows, is a relatively recent concept. As late as the early 1800s, children were viewed functionally as adults with essentially the same psychological as well as physical and physiological construction and capacities. Every characteristic of the adult was present, however indistinctly, at the moment of conception—the homunculus contained within the fertilized egg (Ausubel et al., 1980). The convergence of several discoveries including that of a progressive organogenesis in fetal life as well as Darwin's radical introduction of species evolution (Charlesworth, 1992) called into severe debate these preformed models of development and opened up a study of developmental ontogeny from infancy through adulthood.

Since the arrival of a concept of developmental epigenesis, notions about developmental progression have reflected in part the cultural contexts in which they were proposed. Freud's ideas and psychoanalytic developmental models are no exception; and each shift in approaches to development has carried vestiges of the theory left behind—the epigenesis of developmental theories about development.

By the late nineteenth and early twentieth century, the prevailing view of development of children was that of an innate determinism governed by variously termed biologic, neural, internal, or maturational forces that were programmed from conception (Gottlieb, 1983). Predetermined developmental stages emerged and progressed because of a preset timetable. How the timetable worked was not so well understood or even explicitly considered but that there was a reliable, always active, and probably unitary biologic clock was a given. With the advent of a language of genetics, this inevitable progression was couched in the terms of biologic endowment—that a part of an inherited substrate unique to humans was responsible for the developmental timetable. Children matured in a more or less uniform way in similar patterns and stages across all cultures. Precocities, delays, and derailings of development happened because of the intrusions, excesses, or neglects within the child's environment imbalancing this preset clock and slowing the rate of progression or distorting a given stage of maturation. Individual differences reflected in part the misintentioned or accidental environmental alteration of a predetermined plan as well as the misfortunes of endowment. Freud's initial formulation of psychosexual stages reflected this kind of biologically determined and instinctually regulated developmental model (Freud, 1905). But one of the clearest statements of a predetermined, maturational timetable was made by Gesell (and parenthetically also reflected in the writings of early child analysts working in Vienna).

Strongly influenced by embryologists and early geneticists, Gesell set out to create an embryology of development in which the implicit driving force was an internal program that was highly stable across individuals and relatively impermeable to environmental alteration. Individual differences were attributable to differences in the innately set rates of progression. The fundamental problem was to define the stages of postnatal ontology in which the central assumption was that physical and personality maturation progressed via a single cause— "the net sum of gene effects operating in a self-limiting time cycle" (Gesell, 1945, p. 23).

Thus, the models of development that influenced the earliest child and adult analysts were inherently linear and progressive; defined stages afforded a way to assess progress and failures. Additionally, assuming a single cause or reality, that is, an innate regulatory system as the single driving force facilitated outcome prediction as well as reconstruction. In more modern terms, a single cause carried most of the variance for individual differences and thus, the prediction problem was simple. Symptoms could directly reflect a given stage of development and the time when perturbations in that stage occurred. Importantly, distortions in a given stage dramatically disfigured further stages and might even impede or block any further progression, leaving as it were psychological scars that were relatively easily dated by their stage specific characteristics.

For psychoanalysis, such a unidimensional regulatory theory began to shift with the development of the structural model and with the observations of many child analysts working in nursery schools and orphanages (e.g., Rene Spitz, Margaret Mahler, Anna Freud). By the mid-1930s—after the First World War and as conditions deteriorated toward the Second—"notions of imbalances and the need to restore equilibrium and avoid disorder and chaos began to be incorporated into theories of development. While still innately genetically driven, development moved also on the basis of internal and/or external conflict or obstacle. Conflicts occurred among instinctual demands, ego capacities, and external experiences. For example, distortions or imbalances between the maturation of ego functions and instinctual life or between ego capacities and environmental demands contributed to deviations in the timing of development including regressions, fixations, or apparently precocious maturation.

In these emerging points of view, developmental gains were made more often at a cost or at least with effort, energy, or under the urgency of instinctual drives, not solely because of inherent progressivism; and chaos, dissolution, or even death (as with severely neglected children) were the inevitable outcomes if development was left to emerge independently and without maintenance. It was clear that in order for the innate regulatory mechanisms to run and unfold properly, right and sufficient conditions were required. In many cases, experiential input was critical for maintenance of developmental change, not additional, incidental or unfortunate. For instance, in the case of aggression in children, environmental input was necessary to keep the innate mechanisms properly channeled. Or on the more positive side, encountering novel situations pushed children to attempt first to incorporate these into their world and then to shift their own capacities to accommodate the situations—Piaget's stages of intellectual progression (Piaget, 1952, 1954). In these models, experience was the positive nidus for maturation—that is, experience kept the maturational engine moving.

Similarly, in psychoanalytic theories of development, mental structures were defined through constant interaction with nurturing, depriving, or neglectful forces. Ego defined from id, the stimulus barrier protecting the organism from excessive impingement, increasing ability for anxiety regulation and tolerating strong wishes and affects, developmentally hierarchical defense mechanisms—each matured or appeared not so much in predefined stages but in relation at least partially to the interactions among given sets of internal and external circumstances. Incorporating a more active role for experience in shaping or maintaining maturation meant also that predictions could not be so clearly made based on deficits and flaws in antecedent stages. However, although the prediction might be less accurate, early stages were still viewed as directly causal of later ones, and there was still an implied order to development based on genetic/biologic mechanisms influencing the emergence of structure and function. Nonetheless, an interactive, dynamic, and at times, pessimistic language had entered psychoanalytic notions of development.

The pessimism or at least caution was reflected in child analysts' increasing emphasis on the critical formative nature of infancy and early childhood in which so many capacities appeared to emerge so quickly and were so vulnerable to early accidents or conditions that did not sustain or set necessary developmental trends in motion. Child analysts closely observing children in group settings called attention to the limits of forward prediction and the potential distortions of developmental reconstructions made from adulthood. The earliest psychoanalytic expression of the notion of critical periods emerged from observations of anaclitic depression and mortality among adequately nourished but psychologically deprived institutionalized children (Spitz & Wolf, 1946), and was given further evidence in the studies of children abandoned and severely traumatized in the Second World War (Hellman, 1983).

Perhaps as antidote to the potential bleakness of understanding early vulnerability, evolving analytic developmental theory influenced by the ego psychologists also incorporated notions of adaptation and allowed that some early failures could be adapted to at least in part and development would progress without a clearly evident stage-defined marker of when the failure or deficiency occurred. Adaptation, as defined particularly by Hartmann (1964), meant also that development changes occurred in part because of what the child needed to accomplish psychologically at a given period and that earlier deficiencies might be reworked or reorganized into character later in development (e.g., children who were blind [Burlingham, 1961] or overly sensitive to environmental stimulation [Bergman & Escalona, 1949; Escalona, 1963]).[2]

2. Parenthetically, the need to have a map of the stages of developmental progression also remained strong (as it still does). At the same time they were developing a more complex and interactive model of development regulated in part by interactions be-

As early as the late 1940s, additional revisions in notions of developmental regulation began to emerge that constructed a more contemporary, interactive, and complex picture of developmental timing. Implicit in these revisions was the beginning of a bidirectional model in which there was a feedback loop and perhaps even inductive role for experiences and existing functions to facilitate and turn on certain genetically regulated developmental processes (Gottlieb, 1983; Oppenheim, 1984; Prechtl et al., 1981; Wolff, 1989). Causal links were as likely to go from experience and existing functions to new structures as from genetically regulated events and biologic substrate, that is, from psychology to biology as well as biology to psychology. Moreover, a more complex level of functioning might not be achieved only by simply adding skills or structures to earlier states, and new levels of functioning were not always so directly traceable to antecedent states. Earlier modes of functioning might be lost, suppressed, or reorganized to achieve higher or more complex capacities that were adaptive for the individual's needs at that moment in chronological maturation and in a given set of external circumstances—so-called ontogenetic adaptations (Oppenheim, 1981; 1984).

In these more interactive frames of reference, several developmentalists including Waddington (1957), Piaget (1952, 1954), and Anna Freud (1963, 1965, 1974, 1981) proposed models for different lines or channels of development in which each was dependent on and regulating of others. Reacting to the apparent reductionism of focusing on one stage or aspect of development, for example, libidinal stages, as primarily causal or regulating of all others, Anna Freud (1965) outlined a more synthetic view in which a child's presentation at any given point in time was seen across multiple domains—the contribution of developmental lines (1963, 1981). There was no special emphasis on any one period or event as pathogenic nor was one area of development (e.g., object relations) primary to others. Rather, development involved continual interactions among various lines or functions such

---

tween biology and experience, child analysts (and their colleagues in related developmental fields) actively worked to define specific developmental phases or tasks that would provide an implicit metric against which to measure relative success or failure and the regularity at any given stage. As theories of developmental regulation took on the more complicated notions of adaptation and a constant interaction among endowment, biological needs, and environmental conditions, tests and measures of developmental competency appeared in remarkable number, at least one purpose of which was to provide a predictive frame against which children could be compared to themselves and others and through which stages of development might still be measured (for a review of such measures, see Francis et al., 1987).

as "dependency to emotional self-reliance" and "responsibility in body management."[3]

At any given moment, progression along individual lines or channels of development might be synchronous (e.g., harmonious) or imbalanced. For example, self-care and tolerating separation are often parallel developmental achievements whereas language delays may complicate children's capacity to tolerate frustration. Periods of imbalance are markers not only of potential developmental problems, but also (under proper environmental conditions) encourage efforts toward self-righting and thus provide an impetus to move development along. Imbalances are possible in many directions. There may be imbalances across different lines of development related to disparities between instincts and ego capacities, between environmental demands and biological endowment or ego maturation, or among competing environmental conditions. In this model, efforts toward adaptation and reachieving equilibrium among lines of development are, metapsychologically, part of the fuel that pushes development on.[4]

Viewed from a contemporary perspective, developmental lines may be thought of as superordinate psychological regulatory functions that account at least in part for the varying rates and timing of development and as prototypes of gene-environment interaction (Cohen & Leck-

3. Note that developmental lines are cast in a terminology suggestive of functions superordinate to more molecular capacities. The developmental line for "emotional self-reliance" involves affect differentiation, perspective taking, arousal and anxiety regulation to name only a few more specific functions required.

4. The adaptationist point of view potentially brings several conceptual confusions that, at the least, need to be made explicit. First, and perhaps most obvious, adaptation as used in this text refers to an individual in a specific context and a specific phase of development, not the adaptation of groups or species across generations with possible concomitant alterations in genetic substrate. Second, as analysts, we are most concerned with psychological adaptation, that is, the adopting of a set of behaviors and/or psychological states (e.g., beliefs, feelings, defenses) in response to internal feelings, wishes, memories, and experiences. What is internally adaptive may appear maladaptive against an external context. Third, in all instances, adaptationist thinking carries the risk emerging from retrospective explaining—what in the case of evolutionary adaptation, Dennett (1995) has called "reverse engineering"—assuming that a set of behaviors exists in order to optimize, in our case, an individual's development or that those behaviors must be the best solution to internal and external experiences. Particularly in the case of developmental or ontogenetic adaptations, it is important to keep in mind that a set of behaviors or mental states may be only one of many possibilities in response to a given environmental context or developmental need. While it may seem "obvious" in retrospect why a given choice was made, which choices win out may be somewhat unpredictable or at the least irreproducible if the tape of an individual's life events could be replayed.

man, 1994; Plomin, 1985; Rose, 1995), the most contemporary developmental paradigm. In models of gene-environmental interaction, a given genotype has a phenotypic range of reaction, that is, a gene may be fully or only partially expressed depending both on the expression of other genes and on environmental conditions and/or external events (e.g., the phenotypic expression of the genetic endowment for height). Further, the timing of these external events may alter other regulatory processes involved in the full expression of the genetic substrate related to the function in question (e.g., for height, the timing of puberty). The model of gene-environment interaction is equally appropriate when applied, at least as a working metaphor, to psychological structures. For example, complete expression of capacities for full and intimate relationships with others may be limited by early deprivation that alters the development downstream of a full range of capacities for empathy and an integrated sense of self and other. In terms of developmental lines, the regulatory process of moving from "dependency to emotional self-reliance to adult object relationships" is modified by early deprivation. Alteration of this regulatory line also modifies the regulation of progress along other lines (or, in the genetic metaphor, the expression of other genetic substrate and the subsequent activation of other regulatory genetic systems). For example, failure to progress toward emotional self-reliance is paralleled by disturbances in the child's care of his own body.

In these bidirectional, gene-environment interaction models, experiences and existing structures may facilitate the emergence of other structures, maintain existing functions, or induce new ones (Gottlieb, 1983). For example, early in brain development, the amount and site-specificity of synaptic loss or connectivity is dependent on perceptual input from experience (Greenough, 1986, 1991; Greenough et al., 1987; Huttenlocher et al., 1982). The function of perception and the degree of stimulation in the environment maintains and facilitates in varying degrees synaptic connections. Similarly, under conditions of extreme stress or early toxic exposure, trophic factors in the brain are altered that also influence synaptic remodeling. In turn, functions enhanced or diminished during the period of synaptic remodeling facilitate, maintain, and possibly induce other timed processes to begin that will be evident in the infant and young child's behavioral repertoire. In these ways, experience shapes the function and emergence of basic neural processes, and psychology becomes "hard-wired." Altered expression of one line of function changes the timing of various other events downstream; and that initial alteration may reflect any number of psychophysiological conditions such as the chronic stress associated with traumatic events including parental neglect or abuse, serious illnesses, or toxic exposures. Developing systems are then turned on or off earlier or later than might have been true with another set of conditions, and there results a different organization of the functions subserving, for example, affect regulation.

Two aspects of these additions to notions of development define a paradigm shift in the study of epigenesis that carries important implications for psychoanalytic models of development. First is a shift from a view in which developmental changes are defined in reference to what is to come or to the presumed final stage—adulthood—to a perspective in which level of functioning is interpretable in terms of itself on the basis of its individual adaptive utility (Gottlieb, 1983; Oppenheim, 1981, 1984). Adaptation increases the individual's chance to move to subsequent stages of development and to maximize gains from the environment based on a given endowment. In this way of viewing development, psychoanalytically defined stages such as the oedipal period not only define a specific period of development but also represent a time when several lines of development are reorganized into a different pattern of adapting to internal and external conditions—moving to triadic relations from a predominantly dyadic mode of relating at a time when that reorganization is most adaptive to external and internal conditions and most likely to facilitate ongoing reorganizations. These adaptations may require suppression and destruction of antecedent functions as well as construction, revision, and maintenance. Ontogenetic adaptations, exemplified by earlier cited examples of synaptic pruning and connectivity, reflect the constellation of genetically timed events, biologic endowments, previous experiences, and current situations. While there is a general age-based regularity to patterns of adaptation, there is also the possibility for enormous individual variability in the specifics of capacities lost, reorganized, or maintained in order to maximize adaptation. Failure to remodel and reorganize appropriately a given set of functions results in maladaptation when internal and/or external conditions change. And this kind of continual reorganization and modification continues throughout the lifespan. Albeit with the more complex psychological functions of adulthood, rates of development may be slower and there are fewer degrees of freedom or pluripotent options for change. Nonetheless, gene-environment models allow for the still present possibility of psychological remodeling and reorganization to optimize adaptation to, for example, psychobiological events such as pregnancy, parenting, or menopause or to psychological interventions such as analysis.

The possibility of enormous individual variability in any given developmental adaptation or series of interactions represents the second feature of the contemporary developmental paradigm shift—from a predetermined to a more probabilistic view (Wolff, 1981, 1989). Development is neither linear, stage specific nor predictable, for different areas of function proceed at different rates and their interactions at any one point affect the child's adaptation and development in all other areas. A genetically based algorithm may set a series of processes in motion, but these are then influenced by myriad experiences that converge in varying intensities and durations and potentially influence all other events chronologically downstream. Developmental regulation while surely dependent on a regulatory genetic substrate in the most general of ways nonetheless involves some random or chance events that alter the timing of subsequent events. Loss, suppression, and reorganization is the rule, and any one level of functioning may contain only few, if any, *unaltered* traces of earlier ones.

In this more probabilistic developmental perspective, no one maturational event is ever quite like another, and there is little way even given identical genetic substrate and what appears identical experience to reproduce exactly the same pattern or rate of development a second or third time for any one individual. The later appearance of timed events reflects circumstances set in motion by previous ones and thus even the exact timing could never be reproduced. There are too many possibilities—too many genes to be expressed in slightly different patterns, to interact in different ways, or to be expressed in a phenotype that is a few degrees different—too many branch points at any one stage to even assume that the same path would be followed even given the same conditions.

These interactive models redirect psychoanalytic theories of development toward a focus on individual patterns of adapting and maladapting and on the possibility that individuals may move back and forth between normal and abnormal modes of functioning as a consequence of differing developmental stressors and environmental conditions (Cicchetti, 1993; Cicchetti & Cohen, 1995). Development in this more contemporary view is driven in part by self-correcting forces occurring in the face of unforeseen environmental contingencies, and the individual capacity for self-correction in and of itself reflects genetic endowment and past gene-environment interactions. Instead of stages that contain the history of each preceding stage, any one pattern of ordered or disordered behavior reflects multiple transactions between biological or genetic factors and external environmental conditions and the selective loss, suppression, or enhancement of functions. An emphasis on prediction is replaced in part with an emphasis on understanding the functions that a given arrangement of behaviors attempt to serve at any one point in development. The assumption of a regular, sequenced, unfolding while still true holds less explanatory power than a model of probabilistic change in which no one event or state is primary and past history is, at least in part, rewritten at each new stage.

CHILDREN'S AND ADULTS' FANTASIES OF HOW DEVELOPMENT HAPPENS

Discussions with groups of young children and with children and adults in analysis reveal many of the themes reflected in the epigenesis of a theory of developmental regulation. In particular are the often considerable tensions among the fantasies of an inevitable thrust (or lack thereof) to maturation, change that is of the body and the genes and not controllable, the wish not to go forward or even to turn the clock backwards, and adulthood as the final stage with no room for further change. There is frequently the deeply held belief and wish that knowing what one knows now, if the clock could be turned back and one or more events changed, the outcome would not only be better but assuredly one hundred percent predictable; and each of us may spend much time wondering with mixtures of awe, remorse, and joy how we got to where we are, where we will be at some time later, and by what means and with whose help and care.

Literature for children and adults reflects in part the universality of certain fantasies about regulating development. Stories are filled with fantasies of staying young forever (e.g., Peter Pan), postponing aging, growing up fast, looking ahead or backwards to know who we will be (e.g., *Back to the Future, Time Machine*), or acquiring some magic power, potion, or machine that will grant eternal youth. Many of these stories are predicated on the inherent idea that development is something exquisitely and closely regulated and predictable or that development involves constant conflict and struggle—progress gripped from the fire and pain of growing. Three perspectives from clinical material on how development happens provide illustrations for the following fantasies—development as an inevitable, progressive change, development that can be stopped and that involves loss as well as gain, and development as metamorphosis or transformation accomplished through the power of others.

Conversations with young children capture in particular the fantasies of a dynamic, inevitable thrust to development with a clearly predictable outcome. When asked, "How long does it take to grow up?" a four-and-a-half-year-old boy, showing off his emerging capacities to leap like a frog, answered assuredly, "14,000 years." Responding to his teacher's wonderment at such a long time, he nodded seriously as he hit ground with a loud thump and said, "Yes, that's just the way it is." When another five-year-old girl was asked what things help one grow up, she pondered the dilemma only briefly and answered with the confidence of a tenured professor, "You have to get a lot of sleep and eat a lot of healthy food—that's all it takes." A third child offered that growing up happened because her mom and dad were grown-up—it had happened for them so it was a given that it would happen for her. How was of less immediate concern since it was just going to do so.

Asked what changes when you get older, one four-year-old said "you get breasts," another "well, you just get bigger," and another "you can use a chain saw," which turned out as he talked to be fraught with the inevitable dangers of losing limb and life—and as his teacher later revealed, with his search for a father he had never known. Several children vigorously agreed that the main way you knew you were grown up was when you could drive a car. Baby sitters who could drive were surely at the cusp of adulthood much more than those who had to be brought by their own parents. Adulthood, though perhaps inevitable, was not necessarily an enviable or desired state even if it promised breasts, cars, and chainsaws. Adults, in the vision of one group, were forever barred from being able to jump like a frog and laugh so long and hard that the world seemed to be all foggy and turned upside down. Adults surely couldn't blow bubbles with their apple juice and could never go back to being a baby—even if that might be desired to which all, of course, vigorously asserted "No way."

What development would bring was a prevailing concern for these children even outside the stimulation of these group discussions. A petite, quietly solemn four-year-old girl sitting very close to her teacher had recently been weaving over a week's time a story about getting bigger and having a baby that she would bring back to her nursery school. She would be the mother then and maybe the tree by the back steps would be so much taller that she would have to stand on her tiptoes to look around and see her own baby playing in the yard. She fell silent as her teacher commented on how much everyone changes as they grow older and wondered aloud how it was that those changes happened. Suddenly, she smiled, saying she knew. When she turned five, her father had promised they would plant a tree together and that she would then grow right along with her tree. The tree, and implicitly her father's devotion, was what would help her grow up. Of course, she added being five was pretty close to being grown up. At the very least, she was surely older than her baby brother—she could walk, talk, get herself dressed, knew the ins and outs of bathing, toileting, how to make her own breakfast. How could there be much more to learn in this push toward being grown up? But that it indeed was a push and an imperative that had the quality of something that simply happens was clear.

Another group of five-year-olds were rolling over each other in group glee and scorn, giggling at the thought of how babies knew so little about the real world and at the similar thought that their moms and dads had once been babies (not of course mentioning that they had too). When their teacher asked whether it was possible to decide just not to grow up, the group laughed loudly and a little anxiously at such a silly thought. Like jumping off a roof without falling, like falling in a pool without getting wet, like . . . well, like wishing really long for something nearly impossible to happen . . . but . . . maybe, just maybe it was possible. Maybe it was possible to go back, to stop development, to grow more slowly or faster, to be grown up at five, to not grow up for 14 millenia—in whichever version with whatever colors, how development happens was both a conundrum for these young children and one they pondered with enormous preoccupation. At least one solution to their preoccupations seemed to be the assurance that because development had occurred for their parents as well as because of their parents' love, they too would grow up. But their concerns reappeared many times with only the slightest stimuli and reflected in part worries about what would have to be given up as well as gained as development progressed.

Preoccupied and burdened with the hidden risks of getting older, a three-year-old girl in analysis approached her fourth birthday with a painful struggle centered around her wish to stop development and not to grow up—she wanted to stop the clock. As gloomy and morbid as a thirty-nine-year-old nearing forty, Sophie sadly reported she simply did not want to be four years old, and it would just not happen. For many sessions before her birthday, she tried to fit herself into small corners or curl under or on top of very small cabinets and tables to show me (and convince herself) that she really was not growing any bigger. She grumpily rejected any of her parents' or relatives' enthusiastic temptings of the many rewards maturity would bring—new clothes intended for more grown-up girls, a bigger bed, a wonderful party, even the opportunity to spend afternoons and evenings with friends from her nursery program. Instead of offering comfort, these enticements only increased Sophie's near terror that once she became four, she would not only be forever changed and surely not for the better, but that she would also lose things she could not quite find the words for.

Always prone to save scraps of paper she found in the play room, she became ever more vigilant to hold onto any scrap however tiny that crossed our table and our work. Separations from her mother to attend nursery school—always difficult—became more prolonged and intense with Sophie often dissolving in tears as she held onto her mother's leg. She was deeply preoccupied with the ages of different persons and pondered the puzzle of the age differences in her siblings and relatives and how could one really tell how old someone was.

The implied maturity of four surely seemed to threaten a loss of a close tie to her mother, but it also seemed to carry with it the frightening possibility of becoming a different person—changed by a process she had no control over. Kicking, screaming, and terrified, Sophie was being pulled along by a maturational tide. She captured the dilemma of becoming a changed person on several occasions when she used her beloved blanket as a sacrifice, throwing it symbolically away during our play to see what would happen if she gave it up even briefly as a gesture to her impending watershed day. Her actual birthday came and went with little mention from her as if no real event could be quite as dramatic as her fantasied dread. In the days after her birthday, Sophie made few references to the transformation she had so dreaded until she announced at the beginning of a session that she had moved into her "big girl bed." With a mixture of remorse and excited curiosity, she described rearranging her room to accommodate all of her new furniture that had come for her birthday. These tentative steps into four years seemed to usher in a long period in her analysis of her showing me what she could do now with her maturationally granted prowess— she could jump from taller chairs and steps and balance gracefully on one foot. She studied her new found skills closely in the mirror in our room and simultaneously wondered what had she been like as a baby but not so much what she would be like as she got older. Long, dreamy hours were spent weaving stories of what she had been like a long time ago—how did one know time was passing? What was it really like to grow up? Why and how did it happen? Her favorite book for us to read together described a little girl's year of holidays that surprisingly came around again the next year and the next with a stable and comforting predictability.

In the months that followed her fourth birthday, Sophie made many developmental gains and adaptations that were apparent at least to an outside observer. Her school noted her changes and even described her as more assertive, becoming a leader among her peers. But almost all changes were accompanied by an often agonizing preoccupation about stepping forward and the inherent loss hidden within gain. Inevitable developmental change, not always seeming hers to master, at times continued to master her particularly around moments of maturational transitions—birthdays, changing schools, new teachers, and even the end of her analysis. On the last day of her analysis, Sophie carefully surveyed the room and identified items by their place in the developmental epochs of the work with her analyst—always been here, had this toy a little while, this is new. As the end of the hour and the moment symbolizing yet another developmental transition approached, she identified a toy bear as the captain who would stay at the helm in the playroom watching over everything and keeping track of who and what changed and got older. The bear acquired an ageless, ever-present, and always-the-same quality as it gained the responsibility of watching over everyone's developmental changes, their gains, and their losses.

Ontogenetic transformations or complete metamorphosis were captured in the deep fantasy of a young woman, R., in analysis that there would come a moment within, or even in spite of, the analysis when she would be miraculously changed. R. would shed her old self, marred by losses and a persistent mix of sadness and rage, and emerge with a clean slate, the full complement of future promise, and with no sense of time lost, regrets owned, or responsibility for the future. How this change would happen involved not so much the result of her work in analysis or even the promise of endowed maturation. Indeed, for her too maturation in and of itself seemed fraught with risks and inevitable loss. Instead, for R. moving forward and making developmental transitions were the responsibilities of the myriad people she pulled into her world—each held the promise or perhaps the magic formula to remake her. Albeit unknown to them, they were the regulators of R.'s development; and they inevitably and repeatedly failed to help her move forward and feel complete, which left her manifestly rejected and sad and, more deeply, rageful and destructive. No person was ever sufficiently able to set things right or to fill in what had been lost or never obtained so that R. could move on; and thus, she remained stuck, unable to move ahead and with a deep sense of being nearly paralyzed.

Alternating between frantic activity to ward off stagnation and quiet, despairing isolation, R. tried to fill in with others what she experienced as marked early failures in parenting and need satisfaction. Further, not only were others responsible for changing and transforming her, but they were also granted the near magical capacity to understand exactly who she wanted to be in her transformed state. Within her analysis, as R. came closer to allowing herself to recognize that no transformation would rid her completely of her past and that persons lost would not return to remake her, she became more overtly rageful, briefly self-destructive, and ultimately she made a series of decisions that led her to a more adaptive life, albeit still incomplete and marred, closer to her family and the home of her early childhood.

METAPSYCHOLOGICAL FUNCTIONS OF DEVELOPMENTAL FANTASIES

The very persistence of these and other fantasies regarding how development happens gives evidence to their utility as clinical material as well as their cultural fixity and raises the question of what functions they serve in mental life. Surely, for both Sophie and R., their respective central fantasies can be viewed from multiple perspectives. Sophie's dilemma reflects at the very least the implied object loss that getting older might bring: her predisposition to anxiety, her concerns about separation in many guises, and her partial failure to move ahead to triadic relations and a fully oedipalized inner world. Similarly, R.'s fantasy of a metamorphosis in the course of an analysis orchestrated by the analyst is not an uncommon wish and might be viewed as reflective of earlier modes of relating, an intolerance of ambivalence, or old omnipotent wishes. However, for both as well as for the other examples cited, couching these fantasies in terms of developmental regulation highlights the psychological functions served—their role in the creation or maintenance of ties to others and in defense and ego/super-ego function.

For Sophie, development moved in spite of her—and even in spite of her powerful wishes—and in that progression she lost rather than gained. By stopping the process in her fantasy, she could at least hold her ground—no gain, no loss. That such was impossible in reality only increased her determination to hold on and move at her own pace, lingering and remembering as long as she could. The fantasy kept her close in her inner world to an exclusive tie with her mother and to others she did not want to abandon as she moved out into the world. In contrast, for many children and adults, the potential gains overshadow the certain losses; and the fantasied possibility of a complete developmental transformation, or at least of better things to come, lures them into the maturational unknown. Being able to be with someone much admired or desired, to have greater skills with which to impress them, to possess, engage, and be more in control are some of the gains offered by maturational shifts and transformations.

For R., fantasies of developmental transformations also involved the action and presence of others—transformed by another's love, power, knowledge of what is best or right, growing and developing under the romantic attachment, admiration, and support of another. In this way, the other person, real and in the internal object world, motivates aspects of developmental change. In children, this relation may indeed be experienced in reality and far more globally and somatically as manifest in the failure to grow in many deprived children, but the link between developmental change and ties to important others is evident in all children and adults in many different settings—romantic relations, teacher-student, parent-child, therapist-patient. Indeed, in the dialectic of gene-environment interactions, the critical "environment" is more often than not relationships with others that are developmentally sustaining, facilitating, and perhaps even at times, inductive of other biological and psychological processes of change and adaptation. Love for another may very well set in motion a number of other processes that allow an individual to make room mentally for another person and to move to another level of relatedness that in turn interacts with and regulates other lines of development. Conversely, deficits in the ability to be with, search out, and take in relations with others, reflecting whatever mix of endowment and experiences, impair subsequent capacities to use others to facilitate ongoing development. In other words, the fantasy that developmental progressions require or demand another person captures something that is structurally necessary and true about all developmental change and regulation.

Both Sophie and R. struggle in their different developmental phases and with their very different endowments and experiences with the dilemma of development as a process involving loss as well as gain and the risk that changes are not guaranteed to be better and may perhaps be destructive and chaotic. The regulatory engine may run wild or stop—the genes may fail. Sophie struggles to hold the tide back. R. wishes for a metamorphosis that by implication is the emergence of something or someone more beautiful and capable than before. Others may wish for a development that never closes down any options, everything gained in one period is carried always ahead and is always available to be activated. In any case, fantasies of stopping development, returning to earlier stages to try again, leaping forward to peek into the future, or never relinquishing any developmental function to permit building another serve to deny the risks inherent in development, the possibility of accidental or unforeseen outcomes, and the chaos that may be implicitly a part of change. They protect against acknowledging events we fear we can never adapt to and options we never want to give up.

Further, fantasies of transformation or development by metamorphosis serve to deny the past and what has come before developmentally. They protect against regret and persistent disappointment. Such fantasies involve the wish to start over, implicitly to go back to the beginning, if not as an infant at least as an individual with no developmental history. In this way, the fantasy of transformation as an attempt to regulate development allows for perpetual opportunity for another chance and for change with no responsibility for, or relation to, what has happened before. Indeed, expecting a complete transformation, or accepting a staged theory of development in which early failures impeded later progress, allows the individual to escape reflection and awareness of his or her own contribution to developmental change. For example, a college-aged adult, struggling to move into what she viewed as real adult life and responsibilities, tried on for size the idea of developmental arrests and failed epigenetic stages at a time beyond immediately available memory. As she observed, something must have happened very early on that altered, maybe even permanently changed, her capacity to move forward, to grow and change. Or a young man, remembering his college-learned understanding of stages of development, felt he had only a short time to complete the assigned developmental tasks before he reached another decade and the clock was reset. What wasn't done at that point would never be achieved and would always be found lacking, a permanent scar. In these instances, development occurred by installments, granted and regulated by processes outside an individual's control and awareness and giving in each installment more or less of what was required to move ahead or not— fate as much as chance.

To hold that development is regulated outside of us whether by the wish to hold onto or be close to another or by an unseen but all-powerful force in the guise of a clock, engine, or gene is to accept regulation outside of our charge and our responsibility. We might wish to stop the clock or tinker with the process but implicit in these wishes is the sense, or conviction, that the process really is just beyond our control. Like aging, it just happens. In these and myriad other examples is reflected the presently curious but historically once-held notion that developmental regulation is fixed, a quota granted in our genes beyond our capacity to change or shape and for better or worse, that which regulates us. Paradoxically, because they invoke immutability and control by processes other than ourselves, such fantasies serve the wish to disavow a continually interactive genetic endowment, to exist outside the body, and in a sense to live outside an awareness of mental life and the possibility of change and revision and of continual adaptation to internal and external circumstances.

To accept a responsibility in the role of regulating our own development implies neither a moral accountability for who we have become nor an active, conscious control of all developmentally shaping experiences. Rather, like accepting responsibility for our unconscious lives and own histories (Loewald, 1978), to be responsible for our own developmental regulation is to acknowledge the interactive admixture of genetics and experience that is constantly a part of our biology and psychology and to accept a process that is continually in flux, rarely predictable, and sometimes chaotic and irregular. We do not become who we are solely by the genes we were given, the children we were, or the lives we have experienced. In a sense, what makes development happen or continue as adults is how much we are able to accept a reflective inner responsiveness toward those present, past, and future times of developmental reorganization and adaptation made necessary by the internal demands of our biology and psychology and the external circumstances which we both choose and find ourselves in. The effort to reflect upon how development happens lifts us a little above day-to-day happenstance and timed inevitability into the tragic grace of self-awareness.

BIBLIOGRAPHY

AUSUBEL, D. P., SULLIVAN, E. V., & IVES, S. W. (1980). *Theory and Problems of Child Development,* 3rd ed. New York: Grune and Stratton.

BERGMAN, P. & ESCALONA, S. K. (1949). Unusual sensitivities in very young children. *Psychoanalytic Study of the Child* 3/4: 333–52.

BURLINGHAM, D. T. (1961). Some notes on the development of the blind, *Psychoanalytic Study of the Child* 16:121–45.

CHARLESWORTH, W. R. (1992). Darwin and developmental psychology: Past and present, *Developmental Psychology* 28:5–16.

CICCHETTI, D. (1993). Developmental psychopathology: Reactions, reflections, projections, *Developmental Review* 13:471–502.

CICCHETTI, D. & COHEN, D. J. (1995). *Developmental Psychopathology* (New York: John Wiley & Sons.

COHEN, D. J. & LECKMAN, J. F. (1994). Developmental psychopathology and neurobiology of Tourette's syndrome, *Journal of the American Academy of Child and Adolescent Psychiatry* 33:2–15.

DENNETT, D. C. (1995). *Darwin's Dangerous Idea: Evolution and the Meanings of Life.* New York: Simon and Schuster.

EDELSON, M. (1984). *Hypothesis and Evidence in Psychoanalysis.* Chicago: University of Chicago Press.

ESCALONA, S. K. (1963). Patterns of infantile experience and the developmental process, *Psychoanalytic Study of the Child* 18:197–244.

FRANCIS, P. L., SELF, P. A., & HOROWITZ, F. D. (1987). The behavioral assessment of the neonate: An overview, in *Handbook of Infant Development,* ed. J. D. Osofsky. New York: John Wiley and Sons, 723–79.

FREUD, A. (1963). The concept of developmental lines, *Psychoanalytic Study of the Child* 18:245–65.

———— (1965). Normality and pathology in childhood, in *The Writings of Anna Freud*.

————(1974). A psychoanalytic view of developmental psychopathology, in *The Writings of Anna Freud*, 57–74.

———— (1981). The concept of developmental lines: Their diagnostic significance, *Psychoanalytic Study of the Child* 36:129–36.

FREUD, S.(1905). Three essays on the theory of sexuality, in *SE*, 130–243.

GESELL, A.(1945). *The Embryology of Behavior.* New York: Harper.

GOTTLIEB, G. (1983). The psychobiological approach to developmental issues, in *Infancy and Developmental Psychobiology*, ed. M. M. Haith et al., *Handbook of Child Psychology*. New York: John Wiley and Sons, 1–26.

GREENOUGH, W. T. (1991). Experience as a component of normal development. Evolutionary considerations, *Developmental Psychology* 27:14–17.

———— (1986). What's special about development? Thoughts on the bases of experience-sensitive synaptic plasticity, in *Developmental Neuropsychobiology*, ed. W. T. Greenough et al. New York: Academic Press, 387–407.

GREENOUGH, W. T., BLACK, J. E., & WALLACE, E. S. (1987). Experience and brain development, *Child Development* 58:539–59.

HARTMANN, H. (1964). Psychoanalysis and developmental psychology, in *Essays on Ego Psychology: Selected Problems in Psychoanalytic Theory*, ed. N. York. New York: International Universities Press.

HELLMAN, I. (1983).Work in Hampstead War Nurseries, *International Journal of Psychoanalysis* 64:435–40.

HUTTENLOCHER, P. R., DE COURTEN, C., GAREY, L. J., & VAN DER LOOG, H. (1982). Synaptogenesis in human visual cortex: Evidence for synapse elimination during normal development, *Neuroscience Letter* 33:247–52.

JOHNSON, T. H. (1958). *The Letters of Emily Dickinson:* Letter to T. W. Higgins, April 25, 1862. vol. 2, pp. 404. Cambridge, Mass.: Harvard University Press.

KESSEN, W. (1990). *The Rise and Fall of Development.* Worcester, Mass.: Clark University Press.

LOEWALD, H. (1978). *Psychoanalysis and the History of the Individual.* New Haven, Conn.: Yale University Press.

OPPENHEIM, R. W. (1981). Ontogenetic adaptations and retrogressive processes in the development of the nervous system and behavior: A neuroembryological perspective, in *Maturation and Development: Biological and Psychological Perspective*, ed. K. J. Connolly et al., Clinics in Developmental Medicine, no. 77/78. London: Spastics International Medical Publications.

———— (1984).Ontogenetic adaptations in neural development: Toward a more 'ecological' developmental psychobiology, in *Continuity of Neural Function from Prenatal to Postnatal Life*, ed. H. F. R. Prechtl, Clinics in Developmental Medicine, No. 94. Oxford: Spastics International Medical Publications.

PIAGET, J. (1952). *The Origins of Intelligence in Children*. New York: International Universities Press.

———— (1954). *The Construction of Reality in the Child*. New York: Basic Books.

PLOMIN, R. (1985). Behavioral genetics, *Current Topics in Human Intelligence* 1:297–320.

PRECHTL, H. F. R., CONNOLLY, J., & CONNOLLY, K. J. (1981). Maturation and development, in *Maturation and Development: Biological and Psychological Perspectives*, ed. K. J. Connolly et al., Clinics in Developmental Medicine, No. 77/78. London: Spastics International Medical Publications, ix–xii.

ROSE, R. J. (1995). Genes and human behavior, *Annual Review of Psychology* 46:625–54.

SPITZ, R. A. & WOLF, J. M. (1946). Anaclitic depression: An inquiry into the genesis of psychiatric conditions in early childhood, *Psychoanalytic Study of the Child* 2:313–42.

TYSON, P. & TYSON, R. (1990). *Psychoanalytic Theories of Development: An Integration*. New Haven: Yale University Press.

WADDINGTON, C. H. (1957). *The Strategy of the Genes*. London: George, Allen, and Unwin.

WOLFF, P. H. (1981). Normal variation in human maturation, in *Maturation and Development: Biological and Psychological Perspectives*, ed. K. J. Connolly et al., Clinics in Developmental Medicine, N. 77/78. London: Spastics International Medical Publications.

———— (1989). The concept of development: How does it constrain assessment and therapy? in *Challenges to Developmental Paradigms: Implications for Theory, Assessment, and Treatment*, ed. P. R. Zelazo et al. Hillsdale, New Jersey: Lawrence Erlbaum Associates, 13–28.

WOLPERT, L. (1994) Do we understand development? *Science* 266:571–72.

The Interaction between Self and Others

A Different Perspective on Narcissism

RONNIE SOLAN, Ph.D.

This paper explores a perspective that expands the scope of the "healthy" narcissistic function to include the narcissistic preservation of self-identities during interaction between self and others. After a brief review of the literature from Freud to current views on the subject, the author describes the mutual influence of narcissistic processing and object relation and goes on to theorize that self-preservation is accomplished by the narcissistic envelope through immunization and defensive processing. Narcissistic immune processing provides familiarity, cohesiveness, equilibrium, integrity, and continuity to the self's separateness in an affective state of stability, which may make the libidinal need for object relation and interrelation with the world possible without undermining the constancy and safety of the self. The defensive processing preserves the self from incohesiveness and vulnerability during exposure to the unfamiliar (by creating a false self-identity, withdrawing into a narcissistic state, or preventing new interactions). The theoretical implications of this argument and their practical application are illustrated by several clinical vignettes.

IN GREEK MYTHOLOGY, NARCISSUS IS A YOUTH WHO FELL IN LOVE WITH his own image when he saw its reflection in a pool. Narcissistic well-

Psychoanalyst, clinical psychologist, member of the Israel Psychoanalytic Society; training analyst; supervisor and lecturer in the Israel Psychoanalytic Institute, lecturer in Postgraduate Psychotherapy Section, Sackler School of Medicine, Tel-Aviv University.

The Psychoanalytic Study of the Child 54, ed. Albert J. Solnit, Peter B. Neubauer, Samuel Abrams, and A. Scott Dowling (Yale University Press, copyright © 1999 by Albert J. Solnit, Peter B. Neubauer, Samuel Abrams, and A. Scott Dowling).

being and self-love are textured primarily by familiar bodily and sense perceptions experienced within the primal object relation, and they are linked to psychobiological homeostasis.

When Freud first elucidated the concept of narcissism, he identified two phenomena that seem characteristic of narcissism—namely, "self-love" and "narcissism of minor differences": "In the undisguised antipathies and aversions which people feel towards strangers with whom they have to do we may recognize the expression of self-love—of narcissism. This self-love works for the preservation of the individual, and behaves as though the occurrence of any divergence from his [or her] particular lines of development involved a criticism of them and a demand for their alteration" (Freud, 1921, p. 102). It is precisely the minor differences in people who are otherwise alike that form the basis of feelings of strangeness and hostility between them (Freud, 1917, p. 199).

These concepts bring to mind the two "faces" of narcissism: the narcissistic need for sameness and familiarities when facing interaction with others, and the narcissistic vulnerability triggered by interaction with the unfamiliar or nonself. The following exploration of the concept of narcissism as related to these two aspects will serve as a basis for viewing the interaction between self and other in a somewhat different perspective. I will introduce the subject of my paper with the following analytical fragment:

Dan, a ballet conductor and choreographer in his mid-forties, came to analysis seeking to clarify some difficulties related to his artistic creativity. He mentioned that he had decided to introduce some new steps and variations into the familiar dance program of his ballet ensemble, which he had not changed for quite some time. When the dancers began rehearsing the new arrangements, Dan noticed that feelings of strangeness were affecting his work, especially when he led the dancers through the new routines, which disturbed his sense of unity as conductor and choreographer. He felt as if the earlier music and dance rhythms were still in his body—side by side with the new ones—disrupting the quality of his work. He often spoke of the great joy he felt at leading the company in a harmonious, unified, and coherent rhythm. Now, he suddenly felt a strange vulnerability at the dancers' mistakes, as if he feared that instead of the new variations they would mistakenly revert to the old familiar steps and rhythms, undermining his own and the group's cohesiveness and unity.

Dan came to acknowledge his fears of losing the familiar

rhythm, which until then had seemed to preserve his rhythmic identity, by working through his associations with his mother, who loved to sing and led the whole family to create a unified rhythmic unit. These family gatherings were very dear to Dan. When I commented that losing the familiar rhythm was for him akin to losing the family unity or identity, he said he could almost feel the physical anxiety he experienced as a child when he sang out of tune, and the distress of being an outsider at these musical events, which symbolized family cohesiveness. It took time before Dan and his dancers could accept the strange new variations, but they eventually came to love them as well as the original creation.

Whereas affects of uneasiness that make us feel temporarily alien or "uncanny" (Freud, 1919) reflect a narcissistic state of pain or injury related to minor or major differences, affects of well-being are related to identifying the original, genuine, and familiar. Bollas (1992) suggests that repetition of the familiar gives us comfort, whereas a surprising and unexpected variation may change the familiar into the strange, undermining the feelings of coherence and well-being. Minor divergences from the familiar are eased by repetition and familiarization and may eventually even bring pleasure. We can say that minor divergences refer to differences from the self-love of narcissism in sameness. The process also clarifies our interaction with others: Some people adopt a separate self-identity, different from their usual self-identity (e.g., the self-identity of rhythm), in interacting with others; they even come to enjoy this different identity while they also manage to preserve their original self-identity throughout the process; for others, such interaction involves forgoing their well-being and self-identities; still others fear whatever is strange to their self-identities to the point of withdrawing into themselves rather than facing any interaction with others.

THEORETICAL BASES OF CURRENT VIEWS ON NARCISSISM

Ever since Freud (1914) first probed the concept of narcissism, it has been a source of fascination for many psychoanalysts (e.g., Morrison, 1986; Sandler et al., 1991). The pathological aspects have attracted special interest (Freud, 1914; Grunberger, 1971; Kohut, 1971, 1977; Kernberg, 1974). Rather than reviewing the extensive literature on the subject, I will briefly mention some aspects of self-preservation that are related to narcissism.

As early as 1895, Freud was already scrutinizing questions of permeability and impermeability in the neuron system and their relation to perception, memory, and sensitivity to the cathexis of experience. The concept of a "protective shield against stimuli" (1914, 1920) was further studied as the need to safeguard the psychic apparatus from external stimuli and quantities of excitation that could not be discharged or controlled (1926). Freud claimed that narcissism acts as "the libidinal complement to the egoism of the instinct of self-preservation" (1914, pp. 73–74). This phenomenon, which Freud referred to as "self-love—of narcissism" (1921), makes one wonder whether, even at that early date, he might have been referring to narcissism as being in charge of self-preservation against the "minor differences." At any rate, Freud assumed that the self-preservation drives were subordinate to ego interests, and he conceived of the "bodily ego" as "the projection of a surface that contains and maintains contact with the outside world" (1923, p. 24).

In the past thirty years, a number of authors have dealt with similar protective concepts by using such metaphors as the "container object" (Bion, 1962); the "holding mother" (Winnicott, 1965); "psychic skin and second skin" (Bick, 1968); "ego-skin and psychic envelopes" (Anzieu, 1985, 1987); the "screening mechanism" (Esman, 1983); the "protective shell" (Tustin, 1990); the "membrane, the family envelope, and structural stability" (Houzel, 1990, 1996). They all seem to agree that the psychic apparatus is fragile and needs to be protected, regulated, and equilibrated by a "shield" or envelope in order to avoid overexcitation and the traumatic experience of being overwhelmed by unorganized sense data (Sandler, 1987).

Permeable "raw sensations" (Tustin, 1990)—e.g., rhythm stimuli that seep in within the sensorimotor and proprioceptive surface (Anzieu, 1985, 1987)—are processed via perceptions of bodily and sense data (Sandler, 1987) and are then encrypted with "psychic texture" (Bollas, 1992) and "specific shapes" (Tustin, 1990, p. 51; Emde, 1988; Stern, 1985). Thus, familiar meaning is attributed to self-experiencing (Bollas, 1992; Ogden, 1992; Modell, 1993), to the "core self" (Stern, 1985), to the self-identities, and to virtues concerning the self's relations to others (Solan, 1991). The sensorial "floor" of self-experiencing is generated by the most primitive meaning "on the basis of the organization of sensory impression, particularly at skin surface (autistic-contiguous position)" (Ogden, 1992, p. 4). The process of sensory integration acts as a safety principle that regulates the feeling state of affects, sensations, and body reactions (Sandler, 1987). Stern (1985) called this processing "representations of interactions that have been generalized" (RIG) and asserted that "infants appear to have an innate general capacity ... to take information received in one sensory modality and somehow translate it into another sensory modality ... it involves an encoding into still mysterious amodal representation, which can then be recognized in any of the sensory modes" (p. 51).

Narcissism as a "primary agency" (Grunberger, 1971) is activated to reserve the sense of self as an invariant, that "which does not change in the face of all the things that do change" (Stern, 1985, pp. 70–71). This means that while the self is exchanging excitations (vibrations) with the nonself in the external world ("structural stability," Houzel, 1996), both interacting partners may preserve their self-sense as invariant. "Object constancy is a developmental capacity that provides the child with a sense of himself and his parents and enables him to become increasingly independent in forming new personal relationships, which in turn increasingly enable him significantly to shape his own social environment" (Solnit, 1982a, p. 217). By sharing a "medium" (Solan, 1996) for their interrelation and mediating their "jointness," which "represents an encounter between mother and infant or any partners experiencing ... mutual satisfaction while concomitantly safeguarding separateness" (Solan, 1991, p. 337), both parties might decipher textured stimuli similar to those already encrypted as perceptions. This deciphering might bring about experiences of familiarity and sameness (Moses & Bene-Moses, 1980), of affective states of well-being, and of the "self-love of narcissism" (Freud, 1921).

Perceptions and symbolizations of stimuli are infinitely experienced in motion (Rosenfield, 1992) by being connected to a familiar "representational world" (Sandler, 1987, 1990; Kernberg, 1983). This "organizing activity" of sensory integration is "an attempt to add meaning to incoming excitation ... in terms of past experience and future activity ... [that] constitutes an internal frame of reference by which the outside world is assessed" (Sandler, 1987, p. 3). It immunizes the innate ability to differentiate self from nonself, maintain a relation with the other, and even enjoy it (Winnicott, 1960; Stern, 1985; Emde, 1988), as well as to "contain and convey our growing knowledge of the world ... improving our attempts at making sense of the world ... [and our] clarity and precision of expression and communication" (Laor, 1990, p. 147). Thus, "Memories and psychic representations of primary relationships, especially those with continuing influence, are modified and reshaped by ongoing development, by the never-ending resonances between current perception, experience and motives and the abiding residues of past perceptions and experiences. These resonating, changing, but persisting genetic (historical) influences explain how each individual retains his unique integrity at the same time as he changes, develops and becomes increasingly unique and constant as a personality" (Solnit, 1982b, p. 34).

The processing function of the narcissistic envelope may be considered along the line proposed by Anzieu concerning *psychic envelopes* that serve as ego skin, sensitive membrane-like surfaces or sensorimotor tonus, which are permeable to proprioceptive and other sensorial images that leave their footprints on them. These footprints then draw on images that act as reference points to give sense to nonverbal communication and promote self-individuation (Anzieu, 1985, 1987).

NARCISSISTIC PERSPECTIVES ON INTERACTION WITH OTHERS

I propose to consider narcissism as one of the psychic envelopes that function as the "immune system" of our familiar sense of self while being permeable to excitations with the nonfamiliar other. Familiar self-identity is a symbolic representation of generalized phenomena that synthesizes a continuity of self-experiences and affinities (or sensitivities) intensively linked to our senses (taste, smell, vision, etc.).

Sensorial and proprioceptive impressions excite the sensitive membrane-like spaces of the self. They are encrypted within the sensory motor tonus and give rise to self-experiences, which are demarcated by unique data of familiar sensorial narcissistic characteristics, such as rhythmic identity, taste identity, posture and sex identity, etc., and are interconnected with perceptions of drives and affects in object relations. Then they are agglomerated, condensed into codes and symbols, demarcated, classified, and organized into coded networks before being incorporated into the self-continuum.

Thus, the narcissistic envelope contains data concerning self-experiences that are always subjective psychobiological-narcissistic perceptions increasingly vulnerable to any nonfamiliar sensorial excitations. The data concern the self, the objects of the self, its environment, and familiar object relations, all textured as narcissistic attributes that are clearly differentiated from one another. Its coded network represents a dynamic schematization of constant associations, differentiations, and interconnections of stimuli via the continuous integration and regulation of these attributes. Hence, the narcissistic envelope functions as a distinct framework for the familiar belongings of the self.

Any new perceptions experienced in interactions are gradually and systematically classified into the coded networks by means of associations and symbolizations to the familiar codes. Sensorial images often change their interconnections and regroup differently into self-cohesiveness by a perpetual motion that acts as mediator between self and nonself, separate and united, absent and present, external and internal, individual and universal object relationships (Solan, 1989), and social interactions. This sequence balances the "substantial discrepancy between the mental representation of the actual (state of the) self of the moment and an ideal shape of the self" (Joffe & Sandler, 1968, p. 189) and brings equilibrium to those narcissistic attributes recognizable as familiar-ideal self-belongings as well as to attributes perceived as slightly different and those more or less strange to the narcissistic network. Consequently, deciphering associations of familiar experiences (whether new or predicted) will rarely be identified in sameness, but whenever this occurs we feel a narcissistic libidinal elation, a self-love of narcissism (Freud, 1921), an "identity of perception" (Sandler, 1990), or the fulfillment of a wish. Minor differences experienced as only similar to familiar stimuli produce an affective state of familiarity and safety.

From a narcissistic point of view, interaction means mutual experiencing between separate units of self-identity that seek in each other the libidinal gratification of similar textured stimuli. While exchanging excitations (proprioceptive and other sensorial images) with the other, each unit is protected by its own narcissistic envelope, which features different sensorial identities that seep in (mutually) and leave their footprints in the self-spaces of each. Thus, the sensitive narcissistic envelope might easily decipher familiar or unfamiliar particularities of rhythmic interaction (as a prototype of the other senses), concerning self-rhythm, object rhythm, and mediated rhythm. It relies on the distinct separateness of the narcissistic boundaries of each of the interacting self-identities, so that their differentiation, on the one hand, and their interconnection, on the other, will preserve the uniqueness of each.

The object (who by definition has a different rhythm), which is perceived through the narcissistic envelope as a nonself whose rhythmic stimuli filter into the space of the self, responds in turn with vibrations that stir up waves of reference, upsetting the balance of familiar rhythms of self-identity. As early as 1914, Freud had observed that narcissism was constantly being battered by reality and that man was forever striving to restore the sense of wholeness of which he had been robbed. Indeed, given the amount of excitations that threaten the sense of self even in the earliest developmental experiences, one may wonder how the self can possibly be immunized against the alien stimuli bursting forth in any interaction. This immunizing mental activity may be considered narcissistic "to the degree that its function is to maintain the structural cohesiveness, temporal stability, and positive affective coloring of the self-representation" (Stolorow, 1975, p. 198).

Processing by the narcissistic envelope involves the following simultaneous yet antagonistic functions: (1) deciphering and integrating familiar affinities among those that filter in; (2) deciphering and resisting unfamiliar or alien sensorial images; and (3) differentiating self-like particles in the nonself via familiarization. The immune system requires permanent regulation of the tensions stirred up by antagonistic feelings, which are created by these narcissistic functions—e.g., nonfamiliarity versus familiarity, nonself versus sense of self, or even accepting the nonself versus rejecting it. It may resemble the conflicting forces in object relation between narcissistic libido and object libido. Unless these functions are integrated, they will lead the individual to experience minor differences as major or alien, threatening self-cohesiveness and arousing resistance to any new situations.

The following example illustrates the transition between resistance and integration of these functions: A psychoanalytic candidate in analysis has three supervisors who differ in their psychoanalytic approaches. For a long time he resisted what he experienced as major differences between the supervisors' interpretations and that of his own familiar personal analyst. Yet he recently began to discern familiarities and similarities between those approaches and his personal analysis. Somewhat later he was astonished to discover he could now differentiate the interpretations of the supervisors and even enjoy the new understanding he gained from each theory: "Once I could really implement processing analysis with my patients from within myself, my technique improved and I came to appreciate the value of my supervision and of my personal analysis. My attunement to my patients was also greatly increased."

Narcissistic immune processing, which integrates and regulates the three functions of narcissism, provides the necessary cohesiveness in familiarity, integrity, and stability to self-separateness in an affective state, from which interrelation with the world becomes possible without undermining equilibrium and safety. Cohesiveness in familiarity is linked to the familiar characteristics of inner experience of object constancy, self constancy, the familiar characteristics of object relationships. In healthy development of these constancies "the aggression is bound by libido and is in the service of affectionate object relationships and representations; conversely, in unhealthy development, as in the sadomasochistic relationships that characterize many of the attachments in abused children and their parents . . . object constancy is associated with an aggressive, pain-inflicting constant object. In these instances, tension reduction is preceded by sudden storms of painful aggression as compared or contrasted to gradual tension reduction associated with object constancy in which the love object representation is predominantly cathected with affectionate, pleasurable, self-esteem–promoting libidinal energies" (Solnit, 1982a, p. 209).

Whenever the narcissistic functions fail to recognize the familiar, strangeness is experienced, and the self is threatened with incohesiveness. The result is felt as an attack on the bodily and sense data, its identities, values, and self-attributes, or as an injury to its affective-state of narcissistic familiarity. *Defensive processing* is then activated by the narcissistic envelope (by splitting, denial, encapsulation, depletion, or narcissistic withdrawal), in order to preserve the self from incohesiveness and vulnerability during exposure to nonfamiliarities in interaction (by creating a false self-identity, by damage to the self-identities, by withdrawal into a narcissistic state) with a propensity for overwhelming helplessness and dissatisfaction within oneself. Activation of the mechanisms of adaptation and defense by the ego is comparable to the immunizing and defensive mechanisms in narcissism.

I believe the following clinical fragment sheds light on the connection between the narcissistic envelope and object relations, which is responsible for integrating most of the self-identities while interacting with others. It also illustrates how, when the immune narcissistic function fails to recognize minor differences as familiar particles, vulnerability emerges accompanied by narcissistic defenses and disturbances in object relations.

Tamar, an attractive woman in her late thirties, has achieved success in her familial and professional functions. She came to analysis complaining of progressive isolation from her husband and three children and dissatisfaction with herself. After many months of analysis, the subject of jealousy toward her sister came up. Although we dealt extensively with the subject through transference, neither of us could understand why she was still stuck in a repetitive cycle of feeling "awareness of childishness" and "my sister is always childish."

In the session detailed below, we explored those feelings in the context of her narcissistic vulnerability. It began with Tamar's associating as she described her family's weekend outing: "I've mentioned the great pleasure I feel whenever I see my husband hugging my daughter softly. But I also feel sorry for being unable to express my own tenderness for her, and I'm uneasy with this inner voice telling me that with such softness, my little girl may remain childish. I've known since early childhood the importance of being considered a mature person."

She paused briefly, as if to catch her breath, and continued: "Yesterday afternoon we took the children for a ride in the car. As we drove we joked, played games, and sang; I was familiar with most of the songs, which I sang as a child, and we were all enjoying our singing together in the car, it was lovely. But then I saw my husband glance at my little girl with such softness, and I felt a sudden need to be appreciated for being mature. That was the way my father always looked at my younger sister, whereas he'd look at me with love and appreciation in his eyes when I behaved maturely; this was how he reassured me that he loved me. But there in the car, I suddenly felt I needed that sort of fatherly glance, and became painfully aware that I could not give my own children this warmth that I so yearned for myself."

This very special moment shed light on Tamar's repeating over and over her childish expressions of love. Clearly, Tamar's narcissistic integrity found expression in her mature handling of relations with others—professional, social, and familial relations—as autonomy, self-esteem, and feelings of safety. But narcissistic tension and vulnerability arose whenever antagonistic deciphering could not be regulated and integrated: Deciphering the familiar in the paternal expression of love for her versus the strangeness of her father's expression of love for her sister. I clarified what she had just said: "You seem to have this need to be loved and appreciated for your matureness—this is your identity-frame for your father's expressions of love for you. But at the same time you also seem to be aware of the subtle difference in your father's soft glance for your sister. You've discovered that you yearned for this glance but also feared losing your unique self-esteem for being so mature."

The little girl who had wanted her father all to herself (oedipal object relation) was jealous of her younger sister for the differences (narcissistic deciphering) of love expression. While oedipal wishes of soft intimacy were inhibited by her superego, she defended herself narcissistically by denying her yearning for a soft glance and encapsulating the codes of warmth, excluding them from her narcissistic belongings and dissociating their code from the continuum of her love experiencing. She also protected herself by splitting off her self-identities: While preserving the integrity of a mature identity, she safeguarded her oedipal object relation in the space of mature love expression and split off the childish self-identity connected to the sister-father relation (which continued to move in her self-space). Any association hereafter with softness (e.g., whenever she wished to hug her children), threatened to undermine her integrity and triggered the sense of warmth as something unfamiliar, and with it the repetition of a familiar yet painful resistance against softness/childishness. I elaborated this point by saying: "You fear that your yearning for a soft glance is childish and view it as your separate code of identity for your sister."

This interpretation of her narcissistic defense liberated a flow of associations, including the need for that "soft glance," which was now generated by the familiar meaning of love, and many other experiences of loving parental warmth toward her during her childhood. She could now integrate and regulate "softness" into the continuum of love self-experiencing. In other words, her identity was sufficiently immunized for her to dare exposing herself to new interactions and object relations—so much so that she recently reported with pleasure that she was finally able to hug her children with all the softness she had always felt for them.

The narcissistic attribute of being loved is not a universal invariant but a unique and personal narcissistic feeling. By this I mean that feeling an expression of love may be a familiar affective-state for one person and an unfamiliar and intolerably painful state for another. The interacting self-identities must synchronize their separate love expressions and create a new narcissistically textured space-experience. In this common space of interaction demarcated as "media . . . by the mutual investment of the partners in a joint object, phenomenon, or idea cathected and meaningful to both" (Solan, 1991, p. 337), the separate self and separate other may differentiate, mediate, and enjoy each other.

CLINICAL IMPLICATIONS

The same can be said of the analyst/analysand relationship that unfolds in the analytic situation: it is indeed a microcosm and a stage for exploring the interaction between self and other (nonself). As such, the analytic interaction must include the three narcissistic functions of immunization mentioned above: namely, identifying the familiar and the unfamiliar and enjoying the minor differences in the separate other.

In the analytic setting, analyst and analysand share a common language of working through a mediating space, in which they mutually and simultaneously synchronize their efforts and invest in the common goal of enabling the analysis of unconscious expressions in the analysand (Solan, 1983, 1991). To achieve this goal, both parties must move jointly via their proximity and separateness, through exchanges of excitations that are linked to verbalized associations. While screening and differentiating the vibrations of each other and their common spaces, their narcissistic sensors may decipher in the atmosphere of the session what is familiar for each of them and may also differentiate unfamiliar particles, detect discrepancies, and work through them together by familiarizing themselves with the minor differences.

During this sharing of emotions and experiences, both self-identities need to be immunized in order for each to keep its self-spaces and characteristics from being confused with the other's, so as to protect their shared working alliance at times of separateness and vulnerability. This immunization enables both analyst and analysand to leave their self-spaces open to interaction. The process is a mutually rewarding experience; both self-identities are enriched by the reciprocated symbols and codes of their minor differences. (It may be compared to internalization.) The interaction leads to a similar narcissistic encryption of their new common "media" spaces of interaction, which will be demarcated, symbolized, and similarly shaped within both narcissistic envelopes, creating what is usually called a "common mind" or "outlook" when we encounter the other. The new intimate joint interaction will of course not be identical to any earlier interaction, object relation, or transference; it will only resemble them.

Through the intimate interactions that take place in psychoanalytic settings, where analyst and analysand can hear only each other's voice, they attune to each other and to each other's senses, regulating their associations and interpretations in their common space. The ongoing synchronization leads to affective and harmonious states of familiarity, safety, mutual trust, and reliance.

For instance, Tamar once reacted to an unsynchronized interpretation of mine that triggered her vulnerability by saying: "You are different today from what I expected. I wonder what happened to you. I feel your impatience and don't like it, but at the same time I like sensing that you are human and not always so tolerant." She had dealt with her narcissistic injury by sensing these minor differences and discrepancies, and differentiated them correctly as part of the analyst's belongings. Her comment led me to decipher the tone of my interpretation as resulting not from her material but from my countertransference. She thus gave evidence to my separateness from her, safeguarded her self, reestablished her safety-feeling in the object relationships, and kept the setting for our ongoing sharing and processing.

Failure in narcissistic immunization might damage a trusting relationship, upset the ongoing psychoanalytical processing, and even "block and nullify enriching experiences, turning potentially new situations into repetitions of old traumatic experiences" (Badaracco, 1992, p. 210). Thus, interpretations, minor changes in the psychoanalytic setting, or any deciphering of the unfamiliar might result in feelings of strangeness and rage toward the disappointing object (analyst/analysand) who "let" the self down. The analysand might then experience (by splitting) the analyst—or vice versa—as a nonself stranger who is responsible for his/her affective-states of injury (alienation). This may lead to avoidance and actual damage of the working alliance, destruction of the alien as analyst-object, or withdrawal into a narcissistic state.

This sequence of vulnerability disturbs the narcissistic state of inner equilibrium and integrity. For me, the crucial question at this time is, how will the analyst and analysand work through in order to preserve their self-identities and the shared space of interaction? How should each one deal with the narcissistic vulnerability that appears? How will each consider the other, who symbolizes many similar yet also strange sensorial images? How will they maintain their own uniqueness in object relations? How will they recover their equilibrium, enable new self-exposure to interaction, and open the self-spaces to further and mutually gratifying attunement with each other and others? I am not proposing a new clinical approach as the answer. However, when narcissistic vulnerability appears, I do suggest that we analyze—within the framework of these questions—the processings of self-immunization, self-defense, and renewal of the capacity for object relations.

The two vignettes presented below illustrate a common experience of analysand and analyst as well as that of many Israelis in relating to the assassination of Prime Minister Yitzhak Rabin in November 1995 and to the ongoing peace process. Many of my patients expressed themselves at the time in almost exact (yet also different) terms of vulnerability on both issues. In this paper I concentrate on those aspects that are akin to narcissistic vulnerability in the interaction between self and others, and on the mutual influence of the narcissistic immunization process and object relations. Although both clinical cases focus especially on the paternal object relation, other important psychoanalytical aspects, particularly the maternal and oedipal object relations, were also thoroughly worked through, as is customary in analysis.

CASE 1: MICHAEL

Michael is thirty-five years old, married, and the father of two young children. He is a pleasant person, with generally good family relations.

He is responsible, very punctual in attending his four sessions a week, and very successful at work. He is a reserve officer in the army, just like his father who was killed in the war when Michael was about ten years old.

Michael came to analysis complaining of frequent narcissistic vulnerability and sleeping difficulties. The following vignette took place after two years of analysis, following a period when we worked through his sharp longings and mourning for his father. We then focused on Michael's encapsulated anger for his father, who left him before he felt capable of undertaking the familial responsibilities. Through his transference, we worked on his apprehension concerning some disappointing aspects of the father's personality, which Michael so admired.

The father died when Michael was in his latency, a crucial stage of identification and internalization of cultural values. During analysis, he frequently repeated that his father "was a real hero who had great respect for his enemies." Michael succeeded in fulfilling his father's legacy of cultural human values by assuming responsibilities and by encapsulating "cursing" as if it were not part of his belongings. But whenever he sensed signs of aggression, his immune system failed, he felt criticized and discredited, as if he was a disappointment (by the paternal standards), and again complained of sleep problems.

Michael recently described his suffering to me: "Today at work, one of my colleagues asked me if I'd be in tomorrow. I said I would, but I immediately asked him whether he wanted to get rid of me. I felt his astonishment when he answered, 'Quite the opposite; I wanted to invite you to our professional meeting tomorrow.'" Michael suffered with such discrepancies, which highlighted his destructive narcissistic vulnerability.

The vignette detailed below took place two days after the Rabin assassination. I was impressed by the distress manifested by my patients at this time. The assassination, the horror, the mourning and grief, the need for togetherness and for condemnation of the outrage were the subjects discussed in every session or encounter with patients, family, and friends.

Michael was grief-stricken and depressed when he arrived for the session. He hardly said hello and went directly to lie down on the couch as I took my seat behind the headrest. He could not conceive that a Jew would assassinate the Jewish Prime Minister and said, "I and other decent people in this country are about to lose our cultural values and our unique Israeli identity. Is it possible that a law student, an educated man like myself and many other Israelis, can lose his self-control because of ideological differences? For me, this man has lost all human dignity and deserves no mercy."

I was deeply aware that we were all sharing an experience of intense vulnerability in facing any similarity between our own code of human identity and that of the assassin, yet the experience was different for each person. I listened while Michael verbalized his horror and repeated over and over, in agony, "I hope he will be locked up forever." In this particular session I noticed that my attunement to Michael's associations was being disturbed more than usual by my own associations. Having to differentiate his flow of associations from mine, I let myself dive into my own separateness, and a chain of associations led me to my own childhood. I was about seven years old when British tanks occupied Tel Aviv and imposed a strict curfew on the city during the Purim holiday. The streets were deserted except for the British soldiers in their red caps. I remember thinking: "How can it be that these people who look so similar to us and who probably have children like me are such monsters?" I recalled my anger at not being allowed to go out in my Peter Pan costume. Despite the curfew, I did go out (I don't know how I dared) to see for myself the horror of the British monsters while hoping to find human beings who were fond of children. I was almost in a state of shock when some soldiers gently lifted me up to their tank and played with me. I could remember the antagonistic feelings: On the one hand, anxiety and strangeness—I couldn't believe it was true—and on the other hand, feelings of friendly relief. I then ran home and excitedly cried out to my parents, in a victorious tone, "You see, they are nevertheless human beings, and they do love children!"

With these familiar sensorial images that emerged in my separateness, I could now return to the interaction in enough integrity to attune myself to Michael and grasp his flow of associations as he faced his nonself. Just then, I heard Michael say in distress: "This Jewish student who is just like me lost all human dignity by committing this horror." I could now connect this to Michael's father's being killed by those Arab "monsters" he respected but who lost their dignity when they killed him. I asked him, "Can you see any relation between your father's being killed by the Arabs he so respected as human beings like himself and your own agony before this Jewish student, who is so like you but has lost his human dignity?"

My words triggered an immediate reaction, and Michael began to cry: "You've hit the target. I can remember how the day my father was killed I felt he had been betrayed. He who always respected the Arabs was murdered by them. My whole world collapsed then, just as I feel now with Rabin's assassination. I remember how my father couldn't tolerate that my older brother used to curse me. The day he was killed I promised I would never curse anyone, never betray anyone, although my brother was the one who was always cursing. I have always kept my father's words as the legacy of what he wanted me to be as his son: 'To feel you are a man you must keep your dignity, not to impress others but for your own sake.'"

I realized that Michael's vulnerability also stemmed from deciphering his encapsulated and thus unfamiliar need to curse the student-killer. His super-ego had isolated the aggression to uphold the paternal object relation (worked through in the preceding period). I could sense Michael's encapsulation of sensorial aggression images as a narcissistic defense—as not part of his narcissistic belongings—which could otherwise undermine his self, and destroy his personal, paternal, and national ideals of self-identity. With this in mind, I commented, "It is as if you wanted to protect your own familiar identity and your father's gracious values against losing your dignity."

Michael was confused. How could he differentiate himself from this university student-assassin and protect his own and his father's self-identity concerning human values? He was narcissistically injured, as if he himself had lost his demarcated human identity because another student—one just like him—was now perceived as nonhuman, and he cried out, "It's too shocking. Ideological disagreements exist but the important difference is whether we can or can't argue decently. I hate the feeling of having anything in common with this nonhuman Jewish law student. It frightens me to think that this homicidal tendency might exist in all of us, just like the Arabs who killed my father. Where will it all lead us?" he asked in a troubled voice.

We both experienced a strong uneasiness in confronting such unfamiliarities and injury, and in deciphering this student as not one of our human self-belongings. Unlike my experience with the British, we found no relief in knowing that the assassin was one specific Jewish student, not the prototype of all Jewish students. But we did find some comfort in our sharing of common human values. We both probably needed to temper the threat of facing the unbearable alien space of the assassination by means of our jointness and by associating to the familiarities of each. Each of us had to find his own way to integrate the terrible implications of Rabin's assassination and bear the burden of a violent self-identity.

I commented on what he had just said: "You'd rather experience an identity that is free of what you perceive as nonhuman traits—like those of this man and of whoever killed your father." Michael retorted angrily, contradicting himself: "I don't really believe there's anything murderous within me. If I were to judge him I'd simply eliminate him from society right away." I interrupted him: "Do you realize that you just used the word 'eliminate'? Can you recognize this as a sign of violence?" "Yes," he answered, and continued hesitantly, "that's why I vowed to eliminate cursing from my language."

Michael then associated to what he felt when he got angry at his children: "I told you about eliminating cursing, but I'm also ashamed of feeling angry at my children. Funny, but I suddenly remember that I once visited my father at his military camp and saw him shouting at a soldier for disobeying his orders. It seems I'm afraid of losing my dignity-identity, and also of catching my father losing his control and dignity. To be honest, I felt relief when I saw that my father was also human and lost control just like I do." After a brief pause, he voiced his growing confusion: "Just a second, what am I saying? Is losing control human or nonhuman? When is it human and when does it become nonhuman? What about me, am I or am I not self-controlled?"

We both sank into a deep silence. I waited, aware of Michael's bewilderment and of his need to reorganize and immunize his self-identities and narcissistic belongings in integrity, while focusing on his familiar object relations with his father. In this sequence I could really sense an openness to acknowledge his encapsulated aggression and accept my view of him as being a person who contains aggression. After a while I commented: "I feel that accessing the nonhuman parts within you and within your paternal image is very painful, for at the same time you fear destroying the dignity and noble values of your father, like respecting even your enemies. You wanted to fulfill the paternal legacy by denying the nonhuman in yourself, in me, and in your father."

Michael related to my words: "Can I really accept myself with both of these trends coexisting in me? How can I come to terms with these nonhuman feelings in me, with the image of my father shouting, for 'man hath no preeminence above a beast' [Ecclesiastics 3:19] unless one acts differently. Clearly, there's also a violence in me that I was unaware of until now, the nonhuman within me. I feel like Adam and Eve in Paradise, when they sensed their nakedness and tried to cover up; I feel naked, divested of my self-esteem and in need to cover up—but I'm not alone. I feel I can share my feelings with you."

In fact, Michael was one of several patients who during this period associated to the story of Adam and Eve when facing such dramatic differences in their self-identity: Feelings of nakedness often precede the assessing of concealed encapsulated perceptions. Could this return to familiar and common social paradigms and proverbs (Biblical) bring relief to one's self-identity from a vulnerability related to the major differences? It is probably this need to share common feelings that Michael was expressing, and which I had felt before.

Michael seemed greatly relieved and closed the session by saying, "There's no choice: I must accept these inner feelings; but I must also find a dignified way to keep alive my father's last will, which means so much to me." I felt Michael's attempts to integrate these antagonistic feelings and reduce inner tension, but I also knew that it will take us time to work through his immune processing until he is able to open up to object relations of mutual respect.

CASE 2: DAVID

David is in his early forties, married, and the father of three children. He came to analysis because, although quite successful at work, he had difficulty maintaining good relations with his colleagues and often also with his wife. After almost three years of analysis four times a week, his interaction with others was still impaired by vulnerability and suspiciousness.

During the period in question David's analysis was deeply influenced by the ongoing peace-process negotiations. I avoided his provocative attempts to involve me in any political issues and concentrated on working through his narcissistic vulnerability in facing others. David was very suspicious of the Arabs. In one session, he said in a harsh tone: "How can we think of making peace with the Arabs and believing in their promises? When we do, we'll be unprotected, and they'll surely betray us with the worst terrorist attacks. It's crazy to think we can conduct a dialogue with such people. Another thing I can't understand is your refusal to tell me what you think about making peace with the Arabs."

For quite some time David seemed to suspect me of being his ideological adversary. The result was a narcissistic vulnerability toward my interpretations, as if he felt he could no longer recognize them as friendly and continue his dialogue with me. He seemed alienated by my reactions and tried hard to avoid any familiarity despite my interventions, as if I were going to betray him as he feared the Arabs would do if the peace process succeeded. His feelings of danger and repeated warnings in the media of forthcoming terrorist attacks preoccupied him. I asked myself whether these were "uncanny" feelings of danger, or whether his suspicion and vulnerability led him to perceive the prospects of peace as threatening his well-being. I too feared the threat of fanatic suicide bombers who might blow themselves up in our midst and had to curb my own familiar feelings of anxiety and join his particular suspicion, which was so different from mine. I offered him the following interpretation: "For a long time, in our common work here, you have been suspicious of me, as if I were going to betray you with my interpretations, just as you fear that the Arabs will betray you with their promises to make peace. Do these feelings remind you of something else that you are familiar with?"

I could feel his vulnerability as he angrily shook his head: "You are naive if you believe in peace; you just don't know what hell it will bring us. I could convince you if you'd only listen to me. Instead, you're trying to connect me to childhood feelings that have nothing to do with this."

We seemed to have lost each other. Had his vulnerability engulfed us, each in his own separateness? I searched for some familiar space between us that would allow David's self-identity sufficient safety to renew our interaction. I soon felt I could join his fears and anxiety without confusing them with mine and said, "I share your fears of more terrorist attacks in Israel. We are both familiar with such danger, but you also mistrust me because you believe that I'm not sufficiently aware of the danger and fear that I'm endangering you without your being able to protect yourself."

This time David appeared to be listening to me. His vulnerability had a different flavor when he answered, "There's something true in what you just said; I really feel the need to be alert against any attack. Otherwise, I remain unprotected, helpless, and nobody, not even you, will be able to help me."

For the first time, I felt that his words were very personal, unrelated to current political events. His association was the clue to how he managed to protect his self-identity, and I could sense the minor differences between us. For David self-immunization meant sensing the strangeness and being the first to strike when in danger of being attacked—thus, suspicion of anything or anyone alien (other) had top priority for him whereas my priority was to find common and familiar elements with the recalcitrant other. Sharing his uneasiness, I said calmly: "You probably always had to be on the alert for attacks, so you not only avoided feeling helpless but also abstained from befriending others. Is this way of protecting yourself familiar to you?"

In an aching tone, David associated to the time when his father became ill, a year before his death, and to how he felt he could no longer trust anyone: "Now it sounds ridiculous, but then I blamed my mother for not treating my father well enough; I really believed that, had she treated him better, he wouldn't have been ill or died. I know this is silly, but even now I sometimes have the same harsh feelings. I loved my father dearly. Yet, when I approached him gently to play with him, he'd often dismiss me, scold me for no clear reason, or suddenly, when I least expected it, start shouting at me. When I think of it now, maybe he was in such pain that my presence and my games were unendurable to him. I felt that in his illness my father betrayed me, and my mother was of no help." At this point, sensing the close interrelation between his transference of object relation and narcissistic repetition, I decided to interpret his psychic motion on both levels and said: "I feel your pain and disappointment as it was in the past with your father and mother, and as it is now with your feelings for me. Your need to play peacefully with your father also means that you feared being wounded or betrayed by him. It seems as if you must feel that familiar sense of alertness to the danger and pain that your loved ones, or others, may inflict on you with no warning. The need to protect yourself against being wounded by disappointment, betrayal, or attack is so familiar that even when unneeded, you continue to repeat it endlessly."

I felt that David had connected to his general suspicion of betrayal and could sense the strangeness in his interaction with others as well as his yearning for love and affection. He now associated with his children, whom he loved dearly yet treated impatiently when he was nervous. Despite his father's erratic behavior, he was depressed by the thought that, because of his overalertness, he had not been sufficiently aware or appreciative of his father's love for him.

In the following session David spoke excitedly of a television documentary he had seen about an Arab father who had discovered that the youth he had raised like a son was not his biological child. The father assured the young man that he didn't care whether in infancy the child was mistakenly exchanged for his real son, because he loved him, had raised him, and would not give him up now. David was deeply moved: "Can it be that 'they' [the Arabs] feel the same as I do?" he said in a sheepish tone.

Was David undergoing progressive familiarization with the image of the alien Arab and with the tenderness and affection that transcend suspicion? Could he now connect with his encapsulated code of affection, which he repeatedly mistrusted? This was a very moving moment in David's analysis. Now that his narcissistic vulnerability was moderated and his self-identity was better immunized through our interaction, he transferred onto me his need to examine his feelings together and temporarily reduced his level of suspicion.

David's voice interrupted my thoughts: "Before my whole life is wasted, I wish to be constructive rather than defensive, but I'm still hampered by my suspicions and I don't really know if I can trust others."

Our renewed interaction and immunization of self-identities were cut short by three massive suicide attacks perpetrated by Hammas terrorists during March 1996, which left some sixty dead and scores of wounded, and also deeply affected our befriending interaction. The renewed experience of the trauma that undermined our safety principle might cause us to revert to the old patterns of interaction before we had acquired sufficient new codes to recover from our narcissistic injuries. For each of us, David and myself, our narcissistic vulnerability in facing the trauma again might prevent us from relinquishing familiar ways of self-preservation in favor of others, still unfamiliar but perhaps better. Despite the ongoing threats of terrorist attacks, I hoped that we would achieve better "media" spaces of interaction codes through analysis, notwithstanding Freud's (1932) remark that enemies often remain entrenched in their familiar threats and hatreds rather than risk the unknown in the choice of peace.

I believe that these vignettes illustrate narcissistic processing in self-preservation. During interaction with others, the narcissistic quest for sameness and familiarities stimulates an affective state of safety, but it triggers vulnerability whenever any unfamiliarities are sensed. Narcissistic integration and regulation of the three deciphering processings —signs of familiarity, strangeness, and acceptance—immunize the self by means of integrity, cohesiveness, and continuity of sensorial images related to self-identities, object-identities, and their mediating relations (in self-spaces).

As the self becomes immunized, the other, via the interaction, may be narcissistically perceived as a differentiated and separate object with whom object relation becomes fruitful processing. When there is incoherence in the deciphering processing, suspicion is aroused against any strangeness and any new experiences. The object might then be narcissistically perceived as responsible for the analysand's self-injuries. Encapsulated codes that surface in psychoanalytic sessions as unfamiliar perceptions are worked through and might be reintegrated into the continuum of narcissistic coded networks to generate new yet similar meaning related to the object relation and to the actual interaction.

The clinical cases demonstrate the shifts that evolve between narcissistic processing and object relations. Hence, the working through of narcissistic vulnerability might enable analysts and analysands to overcome narcissistic injuries, reach new levels of libidinal gratification in object relations, and recover our affective state so that attunement to others as separate yet similar human beings will open the demarcated separateness to new mediating spaces of meaningful interaction.

BIBLIOGRAPHY

ANZIEU, D. (1985). *Le Moi-Peau.* Paris: Dunod (published as *The Skin Ego* by Yale University Press, 1989.)
———— (1987). Formal signifiers and the ego-skin. In *Psychic Envelopes*, pp. 11–16. London: Karnac Books.
BADARACCO, J. E. G. (1992). Psychic change and its clinical evaluation. *Int. J. Psycho-Anal.* 73:209–220.
BICK, E. (1968). The experience of the skin in early object relations. *Int. J. Psycho-Anal.* 49:484–486.
BION, W. R. (1962). *Learning from Experience.* New York: Basic Books.
BOLLAS, C. (1992). *Being a Character.* London: Routledge.
EMDE, R. N. (1988). Development terminable and interminable. Part I. *Int. J. Psycho-Anal.* 69:23–42.
ESMAN, A. H. (1983). The "stimulus barrier." A review and reconsideration. *Psychoanal. Study of the Child* 38:193–207.
FREUD, S. (1895). Project for a scientific psychology. *S.E.* 1:295–344.
———— (1914). On Narcissism: an Introduction. S. E., 14: 67–102.
———— (1917). The taboo of virginity (contributions to the psychology of love III), *S.E.* 11:193–208.
———— (1919). The "Uncanny." *S.E.* 17:217–253.
———— (1920). Beyond the pleasure principle. *S.E.* 18:7–64.
———— (1921). Further problems and lines of work. *S.E.* 18:100–104.
———— (1923). The ego and the id. *S.E.* 19:19–28.
———— (1925). Negation. *S.E.* 19:235–243.
———— (1926). Inhibitions, symptoms and anxiety. *S.E.* 20:77–175.
———— (1929). Civilization and its Discontents. *S.E.* 21:64–145.
GRUNBERGER, B. (1971). *Narcissism Psychoanalytic Essays.* Madison, Conn.: Int. Univ. Press.
HOUZEL, D. (1990). The concept of psychic envelope. In *Psychic Envelopes*. London: Karnac Books, pp. 11–16.
———— (1996). The family envelope and what happens when it is torn. *Int. J. Psycho-Anal.* 77:901–912.
JOFFE, W. G. & SANDLER, J. (1968). Adaptation, affects and the representational world. In *From Safety to Superego*, ed. J. Sandler. London: Karnac Books, pp. 180–190, 221–234.
KERNBERG, O. F. (1974). *Borderline Conditions and Pathological Narcissism.* New York: Jason Aronson.
———— (1983). *Internal World and External Reality.* New York: Jason Aronson.
KOHUT, H. (1971). *The Analysis of the Self.* New York: Int. Univ. Press.

———— (1977). *The Restoration of the Self.* New York: Int. Univ. Press.

LAOR, N. (1990). Seduction in Tongues: Reconstructing the field of metaphor in the treatment of schizophrenia. In G. L. Ormiston and R. Sossower (Eds.), *The Discrimination of Medical Authority: Contributions to Medical Studies,* No. 27, pp. 141–175. New York: Greenwood.

MODELL, A. H. (1993). *The Private Self.* Cambridge: Harvard Univ. Press.

MORRISON, A. P. (ed.). (1986). *Essential Papers on Narcissism.* New York: Univ. Press.

MOSES, R. & BENE-MOSES, A. (1980). Psychoanalytic perspectives of the Middle East process. *Samiksa* 34: 117–129.

OGDEN, T. H. (1992). *The Primitive Edge of Experience.* London: Maresfield Library/Karnac Books.

ROSENFIELD, I. (1992). *The Strange, Familiar and Forgotten. An Anatomy of Consciousness.* London: Picador/Macmillan General Books.

SANDLER, J. (1987). *From Safety to Superego.* London: Karnac Books.

———— (1990). On internal object relations. *J. Amer. Psychoanal. Assn.* 38:859–880.

———— (1994). The unconscious and the representational world. In *Psychoanalysis and Development,* eds. M. Ammaniti & D. Stern. New York: New York Univ. Press.

SANDLER, J. ET AL. (eds.) (1991). *Freud's "On Narcissism: An Introduction."* New Haven & London: Yale University Press.

SOLAN, R. (1983). Closeness in the psychoanalytic encounter. *Bull. Psychoanal. Europe* 20/21:65–84.

———— (1989). Objet transitionnel—symbolisation—sublimation. *Rev. Franc. Psychonal.,* Vol. 33:(6)1843–1846.

———— (1991). "Jointness" as integration of merging and separateness in object relations and narcissism. *Psychoanal. Study of the Child* 46:337–352.

———— (1996). The leader and the led—their mutual needs. In *Psychoanalysis at the Political Border.* Madison, Conn.: Int. Univ. Press, pp. 237–255.

———— (1998). Narcissistic fragility in the process of befriending the unfamiliar. *Amer. J. Psycho-Anal.,* Vol. 58:(2)163–186.

SOLNIT, A. (1982a). Developmental perspectives on self and object constancy. *Psychoanal. Study of the Child* 37:201–218.

———— (1982b). Early psychic development as reflected in the psychoanalytic process. *Int. J. Psycho-Anal.* 63:23–36.

STERN, D. N. (1985). *The Interpersonal World of the Infant.* New York: Basic Books.

STOLOROW, R. D. (1975). Toward a functional definition of narcissism. *In Essential Papers on Narcissism,* ed. A. P. Morrison. New York: Univ. Press, pp. 197–209.

TUSTIN, F. (1990). *The Protective Shell in Children and Adults.* New York: Karnac Books.

WINNICOTT, D. W. (1965). *The Maturational Processes and the Facilitating Environment.* London: Hogarth Press.

CLINICAL PAPERS

Obsessional Manifestations
in Children

JUDITH FINGERT CHUSED, M.D.

Material is presented from the analyses of three children who developed obsessional behavior during the course of their analytic work. The author's intent is to use a careful examination of the emergence of these children's obsessions to try to understand the unconscious determinants that lead to the development of obsessive-compulsive behavior as a way to deal with psychic distress.

THE PHARMACOLOGICAL TREATMENT OF OBSESSIONAL SYMPTOMATOL-ogy has received much publicity in recent years (Rasmussen, 1993), with early reports of a specificity that rivals that of lithium and the neuroleptics. Enthusiasm also greeted Freud's discoveries, and initially psychoanalysis was hailed as a panacea for the neuroses. But just as medication appears to be less useful than first suggested (Leonard, 1996), so psychoanalysis has proved to have definite limitations, even in the treatment of the disorders for which it was initially intended. Unfortunately, these limitations are often all too evident in work with obsessional neuroses and character disorders. In spite of an intellectual appreciation of the symptoms and the underlying conflicts, many obsessional patients get little therapeutic benefit from psychoanalysis. And although a number of explanations have been given for the unyielding quality of obsessional phenomena, from organic pathology to

Clinical professor of psychiatry and behavioral sciences and of pediatrics at George Washington University School of Medicine; training/supervising analyst (child, adolescent, and adult), Washington Psychoanalytic Institute; editorial board, *Psychoanalytic Quarterly* and *Journal of the American Psychoanalytic Association.*

The Psychoanalytic Study of the Child 54, ed. Albert J. Solnit, Peter B. Neubauer, Samuel Abrams, and A. Scott Dowling (Yale University Press, copyright © 1999 by Albert J. Solnit, Peter B. Neubauer, Samuel Abrams, and A. Scott Dowling).

structural vulnerability, a unifying etiology, a definitive lesion in the caudate nuclei or a specific ego deficit has not been identified.

I do not believe there is a single etiology for all obsessional phenomena, be they ego-alien symptoms or integrated character traits. However, I suspect that some common factors other than unconscious conflict are responsible for their production. The question is how to identify these factors.

In childhood, obsessional symptoms are common. Compulsive rituals or obsessional doubting frequently occur during periods of rapid development—for example, in the rapprochement phase, at the beginning of latency, or during adolescence. Such symptoms often arise and then disappear without treatment. They are understood to reflect the child's attempt to master and control potentially disruptive changes in his physical and psychic state. On the other hand, obsessional symptoms may also herald a more malignant psychotic process, particularly when they are unremitting, with temper tantrums and ego disorganization if interrupted.

Children, more than adults, express their conflicts and concerns through action in the external world. Because of the immaturity of their defenses, the specific motivators and symbolic meaning of their actions are frequently discernible (even if not therapeutically interpretable). It is my hope that exploration of the rituals that develop during children's analyses will further our knowledge of the origins of obsessional mechanisms. For even though obsessional manifestations in children may have a different pathological significance than similar manifestations in adults, the use of obsessions as a compromise formation, dealing with conflict by providing a sense of control over the uncontrollable, is the same.

Child analysis offers us a unique opportunity to study obsessional mechanisms, as not infrequently even children who begin psychoanalysis with no obsessions develop such symptoms over the course of the work. Often this is in response to conflictual material that is emerging through the analysis. However, if one observes the development of the obsessional behavior *in statu nascendi,* before there is a secondary elaboration of meaning and function, the factors eliciting the symptoms and the determinants of the choice of obsessions can be identified.

With this in mind, I examined carefully the process surrounding the emergence of obsessional behavior during the analyses of my child patients. Using material from three analyses I hope to demonstrate the factors that I believe are significant determinants of such behavior. Although only one child presented with obsessional symptoms, during each child's analysis certain actions originating within the therapeutic process were repeated with the urgency and specificity of a compulsion.

CARL

Carl was six years old when he first came to my office. His father and step-mother could no longer tolerate their anxiety over his ceaseless pacing and endless washing rituals, his rage reactions whenever a ritual was interrupted, and his sad, desperate demeanor. Carl's mother had abandoned him when he was three; he was brought to me by his father. Ten years earlier I had evaluated Carl's older brother for depression.

Carl's rituals were ever-present throughout his analysis; from his habitual pacing and counting whenever he felt stressed to more specific rituals around eating and toileting, Carl did little that was not driven, repetitive, and accompanied by multiple explanations and rationalizations. For example, when ending his analytic sessions became difficult, Carl began counting off each second of the final five minutes. He became frantic when the numbers on the clock changed before he had finished with a minute and insisted on unplugging the clock to get it "right."

In the second year of treatment, as Carl struggled between identification with his father (being tough) versus being his love object (which was represented in play by draping his head with a towel to have "girl's hair"), Carl became obsessed with the idea of germinating seeds. He brought in several acorns from outside, and, wrapping them gently in paper towels, he planted them in bathroom cups, which he hid about my office. He talked about what it meant to be able to make seeds grow and spontaneously compared it to making babies. He asked me how many babies I had had—stating emphatically that, as he was younger, he could top any number I had produced. But as he tried to figure out just how many children I had from the accoutrements he had seen around my home office (a basketball net, a dog and cat, school bumper stickers), logic failed him, and he became confused. He tried to connect the basketball net with a little boy he had seen (a girl couldn't have a "real" setup). But the boy was too little to play basketball—maybe the teenager who came before him wasn't really a patient but my son saying goodbye on his way to school. He questioned whether he had really seen the net, left the office to check if it was there, and then as soon as he returned had to hurry back outside because he wasn't sure that the place where he had seen the net (which he had walked past on the way to my office hundreds of times) was really on my property. He finally decided that I didn't have any children yet as he'd never seen me pregnant, said all the talk about "making babies" was making him nervous, and returned to the seeds.

Over the next few weeks, as he continued to plant seeds every day, his technique became increasingly ceremonial and eventually the original connection to making babies or even to making things grow was lost. Two acorns soon became twenty and by the time he was finished with this activity, he had planted over three hundred objects, including pebbles, raisins, and pieces of glass. This activity totally preoccupied him for more than six months.

Over the course of Carl's analysis, we came to understand the genesis of his distress; abandoned by his mother for causes unknown to him, he decided she had left his father (and him) because she didn't like men. As it was women to whom his father turned to share his time in the evening, his bed, and his grown-up ideas, Carl had the fantasy that becoming a woman was a way to prevent abandonment. As might be expected, this fantasy increased his anxiety, not only because of the physical consequences, the reality of biology, but also because women weren't protected against loss any more than men were; after all, his father had already divorced several wives and wasn't particularly satisfied with the current one. As Carl played out his fantasies and the related fears, he was competitive with me, then angry, then bewildered. I, in turn, was impressed by his power to irritate me and simultaneously stimulate my desire to help him. He truly didn't seem to know how he felt about me; afraid to trust, fearful that I would take from him what he wished to extract from me (my ability to procreate), drawn by my acceptance of him to test out some of his phallic and self-asserting impulses, he again and again ended the hour in confusion, attempting to control the world of the office and his conflicting emotions by the most comfortable means, his rituals. Whether seeds or seconds, Carl's hours were filled with rituals; together we were burdened, overwhelmed, and exhausted by them.

The immediate stimulus for the development of his counting and planting ritual was heightened affect within the session, a mixture of longing, anger, and fear. But why it was rituals rather than, for example, play disruption or phobias was unclear. Popular explanations for obsessional phenomenon in children—a strong drive endowment, intellectual precocity, hypersensitivity to stimuli, with the child drawn prematurely to cognitive defenses in response to the threat of being overwhelmed by internal or external stimuli—seem insufficient to account for the "choice" of obsessional behavior.

Prior to her departure when Carl was three, his mother had been withdrawn and depressed for many months. The history, as told by the father, suggested that Carl had never had the opportunity to predictably and consistently engage her. By six, in his awkward approach to me and others, he gave the appearance of being helplessly incompetent in the world of human relationships. An intolerance of strong emotion—not just anger but also sadness and longing, loving feelings—was a major focus in his analysis. He seemed to feel afraid of any emotion; he was as likely to begin counting (or, later, clutch his penis) when he felt understood and appreciated, as when my words produced pain. When affects were stimulated, the psychic sensations themselves seemed to be experienced as dangerous and potentially overwhelming. Anger, particularly anger at a parent and later at me, seemed to be the most frightening. All three parents were idealized, with Carl using denial and displacement to hold his anger in check and to preserve his parents as aggrandized protectors against the angry (through projection) world. At first, it was only in the transference that rage at important objects could be fully expressed.

At the close of Carl's analysis, his sadness and anxiety were reduced, as was the confusion which had been his response to (and defense against) ambivalence and conflicting affect states. Correspondingly, his obsessional symptomatology had disappeared, although a reluctance to join unstructured playground activities at school was evidence of residual character limitations.

A call from his father several years after termination revealed that Carl was "doing well," with no return of the obsessional symptoms but with behavioral standards that Carl himself realized were unrealistically rigid and he talked of "working on" them some day. The phrase, "working on" sounded so much like Carl, a little old man at sixteen as he had been at six.

KAREN

Karen[1] entered analysis at age five because of incapacitating fears of robbers, poison, kidnappers, and ghosts. She was overly attached to her mother, became panicked when separated from her, and was very jealous and aggressive toward her two-year-old sister. An ever-present anticipation of deprivation made her bossy and selfish, completely unable to share, delay gratification, or play with peers.

---

1. I described another aspect of Karen's analysis in *Child and Adolescent Analysis: Its Significance for Clinical Work with Adults,* ed. by Scott Dowling (Madison, Conn.: Int. Univ. Press, 1990), pp. 37–54.

During the course of her analysis, as Karen struggled with her mixed erotic and aggressive feelings for me (part of the transference reenactment of her early relationship with her mother), a ritual developed, a first in the history of this very creative, spirited, and overstimulated little girl. Karen came into my office one day, clearly in a bad mood, and began to ask me to do things that from past experience she knew I would not (read her a story, comb her hair, allow her into the living quarters above my office). She agreed that she only wanted what wasn't available and said that there was no one to play with, her sister was being a baby, and her mother was out of town. With that she fell into my lap. As she struggled to find a more comfortable position, her movements became more and more aggressive, leading me to say, "I think you don't know whether you want to cuddle or fight." With one last elbow thrust to my chest, she jumped from my lap and shouted, "Think, pink—all you do is stink!" She continued to yell at me as she bounced around the office, pointing out one flaw after another in my clothes, the furniture, the toys, the artwork, the plants. Turning to my desk, Karen said, "You're so messy; how can you be a feelings doctor and figure out feelings if you can't even keep your desk straight?" She then proceeded to clean the desk or, more specifically, to clean a multi-compartment box on the desk that contained pencils, pens, paperclips, stamps, etc., exclaiming as she cleaned about how messy I was, how I needed someone to take care of me, and how terrible my mother was for not teaching me to be neat.

Over the next four months, regardless of the topic, Karen returned to cleaning the box whenever strong feelings for me emerged. Her behavior was always the same. First she would circle the desk, glance over at me as if to say, "Don't interfere," and then seize the box and dump its contents onto the floor. Grabbing two pieces of Kleenex and folding them neatly, she would carefully wipe out all the corners of the box and then neatly return the contents to their original compartments. Karen cleaned the box on an average of three out of four sessions, sometimes not touching it for several days, other times "cleaning" it two or three times in a session. As she cleaned she sometimes talked about how messy I was and how important it was to get all the crevices and corners in the box clean. From her talk about my messiness, she moved to how she felt sorry for me because my mother hadn't taught me well. I said she seemed to know a lot about what mothers should do. She responded quickly, "Don't be sad, my mother goes out of town a lot and *I've* learned how to keep my room clean." Not so quick was the exposure of her anger at this often unavailable mother and her fear that she had driven her mother away with her "dirty messiness."

Karen's "cleaning," a multiply determined compromise formation, eventually generated much useful analytic work. But in addition, as an outlet for her drive to action, it permitted her to express the wish to touch and fondle (or hit) me without the associated guilt and shame an actual attempt would produce and allowed her to become aware of her own wishes to be touched without being overwhelmed or frightened by the impulse and the accompanying fantasies.

On the surface her cleaning was similar to Carl's planting of seeds— it was repetitive and ritualistic, always done the same way with the same sequence of actions, and with a subjective feeling of relief from inner pressure once completed. However, when Karen was unable to follow through on her impulse (as happened one day when my desk and the box were covered with papers that I asked her not to disturb), although she was disappointed, and experienced my prohibition as a condemnation of more forbidden, guilt-provoking wishes (becoming quite defensive and retaliatively angry), she was able to give up the action for the moment without disorganization. This was in spite of such intense anger that all semblance of a positive relationship disappeared.

It was different with Carl. When one day he was unable to plant the seeds he had brought because there were no more paper cups in the bathroom, his response was dramatic. He became desperate and confused about what to do with the seeds. As the idea of waiting until the next day was intolerable, he spent the whole hour obsessing about whether to combine the new seeds with old ones he had already planted, wrap the new seeds in wet paper towels, or throw the new seeds away. He tried to coerce me into giving him more paper cups, but when it became clear that I either would not or could not (he wasn't sure which) provide the cups immediately, his anxiety and internal pressure to carry out his ritualized act were so great that he was unable to hear anything I said. It took about 25 minutes for him to quell his agitated confusion and shore up his regressed ego functioning (a frightening time for us). Eventually he began to attend to me. At first all he was aware of was my non-compliance, and as his rage mounted, he became frightened of how angry he was. When I neither yielded nor became angry back, his rage turned to tears. But when he talked about how helpless he felt, how helpless he always felt, and I seemed to understand, the pressure to plant momentarily disappeared.

Karen and Carl had had important yet different experiences with helplessness. Although Karen had been overstimulated and underdisciplined by her immature, self-indulgent mother, she had had no significant losses or prolonged separations during her life; the external dangers in her world were principally projections of her own impulses and fantasies. Carl, however, had suffered major trauma; not only had he lost his mother; he also was prevented from grieving the loss by his father's need to deny her importance. And even though her mother was overstimulating, Karen's fantasy of a negative oedipal victory was never reinforced by external reality. Carl, on the other hand, at times really believed that such a victory was possible, and the pleasure these thoughts provided, though colored by castration fears, increased his guilt over his mother's leaving. His capacity to trust both himself and others was far more limited than Karen's.

As Anna Freud said, "Losing a love object in early life . . . is an experience which can initiate a variety of disturbances. What is significant for obsessional neurosis is not the event as such but the child's belief that it is the result of his own death wishes and the feelings of guilt attached to this interpretation" (1996, pp. 252–53).

DEBRA

The last child I wish to mention is a ten-year-old girl whose preoccupying fantasies were related to chronic overt sexual stimulation by her mother. Debra's conscious erotic fantasies[2] tended to intrude into all her relationships, and by the time she came to analysis she was quite isolated from her peers. Although Debra denied any concern about her lack of friendships, withdrawal from peer activities led to a persistent overinvolvement with her mother and intensified the related conflicts.

Debra was not obsessional in character; her pathology was more in the area of self-esteem regulation. She expected constant praise for her intelligence and talent (which were considerable); any narcissistic disappointment led to sudden rage followed by withdrawal and contempt for her unappreciative audience.

Debra's obsessional activity in the analysis began shortly after a "confession" of masturbation. She made the "confession" while she was decorating a lamp in my office that is in the shape of a glass ball. She and other children I analyze have discovered that this ball (lit by an interior light bulb) melts any crayons pressed to its surface and it had become a means for them to draw, mess, and play out conflicts. The crayon melting for Debra began in this hour as a distraction, intended, I believe, to draw off some of the motor tension she was feeling as she told me of her masturbation. The "confession" had come after many months of

2. Debra was first described in "The evocative power of enactments." *J. Am. Psychoanal. Assn.* 39:615–39.

frustrating silence alternating with polite, clipped sentences. Debra had indicated all along that she had no interest in either being with me or talking to me and that she didn't understand why her parents thought I could help her, particularly since nothing bothered her. Although she initiated the "confession," she began by saying there was something she did that she guessed I might be interested in since *I* was so nosey. Her tone made it perfectly clear that she resented being "forced" to talk, that I, not she, was the one who was interested in problems. It was somewhat defiantly, then, as she melted a crayon, that she said she sometimes stuck her finger "in there" to see if she was clean.

At this point she became aware of a design left by another child and, with competitive vigor, wiped off the other child's work and took over the lamp. The next hour she returned to the lamp as soon as she entered the office, and by the end of the week crayon melting had become her only activity (other than speech). Within two weeks her crayon melting had become as ritualized as Carl's planting of seeds. At first she pretended that the melting crayons were men trying to cross over a barrier that she had to keep clean. This she felt more free to talk about. If they were able to dribble across the barrier before she could wipe them away, they would be free to do evil. She, by keeping the barrier clean (and destroying the dribbles), prevented the evil.

While she melted crayons and told me of the struggles with the evil men, Debra spoke of her dislike of the other children who "dared" disturb her leavings. She claimed indifference to my thoughts about them (or her). However, after she had been at the lamp for several weeks she said she thought I must be very angry about the messing (though I kept it hidden, she said, because I was supposed to "act" like a "good doctor"). Gradually her transference misperceptions and preoccupying sexual daydreams became interwoven, and she developed an erotic fantasy of my spanking her. She imagined that I would act in anger but claim it was "for her own good."

As she began to articulate more directly the fantasy of my spanking her, the "lamp game" lost its specific content and became once again an activity that served to drain off motor energy and make talking tolerable. The crayon melting continued for several more months, ritualistically, but with less interest. Its function had shifted from being a symbolic enactment in play and within the transference of sado-masochistic anal fantasies (not only did she create an incredible mess on and around the lamp, but regardless of the colors other children used, after Debra's hour the lamp was always yellow-brown) to being a means to release enough of the affective tension associated with her aggressive and erotic fantasies for her to tolerate talking about them.

DISCUSSION

In many ways, the rituals these children developed during their analyses were similar. The degree of urgency and their response to interference with their rituals varied, as did, obviously, the conflictual impulses revealed in their actions. And the stimulus was different for each child; Debra, for example, would turn her back on me and increase her absorption in melting whenever she felt I was being intrusive. However, the persistence, predictability, and rigidity of the rituals were the same for each child. Their specific pathology—obsessional or phobic neurosis, narcissistic behavior disorder with self-isolation—was not reflected in the structure of their behavior. In fact, it was the similarity in structure that first made me wonder whether there were non-specific motivators for repetitive, compulsive actions.

With each child, the "analytic ritual" developed when conflictual impulses toward me led to an arousal of feelings that were uncontainable. That is, the tension created by the affective arousal was so great that motor action could not be forestalled through fantasy, thought, or verbalization of conflict. Karen knew that her squirming on my lap was hurting me but also that she wanted to be close to me. Both impulses were experienced as "forbidden"; naming them only increased her tension. They were too strong, and her experience with play, her ability to sublimate, was too limited to make doll playing or drawing a useful form of expression. In addition, conscious thought was still too much an inner parental voice, carrying superego injunctions, for her to derive relief from "figuring out," from cognitively derived "insight." Her need for some form of motor activity was, in part, a reflection of her ego immaturity and vulnerability, of her being a child. However, a motoric restlessness, a need for motor discharge, is evident in adult obsessionals also, when psychic arousal leads to a physical tension that is uncontainable.

Of the children presented, only Carl had an obsessional neurosis. But all of them, during times of ego regression and intensification of primitive impulses and affects (that is, during times of intense transference experience), developed obsessional mechanisms. The common factors that seemed to contribute to their ritualistic behavior were, first, a fear of being overwhelmed by the affect associated with their conflictual impulses; second, a push to action (either motoric or cognitive) when stressed; and, third, *an inability to use others for help in controlling the feelings.*

The inability to use the analyst and the analytic process for relief from immediate psychic stress was related, I believe, to the ambivalence and the intensity of the transference feelings in the child at the time the rituals developed. This perception of affective arousal as *a danger that must be mastered by the individual alone* seems specific to the development of obsessional phenomena (and is unlike phobic or conversion symptoms, in which the patient remains dependent on and interactive with the external world, and depression, in which the attempt to master the danger has been abandoned).

The severely obsessional individual, child or adult, appears to gain little pleasure or benefit from the successful completion of his ritual; all he feels usually is a momentary relief from the urgency, which is all too soon attached to the next compulsion or obsession. During and after the obsessional activity, although the rise in tension followed by abrupt relief has an orgiastic quality, the only conscious gratification is the relief from tension. The power of an obsession to enslave the individual and render reality empty by comparison is impressive. Like masturbation, obsessional activity leaves no room for the other—the individual is both the subject and object, both attacked and attacker. When only the ritual matters, self-reflective functioning ceases, and external reality and human objects have no appeal. And so there arises one of the self-perpetuating problems that seem to characterize obsessional phenomena. Distrustful of objects because of his own ambivalence, the ritual maker must rely on himself for relief from tension. And once a ritual is underway, little in the external world can interrupt it.

All three children had repeated painful experiences in which overwhelming affective arousal, through genital overstimulation (Karen and Debra), interference with autonomous activity (Debra), or inexplicable loss (Carl), developed within important relationships. However, only Carl had a generalized fear of the intimacy in relationships that stimulates feelings. Only Carl used obsessional mechanisms to keep the humans in his environment at arm's length, rendering them helpless to strengthen his ability to deal with the human world. His rituals were the most painful to witness—the urgency to complete, the intense terror when a ritual was interrupted, and the episodes of disorganization were evidence of his fear.

Of the patients presented, only Carl, with a true obsessional neurosis, was convinced that aggression, once expressed, could not be contained and would result in total destruction of the object and complete isolation of the self. It is noteworthy that Freud (1909, p. 235), when he spoke of the obsessional's belief in the omnipotence of thought (particularly of the tremendous power of thought to do harm), emphasized the intensity of affect. And the specific use of obsessional defenses for "affective distancing" was discussed by Sandler and Joffe (1965).

A number of factors, such as neurological damage, constitutional vulnerability, insufficient affect modulation by primary objects early in life, and past traumatic experiences in which helplessness is associated with affect arousal, can lead to intolerance of strong affect. Regardless of the determinants, when strong affect is intolerable, it not infrequently will be defended against by "dehumanization" of the world and the interpersonal relationships within it. Situations that are potentially overstimulating and disorganizing are avoided. Object relationships are avoided because of the affect aroused. And empathy does not exist because of the discomfort stimulated by trial identifications.

The infant and young child use their early object relationships for many things. Identification with objects is essential in the formation of psychic structure, including the structural elements responsible for affect tolerance. However, a child who fears being overwhelmed by affective experiences tends to avoid spontaneous human interaction. And when he utilizes projection and denial (defenses common to all young children) to deal with his own aggression and impulsivity, without the correction provided by experience with a trusted other, the perceived danger in human relationships will grow without check. It is not surprising, then, that a child who resorts to obsessional defenses early in life is at risk for the development of a psychotic process later. With an early avoidance of intimate relationships, not only the development of affect tolerance but also the capacity to reality test, to think, is severely limited. In essence, the development of all ego functions is compromised when receptivity in object relationships and identifications with others are blocked.

Identifications also occur in adulthood. But with an absence of intimate relationships, there is no bond within which identification can develop. In his avoidance of intimacy, which might stimulate unanticipated affects, the obsessional individual loses both the opportunity to increase his capacity for affect tolerance and the experience of pleasure in human interactions.

Affect intolerance is a major problem in the analytic treatment of obsessional individuals. Analysis is a relationship-based therapy; when the experience of intense feelings within the analytic relationship is painful or frightening, early transferences can call forth such strong obsessional defenses that it may be impossible to develop a full analytic process.

Resistance to the transference occurs often with the severe obsessional, with or without overt symptoms. Avoiding intimacy, the obsessional remains self-isolated; in an empty analytic situation, his pathology remains unchanged.

Through my work with obsessional patients I have become convinced that in addition to being precise in the content of my interpretations, I must pay particular attention to the patient's level of arousal and be prepared to talk with him or her about any change in affect state following an intervention. These patients have defended against "outside influence" for so long that unanticipated sensations not infrequently lead to confusion and anxiety, which, in turn, lead to anger against the cause of the distress (the analyst). Such anger is then often projected, producing a paranoid perception of the analyst as intentionally hurtful. At these moments, if the analyst accepts the attributes ascribed to herself and invites the patient to "analyze the analyst," to speculate why the analyst acted as perceived, the patient can often reintegrate and begin to explore his or her experience with less affective arousal. It's as if the analyst's tolerance of the accusations makes the patient's rage less frightening for the patient. Occasionally the behavioral manifestation of the patient's affective reaction to the analyst's interventions is a tightly controlled withdrawal; at such moments the withdrawal must be addressed before the content of the "original" conflicts is explored.

Obsessional mechanisms are not always pathological. In a child or an adult with a history of explosive out-of-control action or ego disorganization when stressed, obsessional mechanisms that develop to deal with the threat of being overwhelmed by affective arousal can be an indication of significant ego development. During early latency, obsessional phenomena are common as the superego of the child becomes increasingly intolerant of id impulses; at that time they contribute to the latency child's increased capacity for cognitive growth. In an analytic patient, struggling with internal conflict, as affect is stimulated by the analytic process, new obsessional mechanisms may herald the emergence of the conflict into the transference. And in the analyst who is "stuck" in a confusing process with the patient, obsessional ruminations may lead to new understanding.

Obsessions can develop in anyone when strong affective arousal is accompanied by a feeling of helplessness. Fortunately, many patients can modify the sensation of helplessness, with increased tolerance for the affect, through their own ego capacities (such as reality testing, memory, cognitive processing) as well as through the temporary use of the therapist as an auxiliary ego. What makes the obsessional patient so difficult to work with are his distrust of others, his fear of losing control, and his disbelief in the reliability of his own perceptions and judgment. When the patient's abhorrence of affective arousal leads to an avoidance of engagement within the therapeutic relationship, the therapist is rendered ineffective, unable to contain and modulate the affect enough for it to be tolerated. And when this patient cannot tolerate the experience of affect, there can be no analytic experience.

BIBLIOGRAPHY

FREUD, A. (1966). "Obsessional Neurosis: A Summary of Psychoanalytic Views," in *The Writings of Anna Freud,* V. New York: Int. Universities Press, pp. 246–61.

FREUD, S. (1909). "Notes upon a case of obsessional neurosis." *S.E.,* 10.

LEONARD, H. (1966). Personal communication.

RASMUSSEN, S. A., ET AL. (1993). "Current issues in the pharmacologic management of obsessive compulsive disorder." *J. Clin. Psychiatry,* 54 Suppl. 4–9.

SANDLER, J. & JOFFE, W. (1965). "Notes on obsessional manifestations in children." *Psychoanal. Study Child,* 20:425–38.

Narrative Performance Mode (NPM) of Discourse

DONALD J. COLEMAN, M.D.

The nature of narrative is explored as well as why narrative has been so natural and so important, universal to people worldwide through the centuries. The function served by stories is explored. Attempts are made to mine the structure of narrative and to answer the reader's question: how will this help me in my day-to-day work as a psychoanalyst? The basic necessities of story are enumerated, and some of the constitutive elements of narrative are contrasted with other modes of discourse. Freud's comments in The Poet and the Daydream *are taken quite literally in this essay, which stresses the influence of unconscious process on changing modes of discourse.*

That moment when the analyst or analysand switches from one mode of discourse to another, here called a juncture, is compared to the pauses, doubts, and changes of venue within the dream. Modes of discourse psychology, dream psychology, and neurosis psychology are studied on parallel or similar tracks.

The analysand's recognition of author, protagonist, antagonist, narrator, and listener (audience) is a new way of thinking about therapeutic action.

A brief synopsis of the technical similarities and differences of a number of discourse modes is given, followed by a survey of recent experimental work on children's theories of the mind and narrative acquisition.

Training and supervising analyst at the Pittsburgh Psychoanalytic Institute in Pennsylvania and a clinical assistant professor of psychiatry at the University of Pittsburgh School of Medicine.

This paper is an aria for Mabel and Buck.

The Psychoanalytic Study of the Child 54, ed. Albert J. Solnit, Peter B. Neubauer, Samuel Abrams, and A. Scott Dowling (Yale University Press, copyright © 1999 by Albert J. Solnit, Peter B. Neubauer, Samuel Abrams, and A. Scott Dowling).

NATURE OF NARRATIVE

PERHAPS TWENTY YEARS AGO I WAS WANDERING THROUGH A UNIVER-
sity bookstore and chanced upon a paperback with the engaging title
How to Do Things with Words (Austin, 1962). My reading of that book, by
J. L. Austin, was the beginning of a journey through linguistics, literary
criticism, poetry, dramaturgy, and the new, exploding discipline of nar-
ratology. As a practicing psychoanalyst, I began to share Percy Walker's
view: "It is a matter for astonishment, when one comes to think of it,
how little use linguistics and other sciences of language are to psychiatrists. When one considers that the psychiatrist spends most of his
time listening and talking to patients, one might suppose that there
would be such a thing as a basic science of listening-and-talking, as indispensable to psychiatrists as anatomy to surgeons" (Walker, 1992).

In my analytic work I had always heard stories, jokes, and synopses of
movies or books. In making a genetic interpretation or construction,
I was telling a story, but it was done in some matter-of-fact, natural way.
Perhaps I had been taught to look through and beyond the story in order to discern what was *really* being talked *about*. Sometimes it seemed
that I wasn't the listener with even-hovering attention, free responsiveness, and free hypotheses-making abilities. It was as if I shouldn't
be the listener. I felt strange and "directed." The patient and I were in
dialogue moving with increasing speed and force with states of strong
feelings toward some destined denouement. There might then be another slight pause or change in voice or affective tone at which I found
myself making a genetic reconstruction or intervention. The talk of the
talking cure has been a neglected object of study by psychoanalysts
(with a few notable exceptions). As far back as 1958 Rado wrote that as
yet "we do not possess even the beginnings of a technology of therapeutic talk."

There are two modes of discourse that entail narrative and will be
highlighted in this essay: Narrative Performance Mode (NPM) and
Dramatic Enactment Performance Mode (DEPM). NPM uses a narrator to tell the story in the past tense. DEPM enacts the story in the recurrent present tense. The Lyrical Mode, the Argumentative Mode,
and the Descriptive Mode are other modes that do not, for the most
part, use narrative.

The Rat Man, in *telling* Freud the *story* of the episodes in his life while
on military maneuvers, embedded the story told by the cruel Captain
of the torture by rats eating their way up into a man's anus and rectum.
Soon we read that he was pacing in front of Freud, gesticulating, gri-
macing, pausing, and addressing Freud as "Captain Freud."

In telling the story of the Rat Man's performing the story told to him of the rat torture, Freud said that the Rat Man was again standing up and gave all signs of horror and resistance. The Rat Man then resumed telling the story. He had returned to the Narrative Mode (NPM) and said, " . . . bored in . . . " There was a brief pause, a silence that I here characterize as a *juncture,* and then Freud said, "into the anus." Freud (in writing up the case) "permitted" himself to complete the story and, in so doing, switched to dramatic-enactment performance (DEPM) with the Rat Man as counter-actor. This was a *mise en abyme,* to use a term coined by André Gide in 1893. This is a reflection of the story that brings out the meaning and form of the work. The device gets its name from heraldry. A small second representation of the full-sized shield is placed "en abyme" at the center of it. Gide (1984) wrote: "In a work of art, I rather like to find thus transposed, at the level of the characters, the subject of the work itself. Nothing sheds more light on the work or displays the proportions of the whole work more accurately. In litera-ture, there is the scene in which a play is acted in *Hamlet.*" Both the Rat Man and Freud turn the narrative back on itself.

In his *The Mirror in the Text,* Lucien Dällenbach (1977) writes: "As for those reflections (by far the most frequent) for which fidelity is con-stricting, rather than seeing them in terms of the 'miniature model' one might better compare them to the figures created by what Freudian psychoanalysis calls the 'primary processes' since they derive from 'condensation' and 'displacement' rather like the 'dreamwork.' Thanks to the *mise en abyme,* the redundancy is diminished; the narra-tive becomes informing and open" (p. 57).

The device looks back to the past and foretells the future. In the past, there was a masochistic soldier who was treated in a sadistic manner by another soldier with a bucket of rats. Then there was the Rat Man, who was treated cruelly by the captain. Then there was a masochistic Rat Man-protagonist seducing and inviting Freud to probe. The various protagonists and antagonists are, by analogy, isomorphic in their ac-tions and motivations to the motivations and actions of the characters back on the military maneuvers.

A BRIEF LOOK AT PRENARRATIVITY

What does the explication of *mise en abyme* (which turns up in many an-alytic hours) have to do with narrative and child analysis? The key metaphor that Gide and subsequent commentators focus on is *reflec-tion.* In one of the many studies that demonstrate the infant's ability to imitate the action of another, Scaife and Bruner (1975) found that infants as young as two months will readjust their gaze contingent on a change in the focus of visual attention of an adult. Butterworth and Cochran (1980) confirmed this work and found babies of 6 through 18 months reflecting their mother's gaze and change in focus of attention. Janet Astington (1991) is one of the developmental workers who attempts to demonstrate that only after age four does a child develop a truly representational view of representation. One also thinks of the mimesis or reflection of their mothers' facial expressions by the youngsters in Emde's cliff experiments (Sorce and Emde, 1981). Time and space do not permit a review of the literature concerning the transformation from transitional space to intersubjective space in which one experiences one's private stories and stagings. Material-reality space is also a container for the child to project his or her reflections. To suggest an answer to the question posed at the beginning of this paragraph, during the acquisition of narrative abilities (around 4.5 years) the reflection of self-reflective thought may have to be in place before the child can use narrative to "endow experience with meaning" (Bruner, 1986).

At first, the child might simply verbalize subject and object ("Mommy car?"). The caregiver often "is ahead" to elaborate the story: ("Yes, you're happy to hear Mommy honk the horn of her car. She'll be here very soon.") From early childhood we listen to stories, enact them in play, and eventually tell ourselves stories either in private or in public. At around four and a half years we can tell ourselves a secret, tell a lie, and *represent* the process of representing *and* recounting.

Russell Meares, in *The Metaphor of Play* (1993), wrote about Edmund Gosse. "A five-year-old child in Victorian England discovered that his father did not know of a misdemeanor that the child had recently committed. Years later he wrote of the immense import of this experience: "Of all the thoughts that rushed upon my savage and undeveloped little brain at this crisis, the most curious was that I had found a companion and a confidant in myself. There was a secret in this world and it belonged to me and to somebody who lived in the same body with me. There were two of us, and we could talk with one another . . . the sense of my individuality now suddenly descended upon me, and it is equally certain that it was a great solace to me to find a sympathizer in my own breast'" (Gosse 1907, p. 58).

This sense of one's individuality is what is fostered by psychoanalysis. I agree with Jonathan Lear that the attainment of one's individuality can be done only in a felt, experiential atmosphere of love (1990, pp. 25–27). Perhaps what makes primary process primary is that there are no splits, no linkages or distinctions. Edmund Gosse discovered that his father didn't know who had broken his ceramic tile. What little Edmund could do was create a split between himself and his story, between the narrator of his story of how things get broken and his listener, between himself and what he knew, and between his father and what he knew. He had put together a series of events, his subjective states, and a revelation or discovery that he lived in his secret world. He realized a split between the meaning he performed in his secret story and the meaning his father might construe from walking around the family grounds.

Within the family, stories pass from generation to generation. A person's story of her/his pathogenesis is a narrative (Renik), and one's personal myth is the screen narrative (E. Kris). Some of our classical logic is constituted by argument using metaphor and falls under the rubric of narrative (Johnson, 1987).

In the *Rationality of Emotion* (1991), the philosopher Ronald de Sousa proposes a set of desires related to a self-representation *within* a "paradigm scenario." He also writes that "by the time toddlers are four or five years old, they have a very good sense of what kinds of stories lead to what simple emotions. Learning these scenarios continues indefinitely" (p. 183). Bennett Simon (1988) adds significantly to our knowledge of stories, how we use them, and, more importantly, how the ability to form stories is ineluctably tied to one's family, kith, and kin: "Tragedy, then, in form and content confronts us with an awesome dialectic between the meaningful and the meaningless, between the linking and connecting of persons, ideals, and values to each other and the breakdown, the dissolution of these links and connections" (p. 16).

THE PURPOSE OF NARRATIVE

We grow into mysteries, movies, novels, soap operas, stage plays, etc., but we never, it seems, grow out of our need for stories. One reason, I believe, is that the making/telling/listening to a story is a semblance of the life of the mind. By "neuronal Darwinism," according to Edelman (1987), we as animals live out a primary consciousness. With its own neuronal network, primary consciousness enables us to live through real time from moment to moment, while exercising the basic functions of a living organism at a primitive, hedonic level. Another level of neuronal networks allows us to live within possible worlds and within narrative time. We are not stimulus-bound. Making/telling/listening to stories reflect both aspects of the embodied mind. We order and reorder our life experiences through stories. We give disconnected moments of experience an ongoing form and meaning. Using stories, we begin to distinguish self and nonself, leave the frame of magical merger, and create an autonomous storyteller. The ego is an organ of recognition and an organizer of time.

We need to build an inner constancy of culture and environment outside the home. Object constancy has been studied and described. By way of stories, we internalize a constancy of world/ideology/culture. Anthropologists, notably M. Rosaldo, teach us that we begin to learn what goes with what as we watch and listen to our family make sense of events. We enjoy the rhythmic, playful repetition of this learning to make sense. In *The Cambridge Encyclopedia of Language* (Crystal 1987), there is a picture of two latency-age girls bouncing balls against the playground wall while signing "I like coffee, I like tea, I like radio and TV."

Within our private inner narrative space, we put our stories of creation, our basic beliefs about time, space, forces of gravity, and other forms of force, destiny, who we are, what we ought to do, death, and where we are going. Narrative enables the basic assumptions about our identity. In addition, the psychoanalyst is in a unique situation to hear and be part of stories and dramas that are compromise formational in make-up. They encompass id derivatives or instinctual wishes, superego derivatives in the form of inhibitions, restrictions, and ideals, as well as many ego functions. The telling of these stories, the structuring of them, is under the influence of the newly created intersubjective space of the psychoanalytic situation.

MINIMAL REQUIREMENTS OF NARRATIVE

Many scholars and narratologists have outlined the bare necessities of a story. Few do so in a more appealing way than J. Hillis Miller (1990). He states that there must be an initial situation, a sequence leading to a change or reversal of that initial situation, and a learning, discovery, or revelation about the previous situations leading to an end. There are at minimum four characters: a protagonist, an antagonist, a narrator who learns and reports, and a listener. There is repetitive patterning involving some locus of ambiguities, which may be a person or an object that enlivens everything that happens. Miller exemplifies these by A. E. Housman's "The Grizzly Bear."

The Grizzly Bear
The Grizzly Bear is huge and wild;
　He has devoured the infant child.
The infant child is not aware
　He has been eaten by the bear.

There is the initial situation of the grizzly bear and the infant child. Then there is a reversal of that situation: by devouring the child, there is a reversal of fortune and the identity of the child. The protagonist learns nothing. The infant child is the good guy, the protagonist. The grizzly bear is the bad guy, the antagonist. The good guy doesn't have a chance against the bad guy. Only the ironic narrator learns something. There is a pattern called *chiasmus,* after the making of the Greek letter *chi,* which refers to a crisscross reversal of the elements, as in Figure 1. The grizzly bear is first at the beginning of a sentence and then at the end. The infant child is at the end of one sentence and then is at the beginning of the next sentence. The story begins with the bear and ends with the bear. The infant child is encompassed by the story as she / he is enclosed within the paws and jaws of the bear. The chiasmal framing of this story by the bear is seen in many novels, operas, movies, theatrical productions, and psychoanalytic hours. In this instance of the story within the poem, we might schematize:

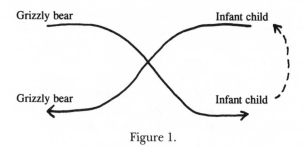

Figure 1.

THREE ASPECTS OF NARRATIVE

Genette (1988) proposes three aspects of narrative for study: (1) the timeless, thematic synopsis of storystuff; (2) the making and shaping of the story out of timeless storystuff; (3) the performance of telling the story in a given situation. The first aspect, known as *recit* or *fabula* in literary criticism, is the timeless, narratorless abstract synopsis of characters and events, as in: "Boy meets girl, girl presents obstacles to boy's goals, etc."

The second aspect of narrative is the shaping and making of the story out of timeless storystuff. Here we can see the two modalities of temporality that characterize narrative: the time it takes to tell and listen to the story. This is within real time, *chronos,* time's arrow. There is also narrative time, *kairos,* the Greek god of opportunity. With the blessing of *kairos,* one creates within the window of opportunity a story/drama with endless possibilities, gaps, chances for errors, and recognitions by way of flashbacks, jumps forward, and repeated events. Within the shaping of narrative are often the iterative, durative, and rhythmic aspects of temporality.

The third aspect, the performance of telling the story in a given situation, is the recitation, or narration. This is the *doing* of a recitation of story within a certain specific situation. In this third aspect there is the control of how soon the listener will hear certain parts of the story. I have called this aspect of narrative the Dramatic Enactment Performance Mode of discourse (DEPM). Any parent who reads a bedtime story to a youngster and "gets into" the character knows about the DEPM. Presuppositions are used in the telling of the story. If someone asks me at dinner, "Won't you pass the salt?" there is the presupposition that I don't want to pass the salt. In the psychoanalytic situation, the storytelling situation is complex, mysterious, and little understood. When does the analysand tell the analyst a story? How is the story told? Will the listener be directed to know that this story is of a genre—say, a piece of autobiographical history, a joke, a political speech, a prayer? Will the story be a *mise en abyme* reflecting a much larger series of relationships in the patient's past, in the present, and in the future relationship between patient and analyst? Will I be made to wait as the analysand tells a story? Will I force the analysand to wait as I tell a story of interpretation or reconstruction? Will I be provoked to ask the question dreaded by all storytellers: What is the point, why are you telling me this story? Will I force the analysand to ask me: What's the point . . . why are you telling me this, Dr. Coleman?

The point varies. Sometimes the telling of the story is the object ("I offer you in evidence . . . or in rebuttal"), as in an argument. The story may be some *exemplum,* as in a parable used in inductive argument. The speech act of "Let me tell you a story" might be: "Let me seduce you, let me threaten you, let me forestall a dangerous situation by telling you a story (à la Scheherazade), let me mock you," etc. An important speech act of the analyst/analysand is to invite the listener's imagination, to hope that the listener will initiate and search for the performance of meanings. Generally, a speech act cannot be conscious. We do not usually say, "I insinuate that John is a bastard."

STORIES IN THE PSYCHOANALYTIC SITUATION

A physician in analysis, let's call him Dr. Deed, recounted a story to me. Like his palindromic precursor, Pip of *Great Expectations,* he traveled back and forth between Deed-the-adult as narrator and Deed the narrator now as inner focalizer—that is, Deed the child. In the story, Deed went to his first day at school and discovered that he was the only child who knew and spoke the word "hysterectomy." There was a quick shift of point of attention to within the mind of the teacher, a character in the story. Deed told this part of the story from the point of view of the teacher. She was pleased and admiring of "this little boy before her eyes." Dr. Deed the adult-objective-narrator quickly shifted back and now was telling me what he saw through the eyes of Deed the child. He saw the other children with dumb and blank faces. He was recreating the sense for me that the other children were *not there*. Deed and his teacher were there alone together. He was in actuality an only child.

Thinking that Deed the adult narrator had provided Deed the child with an adult vocabulary, I said that "hysterectomy" was a big word for a little child. Of course, Deed heard this as criticism and disbelief. He said that he remembered the factual deed, that he *had* used and spoken the word "hysterectomy" on the first day of first grade. I quietly echoed out loud "wreck to me." There was a silence. Dr. Deed's eyes filled. He recalled not knowing what the word meant. He also recalled his mother speaking the word to him, and he added to my echo his mother's heard utterance, "He's a wreck to me."

After my echo there was a silence, as if Dr. Deed had given himself a "time out" in order to sort out and make sense of too much that was going on within him. This was a *juncture,* and we switched from DEPM to his use of the Narrative Performance Mode (NPM). He told stories that he had heard growing up: Deed the baby had caused his mother to bleed and continue to bleed post-partum. He had torn her up inside. She had nearly died and needed a hysterectomy. He recalled an auto accident when he was twelve. A driver ran a red light at an intersection and hit the family car, driven by his mother. Young Deed had been dozing in the front passenger seat. Once again, because he had been sleeping and not on watch, as he put it, he caused his mother to bleed and nearly die.

It was not that his stories located in the past were placing Dr. Deed safely at a distance from himself in the present moment with me. I disagree with Paul Gray's conclusion that "a context in the *past* removes us to a safer distance from the stage where anxiety occurs. The sense of relief that so often accompanies the shift of content away from the current stage of the mind is a familiar and often valuable therapeutic action, but it is a psychotherapeutic, not a psychoanalytic action" (1994, p. 158).

Having felt himself to be the lyrical character who caused his mother's near-death, Deed took responsibility for his feelings and went ahead of me to get in touch with the author of his stories. Rather than be safely distanced, Dr. Deed was in pain, puzzled, argumentative, and amazed that he had not known but did know the meaning of the term. Like Freud's patient Lucy R., he was surprised and amazed that he knew in the past but did not want to know what he knew. He had repossessed, recognized, and owned his lyrical character and linked it to his authored story.

Paul Gray contends that for the patient to tell the analyst a dream lends itself "admirably to the resistance use of the context of the past, as it displaces the analytic focus to some other time and place" (1994, p. 160). This may or may not be so. The dream can be thought of as an attempt to make sense/story in the primary, secondary, and tertiary elaborations. Modell (1988), using backup from the neuroscientist Gerald Edelman, thinks of a constant revision of previous lived experience. The term "remembered present" uses *Nachträglichkeit* of everyday life to convey the process of the past always impacting on the present. There are no archeological finds, no icebergs of repression melting and allowing Titanics to rise to the surface. I think of a surface, a stage floor, an inner theater of the mind in constant motion like a kaleidoscope with our inner characters, events, directors, playwrights, audience, and especially lyrical characters in search, Pirandello fashion, of their authors.

A young lawyer, Gray reports, entered analysis "for anxiety attacks in anticipation of doing courtroom litigation" (1994, p. 162). His mother had grotesquely restricted him in his childhood and threatened that any rebellion on his part would be the cause of her death. The patient gained increasing capacity to recognize patterns of defense. In one hour, he recalled how for "almost a year his mother made his little brother wash his bed sheets every morning because of one episode of soiling" (p. 162). He was remembering these stories in the past tense (NPR), then some anger and disgust began to creep into his voice, and suddenly he became almost inaudible. He stopped and then said, now quite audibly: "Yesterday, I forgot to tell you a dream I had over the weekend. I think I was in a large room with a multitude of people" (p. 163).

Why did the young man decide to tell the story of his forgetting to tell the story of his dream at that particular moment? In the young man's stories, Gray could hear the patient's anger and disgust with his mother. There was a change from the patient's narrative performance mode of discourse (NPM) to a dialogue with increased usage of deictics (DEPM). (Deictics are "pointings" that gain their meanings only within the context of the moment of utterance. These are words like:

"this side of," "on the other side," "*that* object way over *there*," "this," "that," etc. They gain no meaning by reference to some citation in a dictionary. Two people perform meanings in the moment of utterance and the place of utterance in the here and now.)

I agree with Paul Gray's conclusion that "if one is interested in bringing into stable accessibility the ego's unconscious patterns of resistance to unconscious conflict, then it is of ultimate value that greater attention be given to the immediate mental area" (1994, p. 169). To enhance attention to the here-and-now surface in the psychoanalytic situation, it is good for analysts and researchers to learn about the constitutive elements of narrative and drama. Knowing that there was a seachange from the NPM to the DEPM might bring up hypotheses about unconscious conflict. Using the metaphors of instinctual drives, Waelder (1951) writes of a mimetic principle that becomes intraphysic in the person's re-presentation of actions and events apperceived: "if warded-off instinctual drives make their comeback, the return has the same form as the defense mechanism had; they return, as it were, through the same door through which they were ousted [isomorphism]. If the defense mechanism had the form of denial, the return must have the form of an assertion."

Who decides to return the repressed? To my way of thinking, if an author or his/her invented narrator sees that if things continue the way they are going someone will experience physical pain, abandonment, shame, etc., then that inner-stage character will switch to a different author—a playwright, for instance, with invented characters who enact the drama. Roles might be reversed (Kernberg, 1987, Case #3); a protagonist in the prior narrative, a smug narcissistic imposter, might become, in the following drama, a bumbling, humble character. Perhaps the moment that embodies that unconscious conflict is the pause after the young lawyer's narrative and before the drama of "Yesterday I forgot to tell you . . ."

I will now supply the analyst's and the patient's comments without the analyst's asides.

Analyst: In your description of the dream you seem to pick up on the problem you were up against just before you told the dream.
Patient: It was something about my mother . . . the sheets.
Analyst: You sounded as if you were hesitating to speak critically about your mother, and then the memory of the dream interrupted.
Patient: Yes, I remember.
Analyst: Maybe it got unsafe to show me critical feeling toward your mother.
Patient: I don't want you to think I'm being unfair to her.

Analyst: In your memory of the dream you first pictured yourself as a judge, and then you took that away by making . . . etc.
                    (Details within the dream were clarified.)
Patient: Yeah . . . is it that Christ thing again?
Analyst: I guess it suddenly got safer for you to have me see you as sort of Christlike and on the receiving end of someone else's resentment, rather than my hearing your resentment toward your mother.
Patient: Well, I know you won't be critical of me.
Analyst: What I have in mind is the moment when you didn't want me to think of you as unfair to your mother.
Patient: Well, I guess I expect you to be like other people.
Analyst: Could "other people" be one of the generalizations that's a safer way of putting it?
Patient: Well, everyone at home . . . I guess I mean my father [now a freely angry tone] *he never let up . . . Christ! . . . He was always yelling I was being unfair to my brother . . . If he had only been as tough on my mother!*

In his reflections on the material Gray wrote, "I did not overlook that the angry accusation that his father 'never let up' appeared soon after I pressed him a bit about my transference role as inhibiting authority. Nevertheless I could not yet show him evidence, in that hour, that he had found it safe and then conflicted to be aware of even a bit of criticism of me" (p. 165).

This young man had apparently been in the Narrative Performance Mode with Gray, then became silent and switched to the Dramatic Enactment Performance Mode. Neither Freud nor Gray could call attention to the narrative mode, the pause, and then, at least in Freud's case, a felt need to get permission from one of his (Freud's) inner-stage characters and then say, "into the anus." Gray and the young lawyer continue in DEPM dialogue or conversation for the rest of the reported material. In the first intervention, Gray makes an interpretation of the manifest content of the dream to go back to an intuited (by the analyst) conflict within the patient that triggered his remembering the forgotten dream at that moment. In Gray's second intervention, he repeats his first interpretation. The patient by now may be actualizing compliance. He answers, "Yes, I remember" *and even* asks the analyst whether he has it right . . . "Is it that Christ thing again?" In the sixth intervention, the analyst guesses that it suddenly "got safer for you," etc. In the seventh intervention, the analyst tells the patient what he, the analyst, has in mind.

Unconscious irony, it seems to me, occurs through this exchange, especially when the patient says, "Well, I guess I expect you to be like other people." It strikes me as highly ironic when Gray, after pressing the patient through six or seven interventions, notes to himself that the blow up of "he never let up" came after Gray had pressed him a bit about his transference role. This may be an instance in which parts of the unconscious drama (with the playwrights, characters, audience, and directors of *both parties*) find actualization in Gray and the young man. Gray is "induced" (Nielsen, 1994) or, in my terms, directed by the patient's unconscious director into the role of an obsessionally disturbed, internalized mother. The patient's actual mother had been disturbed to psychotic proportions. This man with this mother probably did not enjoy or learn very much about play as a youngster. This is sheer speculation on my part, save for the playroom (courtroom) of the dream. It sounded as if there was little play or leeway within the frame of this dream.

One presupposition in psychoanalytic theory is the continuous, conscious flow, the Jamesian river of conscious mental phenomena. There are, it strikes me, sinkholes, whirlpools, swift/slow currents and backcurrents, silences, and changes in voice and affective tone, which I have termed *junctures*. The patient and I often find unconscious process influencing conflict just before the juncture. There is also difficulty with plausibility. As Gray continued his interpretations, he might have lost credibility in the eyes and ears of the young man's inner "I" positions so that he could not believe Gray was someone different from his internalized mother. Gray's patient continued in the narrative performance using the past tense, recounting stories up to and including his forgotten dream. There was a whirlpool or hole in his story insofar as he had forgotten his dream.

In this young man's stories and in stories in general there is the phenomenon of parallelism of "rhymes of events." A. Kris might call these correlations. There are abundant schemes for rhymes in poetry. In narrative, there are rhymes of events. Italo Calvino (1988) uses the Charlemagne legend to illustrate rhymes of events:

> Late in life the emperor Charlemagne fell in love with a German girl. The barons at his court were extremely worried when they saw that the sovereign, wholly taken up with his amorous passion and unmindful of his regal dignity, was neglecting the affairs of state. When the girl suddenly died, the courtiers were greatly relieved—but not for long, because Charlemagne's love did not die with her. The emperor had the embalmed body carried to his bedchamber, where he refused to be parted from it. The Archbishop Turpin, alarmed by this macabre passion, suspected an enchantment and insisted on examining the corpse. Hidden under the girl's dead tongue he found a ring with a precious

stone set in it. As soon as the ring was in Turpin's hands, Charlemagne fell passionately in love with the archbishop and hurriedly had the girl buried. In order to escape the embarrassing situation, Turpin flung the ring into Lake Constance. Charlemagne thereupon fell in love with the lake and would not leave its shores.

Calvino found this legend in a book on magic collected as unpublished notes by the French Romantic writer Jules Barbey d'Aurevilly. The story is shot through with death while at the same time there is the drive of desire, the form of which is determined by the ring. The love of the young German girl is followed by a necrophilic passion followed by a homosexual passion followed by the mystical union (perhaps, some oceanic feeling) passion for Lake Constance. The Charlemagne legend is an effective and much-loved narrative because there is a series of events that "echo" each other as rhymes do in a poem. The events enlist the listener to order the events as in echo. A reader familiar with the writings of Freud, Greenacre, and others on the fetish and the secret would wonder about the Charlemagne legend, in which the meaning of the ring was kept secret from the characters in the story and from the reader.

By analogy to the Charlemagne legend, the dream of Gray's young lawyer might be considered the "ring," or what Alfred Hitchcock called the MacGuffin. The MacGuffin was something very important in the film story. Alfred Hitchcock warned that the MacGuffin was a red herring placed repeatedly within the narrative to throw the reader/listener/audience off. Within the basic necessities of narrative, the MacGuffin is the locus of ambiguities. The dream was produced and remembered. Then the young man forgot to tell the dream to Gray. The *telling* that he had forgotten *to tell* the dream came in the series of events that have internal "echo rhyme." His telling that he had forgotten to tell the dream came after *telling* that for his brother's one mishap (forgetting? masturbating?) of soiling, mother had the brother wash his bedsheets every morning.

Another technical but important aspect of this clinical vignette is the high density of deictics. Roman Jakobson (1971) called them "shifters" because they shift one's attention away from the story and focus on the speaker and listener, the here-and-now utterance. For instance, compare a mother watching and listening to her child in play who invites the child's playful imagination to a mother who sifts the point of attention to her own mind and away from the child's play.

1. Mother: That's a very interesting look on babydoll's face.

2. Mother: Do *you* think that *I* know what babydoll wants?

The second mother uses "you" and "I" to build an ongoing fabric of dramatic dialogue (DEPM) between mother and child at the expense of the child's playful use of imagination (NPM, or inner, private DEPM of the child). An arguable point is whether the child has 'forced' the mother to intervene and ask such a question. Lou-Marié Kruger and Dennie Palmer Wolf (1994), in an impressive longitudinal study, explore this question. The first mother sits in a darkened theater (in the camera obscura) beside her child, looking at the scene in the inner theater of the child's mind, now externalized to the play toys. She leans over to the child's playwright, producer, director, and actresses and makes her comment.

It would be as if, in the clinical example, the analyst and the patient were sitting in a darkened movie house and the analyst interrupted their mutual gaze at the movie on the screen and asked, "Do you think that the story line in the movie has something to do with the fact that you forgot to buy us popcorn just before we came into the theater . . . and you're afraid I will think that you're being unfair to your mother?" There is, in my mind, something awesome and terribly dangerous in Gray's patient's dreaming, forgetting, and telling of the dream. *Life*-likeness, verisimilitude, failed him. There was too much similarity between the patient's inner object representation of his mother and Gray's activity. One or the other of his dream characters was to be crushed. Annihilation anxiety was about to be dramatized, and he woke up (DeSousa, 1960; Welles & Wrye, 1994). The only escape from observing himself as inhabiting his disturbed mother (and vice versa) was an altered state of consciousness—that is, an awakening from sleep. Again, this is sheer speculation on my part except for the lack of play and/or leeway within the frame of the oneiric courtroom and, possibly, between Gray and the young lawyer in the excerpt.

CLINICAL EXAMPLE OF JUNCTURE

About three years into an analysis with a young, divorced woman, who worked in real estate, I began to feel listless and dull in our hours together. She had made significant gains in the analysis. I gradually began to feel subtle clues within myself that signaled boredom and fatigue. I began to perceive little change in her, and I was definitely feeling distant and, as I put it several times to myself, "on the ropes." She had said that my eyes were blue. Other associations were in the foreground, and our work began to drag on. She again remarked that my eyes were blue. I may have said something like, "I think you may be trying to tell us something by stating that my eyes are blue." She laughingly denied any such hidden communication and simply repeated, "Dr. Coleman, your eyes are blue." Strangely, I imagined my driver's license and my picture and the word "brown" after "color of eyes." I found myself thinking that my father's eyes were hazel but my eyes were brown. There seemed to be some estrangement in my emotional tone, some distance, and yet some closeness as I imagined bobbing and weaving and sagging badly on the ropes.

I said some things that we all have in our kit bag. Perhaps you are trying to tell us something by asserting that my eyes are blue? I asked for her associations to eyes, the color blue, etc. Why now at this time in the analysis had she observed that my eyes were blue? Nothing. Things dragged on. She repeated in a rather casual way that my eyes were blue. Thinking of Fenichel and his notion of "to make a mental note" as well as my feelings of being "out of it and half dead" I said, "I think that at some time in your life you told yourself to remember some scene for the rest of your life and that you need me as part of the scene to be half dead and on the ropes." There was a silence. Then came a sudden and remarkable change in her tone, delivery, and mode of discourse. Unlike the Rat Man and Gray's young lawyer, the switch was from DEPM (drama) to NPM (narrative). She spoke in slow, flat declarative sentences using the past tense and telling stories from a time when she was a little girl. Her mother was looking wistfully at a picture framed in mother of pearl. To the patient then this meant "mother of something special and of great price." Within the frame was a picture of a three-year-old girl, Becky, who had died of spinal meningitis. The patient was born about a year and a half after Becky's death. She told the story of watching her mother look at the picture with sad, loving eyes. Her mother's eyes were glistening and sparkling as she talked to my patient about Becky. The patient told herself that she would never forget that scene.

What she vowed to herself privately was never to think of her private fantasy, in which she was within her mother's womb fighting with her sister, Becky, who was about to be born. She left Becky bleeding to death, and she, my patient, was born. A few years later, she had a close female friend. She would often have sleepovers at the friend's home. They slept in twin beds. Her friend's father would often come in and sexually molest her. By this age she had a baby brother. She returned to her original private story but this time she fought with her "twin," "demasculinized" the twin, and was born a boy-child. She had originally (before the *Nachträglichkeit*) said that she would never remember the rage, sadness, and left-out feelings of her reparative back-to-the-uterus story in which she left Becky dead in the womb and was born a girl-child. Becky's eyes were blue.

What had preceded the juncture was a dramatic enactment in which the patient unconsciously wrote an inner drama, created characters, invented a director, and found ways to interact with people and objects in her environment. She externalized onto me a sequence of characters and events (Sandler, 1976) and unconsciously pressured me with clues and "cues" as a director would do in order to facilitate an actor's getting into a role. The Rat Man had done the same with Freud. For a director to "induce" (Nielsen, 1994) or direct an actor, she would have to be privy to the playwright's drama and the way a scene worked. The curious thing is that in thinking of Fenichel, I was the director to the patient and was recounting a scene. I knew nothing of her inner, private drama. I knew that I remembered listening with my father to the Joe Louis boxing matches on an old Zenith radio. Later I recognized what I didn't want to know and yet did know: how fierce and bloody were my fistfights with my brother. By the iconic actions of feeling on the ropes and half dead, I was in dramatic enactment performance mode (DEPM) of discourse with this lady. I felt estranged. By these iconic actions, I was not aware of old familiar stories in which the patient would help me to keep my father/brother alive by way of idyllic screen memories.

And, of course, when I got better, the patient got better. Fenichel (1929) helped us in recognizing that we often "make a mental note not to ever forget X, Y, and Z." Remarkably, both of us were under the influence of "making a mental note." The mild content of X, Y, and Z (my remembrance of listening to the Joe Louis fights with my father) screened a highly emotionally charged scenario. There was mutual back-and-forth forceful direction. When I said that she needed me as part of the scene to be half dead and on the ropes, I emphasized my "deadness" by iconic actions of speech patterns, I slowed and stretched out the phrase "ha-lf de–ad" (Chatman, 1990). These are iconic in the sense that Chatman uses the term, to denote actions that stand for the bodies and states of mind of the character. I knew that I wasn't half dead, but I was estranged from myself and making iconic actions of speech that signified my half-deadness. My estrangement is the defamiliarization, as the Russian Formalists call it. These are creative movements as in a drama (DEPM) that we are in bemused wonder about afterwards.

THERAPEUTIC ACTION BY RECOGNITION SCENES

It is by way of the therapeutic action that psychoanalytic goals are realized. Therapeutic action takes place when the patient recognizes herself as the playwright, director, and characters of an inner, private drama. If there is inner story and argument, the patient may experience some illusion of "timelessness," hopelessly caught up in oscillation from one position of divergent conflict to another. Therapeutic action is constituted in the patient's recognition that s/he has written the stories and arguments at both horns of the dilemma. For instance, she may have written: "If I enjoy the love of this man I will lose my autonomy and career choices . . . but if I enjoy my autonomy I will lose the love of this man." She recognizes that in writing both scripts she has written in a "heads I lose, tails I lose" dilemma.

If the patient repossesses herself—that is, finds herself to be the unknown author or playwright—then it becomes difficult to delegate to the director the task of finding someone in the environment and in some repetitive, lifeless way to enact or actualize the inner drama by interaction. Sometimes the patient recognizes herself as a lyrical character feeling instinctual wishes, the same strong emotions, over and over again in repeated life scenarios. With the mutual performance of recognition scenes after dramatic enactment, often mutual between analyst and analysand, she recognizes herself as the unconscious playwright who has directed and pressured herself into a certain "lyrical character." Sometimes she discovers a playwright who repeatedly mounts the drama of the maimed avenger getting revenge by being inconsolable.

From a quota of energy to a lyrical character feeling despair or the ecstasy of love, lust, envy, etc. I envisage a transformation. "This transformation of affect has constituted a problem, if not *the* problem, with analysands from the year 1894 to the present" (Lear, 1990). And this transformation from catharsis to signal anxiety has been the beast in the jungle for analysts who theorize. Lear paraphrases Freud's comment in The *Interpretation of Dreams* (1901) this way: "The point of repression, for Freud, is to prevent this causal story from unfolding" (p. 88).

With narrative/dramatic acquisition, the sensations of the body moving, the instinctual e-moting, or the quota of affective charge is transformed to a human lyrical character feeling rage, abandonment, revenge, love, envy, etc. Therapeutic action deals with the recognition of context, the many authors/dramas/arguments/playwrights, for these lyrical characters. One owns one's self feeling within a human situation and by becoming an individual—not as someone experiencing impersonal forces. The lyrical characters are linked to other characters, events, narratives/dramas, authors, and playwrights in a concatenation of causality and meaningfulness.

TECHNICAL ELEMENTS OF NARRATIVE PERFORMANCE MODE (NPM)

Across the top of Table 1 the four modes of discourse are depicted. In the left-hand column are listed some of the constitutive elements

MODES

	DEPM	NPM	Argument	Description
Speech acts	High	Low	High	Medium
Deictics	High	Low	Low	Low
Estrangement	Very High	Low	Low to nil	Low
Tense	Now	Past	DNA	DNA
Engagement	High	+/-High	Medium	Low
Dialogue	High	Low	Medium	Low

(Row label on left side: **Elements**)

Table 1. Attributes of Modes of Discourse

within these modes of discourse. (The constitutive elements of temporality, other than tense, and narrators are not listed in this table; to list them would introduce far too much complexity.)

Speech acts, in the first line, refer to the making of a statement, offer, promise, threat, request, etc. in uttering a sentence, by virtue of the conventional *force* associated with it.

1. I bet you five dollars that the Steelers will win next Sunday.
2. I promise to take you to the park tomorrow.
3. I beg you to stop.
4. I sentence you to five years in prison.
5. I want for us to fuck until we die and arise from the ashes of our lust like Donne's phoenix, as one.

One analysand *implored* me to believe her argument: "I hold these truths to be self-evident: I do all things perfectly and discharge anger in perfectly acceptable ways." She said that she was "a woman under the influence, like a sleepwalker" and trapped in her childish predicament. When we make an utterance, we make something happen in our intrapsychic world and in the environment around us. Like the woman above, the man in example five is enacting the speech act of "I poetize," "I seduce," or "I show off." He acts to persuade his partner to change her ways of thinking and feeling about him. He is bringing about changes within his own private intrapsychic world.

Deictic or shifter is the meaning of a grammatical form that can gain its meaning only by reference to the given utterance of the here and now in which the form appears. The first-person form of a verb, or the first-person pronoun, is a shifter because the basic meaning of the pronoun *you* entails a reference to the listener/reader/audience in the here and now. A child enjoys talking about language. "He recalls the past in this way: 'When I was small, I talked like that, and now I speak differently, like this.' He also sometimes begins to speak in the manner of a baby, either as a game or in order to solicit more tenderness or affection from adults" (Jakobson and Pomorska, 1985).

The importance of deictic and shifter information is best shown in situations when such information is lacking. Imagine being out in the ocean and finding a bottle floating on the surface. We open it and find a message: "Meet us here a week from now and bring a fishing pole this long." We won't be able to know *whom* to meet, *where* or *when* to meet them, or *how long* a fishing pole to bring.

Estrangement refers to the subjective experience of feeling a stranger to yourself. This is, in my experience, less powerful and of shorter duration than dissociative experiences. Like the patient quoted above, the person feels "under the influence" and may be unwittingly ghostwriting an inner scenario in response to another person. When I am estranged in DEPM with an analysand, I am in-between. There seems to be a dialectic between what is represented and what is presumed to be real.

Engagement is most crucial to DEPM. Engagement follows upon estrangement and is best compared to the person in the audience watching an actor recite the stages of man. We are riveted in our seats even as we feel that perceiving his perspiration and make-up might jolt us.

The mark of NPM is its bitemporality. The patient who told the story of watching her mother gaze with glistening eyes at the picture of the patient's dead sister exemplifies (1) the real time in which it took to tell the story and (2) the narrative time it takes for characters to think, feel, do, and say things. In the latter there can be flashbacks, jumps forward, iterative actions, etc. In speaking of her interdicted claustrum fantasy, the patient jumped forward to times when she fantasized that she was a twin and then back again when she realized that she was revising her original story because of her penis envy. NPM is marked by the use of the past tense. Deictics and speech acts are less frequent in NPM than in DEPM. In the psychoanalytic situation, one would expect dialogue, in its overt conscious sense, to be high in DEPM and low in NPM. These "highs" and "lows" are offered more as hypotheses—as orphans seeking homes in some methodological study that could provide evidence.

NARRATIVE ACQUISITION

Recently, while travelling in the Midwest, I saw a T-shirt in a shop. On the front of the shirt was the following legend bordered in red:

Memo from the desk of Toto

Dear Dorothy,

Hate Oz. Took the shoes.

You can find your own way home.

Toto

As my wife and I stood laughing at this shirt, I noticed some young children looking, reading, and laughing too.

There was the red frame, by which it seemed that a page from a notepad belonging to Toto had been found and printed on the T-shirt. This manner of framing a story (within a letter or series of letters found by the narrator) has been used to gain credibility for many years.

The narrator reports the inner feelings of Toto. Initially, Dorothy and Toto were friends with mutual trust. Toto, the protagonist, has wanted to go home. Dorothy, the antagonist, has created obstacles to Toto's going home. Whereas before they were trusted friends, now there is reversal, and Dorothy will come to recognize that Toto has stolen the shoes and has ordered her, like a dog, to find her own way home.

One locus of ambiguities resides in the shoes. The shoes personify one's identity grounded in self-knowledge and knowledge of where one came from. The shoes personify a magical means of finding one's own true self. They personify a person's ability to stand on her/his own two feet, find balance and equilibrium in the upright position, and "push off" from the ground. The powers to walk and to jump are included in the shoes. Plato in the *Laws* noted that play in animals was seen as pushing off from the ground and leaping. This for Plato was the exemplum of play—play with gravity and the lightness of being.

The footprint is the iconic sign. It is a semblance of Toto's foot. It is also the indexical sign for the feet that walked down the yellow brick road and literally plotted or stepped off the land of adventures. Footprint and shoe are metonymy for a whole that was much more than any one *pars pro Toto.*

A narrator takes Toto as the point of attention. Shlomith Rimmon-Kenan (1983) wants us to know that a certain kind of narrator, the "focalizer," not only reports but tells us what he / she sees, feels, and thinks within a character. (It would take us too far afield to report all the reasons that Rimmon-Kenan chooses "focalizer" over the better-known "point of view," "angle of vision," or "perspective.") The focalizer sees through the eyes and heart of Toto. The narrator is saying, "This may *look* and *sound* like my narration, but this is Toto's narrated, interior monologue, *believe* me!" The children reading and laughing do believe. They understand and delight in the fiction invented by the implied author. The children older than 4.5 years can quickly move inside the narrative and see Dorothy through the eyes of a different and changed Toto.

Recent studies have shown that the ability to recognize higher-order intentions to deceive develops at around five years of age (Winner and Leekam, 1991; Leslie, 1987). For the children to laugh they must, at a minimum, be able to recognize that the narrator reports Toto as pretending (not intending) to deceive and that Toto believes his utterance to be false (Coleman and Kay, 1981).

If the author wants us to get the ironic joke, then when did the children learn to distinguish a falsehood intended to mislead (deception) from a falsehood intended to be recognized as false (irony)? Children are not able to assess what it is that the speaker wants the listener to believe until after the age of six (Demorest et al., 1984). These studies all presuppose that the children have gained narrative understanding in a cognitive and emotional manner. These studies have great bearing on reconstructions and the understandings of meanings with regard to childhood seduction scenes in the analyses of young and old adults.

Erikson taught us that the word "theory" relates to *thauma*—wonder, marvel, or that which compels intense gaze. Four- and five-year-olds become able to gaze at the inner, private theater of the mind and make narrative. Erikson (1972) writes about a time when Peggy Penn was play hostess, inviting children, one at a time, to leave their play group and come to a room where table, blocks, and toys were ready for them.

She asked each child to "build something" and to "tell a story" about it. Joan Erikson was recorder in the corner. The story of the five-year-old black boy, Robert, was: "Cars come to the house. The lion bites the snake, who wiggles his tail. The monkey and the kitten try to kill the snake. People come to watch. Little one [black boy] on roof is where smoke comes out."

Erikson spoke of this boy's *performance* "as an example of a five-year-old's capacity to project a relevant personal theme on the *microcosm* of a play table" (pp. 128–30). There are a number of performatives, speech, and dramatic acts done when someone speaks or mimes as Robert did. He may be said to work through a trauma, to perform a new beginning, to confess, to express the exuberance of self-expression, to exercise newly acquired skills toward mastery, to represent the dramatic representation of affect. Children's play can teach us the transformation of "affective charge" that Freud was searching for throughout his career.

Robert's building made of blocks was an erect structure, and he placed himself as the personification of a feeling on top of the building. A teacher of the boy had provided a clue. She said that he could physically compete with older boys and in some "detached" way dance a two-step sideways around the classroom. When she congratulated him, he responded with an affective gesture (head down with shoulders slouched) that corresponded to the doll slumping on the roof, saying, "Yes, but my brain is not good" (p. 130). Gray's young lawyer presented his structure of his night's experiences plus his wanting to tell his story about it ("It was something about my mother . . . the sheets") just as Robert offered his structure and his story about it to the Eriksons.

I submit that for a child to *feelingly* understand, he or she must be able to construct the human drama (with narrative emplotment and lyrical character) within and then to interact with the blocks and toys as well as with people in the environment.

By five years of age, the child has been given a much more mature brain and a gift from her/his mother. Mother has mimed, made up "iconic actions" to bear semblance to inner feelings, and, in all semiotic ways, given the gift of representing a person with motivations, wishes, and feelings *within a narrative.* A mother might invent mimetic actions of her hands and say to her children, "See, the weavers [in "The Emperor's New Clothes"] were just working away." She gestures up into thin air . . . nothing. The children learn to put the subjectivity of the weavers, the courtiers, and the vain emperor within the context of characters *within* the story. When mother read and mimed this part of the story, the children (without knowing the term, *"mise en abyme"*) knew that this reflected the early part of the story, when the emperor spent much time being measured for new clothes in front of mirrors. They would also better understand the end of the story, when the child pointed to the emperor in the street parade and cried out that he was not wearing any clothes.

Robert had learned to play. He had been helped to create a lyrical character who experienced painful feelings in a given story. His affect had been transformed to a lyrical character (a little black boy slumped in despair) "on roof where smoke comes out."

BIBLIOGRAPHY

ASTINGTON, J. W., HARRIS, P. L., & OLSON, D. R. (eds.) (1988). *Developing Theories of Mind.* New York: Cambridge University Press.

AUSTIN, JOHN. (1962). *How to Do Things with Words.* New York: Oxford University Press.

BRUNER, JEROME. (1986). *Actual Minds, Possible Worlds.* Cambridge, Mass.: Harvard University Press.

BUTTERWORTH, G. E. & COCHRAN, E. (1980). Towards a mechanism of joint visual attention in human infancy. *International Journal of Behavioral Development,* 3(3):253–272.

CALVINO, ITALO. (1988). *Six Memos for the Next Millennium.* Cambridge, Mass.: Harvard University Press.

CHATMAN, SEYMOUR. (1990). *Coming To Terms.* Ithaca: Cornell University Press.

COLEMAN, L. & KAY, P. (1981). Prototype semantics: The English word *lie. Language,* 57:26–44.

CRYSTAL, DAVID. (1987). *The Cambridge Encyclopedia of Language.* New York: Cambridge University Press.

DÄLLENBACH, LUCIEN. (1989). *The Mirror in the Text.* Trans. by Jeremy Whitely with Emma Hughes. Chicago: University of Chicago Press.

DeSOUSA, R. (1987). *The Rationality of Emotion.* Cambridge, Mass.: MIT Press.

DEMOREST, A. ET AL. (1984). Words speak louder than actions: Understanding deliberately false remarks. *Child Development,* 55:1527–1534.

EDELMAN, G. (1992). *Bright Air, Brilliant Fire.* New York: Basic Books.

ERIKSON, E. (1972). Play and Actuality. In: *Play and Development.* Ed. M. Piers. New York: Norton, pp. 127–167.

FENICHEL, O. (1929). Communication: The inner injunction to make a mental note. *Int. J. Psychoanal.,* 10:447.

FREUD, S. (1909). Notes upon a case of obsessional neurosis. *S.E.,* 10:153–249.

GENETTE, GÉRARD. (1988). *Narrative Discourse Revisited.* Trans. by Jane E. Lewin. Ithaca, NY: Cornell University Press.

GIDE, ANDRÉ. (1984). *Journals 1889–1949*, tr. J. O'Brien. London: Penguin.

GOSSE, E. (1907). *Father and Son*. Harmondsworth: Penguin, 1983.

GRAY, PAUL. (1994). *The Ego and Analysis of Defense*. Northvale, N.J.: Jason Aronson.

JAKOBSON, R. (1957). *Shifters, Verbal Categories, and the Russian Verb. Selected Works II*. Berlin-New York-Amsterdam: Mouton Publishers, pp. 130–147.

JAKOBSON, R. & POMORSKA, K. (1985). Dialogue on time in language and literature. In *Verbal Art, Verbal Sign, Verbal Time*. Eds. K. Pormorska and S. Rudy. Minneapolis: University of Minnesota Press.

JOHNSON, MARK. (1987). *The Body in the Mind*. Chicago: University of Chicago Press.

KERNBERG, OTTO. (1987). Projection and projective identification: Development and clinical aspects. In: *Projection, Identification, Projective Identification*. Ed. J. Sandler. Madison, Conn.: International Universities Press.

KRUGER, LOU-MARIÉ & WOLF, DENNIE PALMER. (1994). Play and narrative in inhibited children: A longitudinal case study. In: *Children at Play*. Eds. Arietta Slade and Dennie Palmer Wolf. New York: Oxford University Press.

LEAR, JONATHAN. (1990). *Love and Its Place in Nature*. New York: Farrar, Straus & Giroux.

LESLIE, A. (1987). Pretense and representation: The origins of "theory of the mind," *Psychological Review*, 94 (4):412–426.

MEARES, R. (1993). *The Metaphor of Play: Disruption and Restoration in the Borderline Experience*. Northvale, N.J.: Jason Aronson.

MILLER, J. H. (1990). Narrative. In *Critical Terms for Literary Study*. Eds. F. Lentricchia and T. McLaughlin. Chicago: University of Chicago Press.

NIELSEN, A. (1994). Projective identification revisited: Clarification of component steps and relation to countertransference and self psychology. Paper read at the 1/25/94 Meeting of the Chicago Psychoanalytic Society.

RADO, S. (1958). Psychotherapy: a problem of controlled communication. In: *Psychopathology of Communication*. Eds. P. Hoch and J. Zubin. New York: Grune & Stratton, pp. 214–226.

RIMMON-KENAN, S. (1983). *Narrative Fiction: Contemporary Poetics*. New Accents Series. London: Methuen.

SANDLER, J. (1976). Countertransference and role-responsiveness. *Int. Rev. Psychoanal.* 3:43–47.

SCAIFE, M. & BRUNER, J. (1975). The capacity for joint visual attention in the infant. *Nature*, 253:265–266.

SIMON, B. (1988). *Tragic Drama and the Family*. New Haven: Yale University Press.

SORCE, J. F. ET AL. (1985). Maternal emotional signaling: Its effect on the visual cliff behavior of one-year-olds. *Developmental Psychology*, 21, 195–200.

WALKER, P. (1992). *The Message in the Bottle*. New York: Noonday Press, Farrar Straus & Giroux.

WAELDER, R. (1951). The structure of paranoid ideas. *Int. J. Psycho-Anal.* 32:167–177.

WELLES, J. & WRYE, H. (1994). *The Narration of Desire*. Hillsdale, N.J.: Analytic Press.

WINNER, E. & LEEKAM, S. (1991). Distinguishing irony from deception: Understanding the speaker's second-order intention. In: *Perspectives on the Child's Theory of Mind*. Eds. Butterworth, P. et al. New York: Oxford University Press.

Ego Erection

Regressive Perceptual Phenomena in Relation to Psychic Growth

OSCAR F. HILLS, M.D.

Regressive phenomena involving alterations of perceptual and other ego functions are exemplified by the Isakower phenomenon. Originally considered to be a defensive process involving regression to the oral phase in the face of conflict, a number of additional dimensions have been clarified in the literature over time. This paper describes analytic work with a patient who experienced distortions in the perception of his body on the couch. It examines the relationship of these experiences to the Isakower phenomenon. With close attention to analytic case material, it corroborates the oral core, the defensive structure, and the transformational processes characteristic of the episodes. Further, this case demonstrates that orally rooted ego phenomena, arising in response to oedipal conflict, can call forth the analysis of attachment. The vicissitudes of these phenomena throughout an analysis can give representation to the developing capacity for emotional attachment. The capacity for physical attachment, achieved in infancy via the mouth and breast, gives rise incrementally to the capacity for psychic attachment, achieved in adulthood by the waning of the Oedipal complex.

REGRESSIVE EGO PHENOMENA INVOLVING ALTERATIONS OF PERCEPTUAL and other usually autonomous ego functions are well described in the

Assistant clinical professor of psychiatry at Yale University School of Medicine; in private practice in New Haven and Guilford, Conn.; graduate and member of the Western New England Institute for Psychoanalysis, member of the Western New England Psychoanalytic Society, and the American Psychoanalytic Association.
The Psychoanalytic Study of the Child 54, ed. Albert J. Solnit, Peter B. Neubauer, Samuel Abrams, and A. Scott Dowling (Yale University Press, copyright © 1999 by Albert J. Solnit, Peter B. Neubauer, Samuel Abrams, and A. Scott Dowling).

classical psychoanalytic literature. Otto Isakower's (1938) fundamental and evocative characterization of one class of such experiences, originally considered to involve regression to the oral phase, has given us the Isakower phenomenon. A number of additional dimensions of this predormescent perturbation have been clarified in the literature over time. Isakower explicitly stated that the phenomenon is defensive and thus occurs in response to conflict, but having fallen by the wayside in the subsequent early literature, this idea has only recently resurfaced. While most observers now agree that such a phenomenon represents a return to the oral phase at moments of conflict, the more current idea is that later developmental phases and their conflicts can also be represented by developmental transformations of these regressive experiences.

Until very recently, the literature describing regressive sensory phenomena offered little direct analytic data, and contributors frequently cited instances that had occurred outside of the analytic hour. In this paper, I will describe analytic work with a patient who experienced distortions in the perception of his body on the couch, and I will examine the relationship of these phenomena to that described by Isakower. In addition to corroborating the oral core, the defensive structure, and the transformational processes characteristic of the episodes, I will also demonstrate the capacity of regressive ego phenomena to represent adult conflict in an innocent and profoundly infantile mode and at the same time their potential for developmental transformation. They are thus positioned uniquely to reveal to both analyst and analysand the continuing state of the ego along the road of psychic development, from narcissistic isolation to differentiated object relatedness. We will see that orally rooted ego phenomena, arising in response to oedipal conflict, call forth the analysis of attachment. Through this we can observe how the capacity for physical attachment achieved in infancy via the mouth and breast gives rise incrementally to the capacity for psychic attachment achieved in adulthood by the waning of the Oedipus complex.

LITERATURE REVIEW

The paradigm discussion of regressive functioning of the mental apparatus is, of course, Freud's *The Interpretation of Dreams* (1900), in which the dream serves as exemplar of an idea devolved upon its original sensory imagery. Dynamically unconscious, early, and largely visually represented memories influence such topographical regression. These, along with our more occult phylogenetic childhood, of which individual childhood memories are elements of a condensed recapitulation, could be said to attract corresponding present-day thoughts, which are also dynamically isolated, to the regressive pathway of sensory expression in dreaming. The topographical, temporal, and formal components of regression in dreaming derive their primary motive force, at this theoretical level, from the relative absence of the spectrum of sensory input that is present during waking activity. In pathological waking states, however, we encounter regressive phenomena such as auditory or visual hallucinations in spite of the presence of the progressive sensory current. Freud points out that, from the psychological point of view, this finding demonstrates the greater intensity of other regressive motivations in these cases—i.e., the push of topographic censorship, on the one hand, and the pull of visually represented unconscious memories, on the other. In 1914, Freud appended to a new edition of *The Interpretation of Dreams* the felicitous observation that "regression plays a no less important part in the theory of the formation of neurotic symptoms than it does in that of dreams" (p. 548). The psychological laws governing dream formation, then, are also directly instantiated in Freud's formulation of regressive mental functioning, and in fact they underlie as first principles all we know in psychoanalysis.

Isakower (1938) sought to understand a particular class of hypnagogic phenomena in light of these precepts. He paid specific attention to the economic activity and the condition of the ego as it is engaged in the psychic process of falling asleep. During the gradual withdrawal of cathexis from the external world and its redistribution in the ego, there exists a regressive mental configuration, which Isakower likened to the immediately postnatal ego. In this state of mind, perceptions are simultaneously localized as bodily experience and as external phenomena. Isakower's patients described having had such a spell, and most frequently reported it as either a childhood memory or an experience during an illness. They recollected a visual impression of something shadowy and round coming nearer, and often reported a tactile sensation of something crumpled or dry in the mouth and on the skin. In Freud's model of regression, the mental content of phenomena necessarily holds deterministic clues to the meaning of the process. Isakower reasoned that early "ego attitudes" very likely carry with them mental images of the external events of their time. He conjectured that the images described by his patients reflected sucking at the mother's breast and falling asleep there. He further postulated that the conscious quality of these revived early experiences was brought about by psychic conflict and thus amounted to defensive compromise.

He cited as an example an incestuous masturbatory fantasy, repudiated by the superego, for which the experience of infantile suckling,
revived by the ego's regression, is offered up to consciousness as a readily available and gratifyingly innocent substitute (pp. 344–345).

Subsequent notions of the role of early infantile imagery in the constitution of regressive episodes were formulated from all manner of
data. Lewin (1946) described the "dream screen" as representing both
the breast during sleep and the fulfillment of the wish to sleep; he later
explored the oral nature of sleep itself (Lewin, 1948, 1953). Spitz
(1955) re-emphasized the importance of earliest orality in understanding the Isakower phenomenon and saw the classic "approaching
mass" as representing the visually perceived human face, at which he
asserted the infant stares throughout nursing. Kepecs (1952) reported
a man who had interposed a defensive phantom of the maternal breast
between himself and the external world. Finn (1955) saw that the orality of a hospitalized patient accounted for her "blank stage." Almansi
(1958) presented a patient's hypnagogic hallucination of an attractive
cloud with an indistinct beckoning voice as confirmation of Spitz's
formulations. Rycroft (1951) addressed the dynamic significance of
the dream screen, an attempt to re-establish the maternal object relationship in the service of ego development. F. Deutsch (1953) was interested in the object-libidinal underpinnings of regressive sensory
perception. Murphy (1958) reminded us that sensory regression in response to object loss is a narcissistic defense, reflecting a diminution of
ego. In Lewy's (1954) psychotically ill patient, micropsia illustrated the
ego's regressive use of sensory experience and also gave symbolic representation to its own diminishing functional breadth. M. Stern (1961)
noted that "blank hallucinations" appeared in people with the character pathologies associated with oral *deprivation,* the frustration giving
rise to primitive defenses, later revived in response to oedipal conflict
(Stern, 1953). Sperling (1957, 1961) turned his attention to the *technique* involved in the psychoanalytic investigation of hypnagogic hallucinations. He feared that analysts had been too easily misled by the
manifest content of these dreamlike phenomena. It is his *analytic* finding that hypnagogic hallucinations are traceable to experiences far
later than the first six months of life. Fink (1967) presented, with
specifics, an analysand for whom she concluded that the hallucinatory
maternal breast defended against primal-scene memories and castration anxiety associated with the view of the female genital.

The sober gaze of ego psychology turned upon regressive episodes
by the Kris Study Group (Joseph, 1965) offers an experience-near perspective. The emphasis is on disturbances of ordinarily autonomous

ego functions. Clinical examples in the monograph include body-image distortion, perceptual disturbances, and failures of reality testing, as well as difficulties in time and distance judgment, depersonalization experiences, and the classic Isakower phenomenon. Having occurred on the couch, these are amenable to close analytic scrutiny. The group concluded that ego regressions are defensive processes serving multiple functions across the psychic agencies. Castration anxiety predominantly initiates ego regression, but separation anxiety, fear of the superego, and primal-scene experiences are also frequently implicated. The actual predilection for these regressions seems to be linked to early object relations, including identification with a love object also predisposed to discrete ego dysfunction. The Kris Study Group also found that perception, reality testing, and body image were ego functions particularly susceptible to regressive influence. It concurred that the Isakower effect and similar phenomena can be understood as regressive ego phenomena, the analytic exploration of which can yield the same richness of understanding as the investigation of the classic neurotic symptoms.[1]

In both the Isakower phenomenon and the *déjà vu* experience, the oedipal compromise formation involves an infantile and thus innocent union with mother in which the Oedipus complex is conspicuous by its negation. Yet another psychoanalytic observation drawing upon early orality and the nursing situation for its theoretical foundation, and also presenting the Oedipus complex in regression, is Lewin's (1933) "body-phallus equation." The unconscious fantasy that the whole body is a phallus is well described in psychoanalytic writing from Freud to the present, with Tausk's (1919) "influencing machine" and Ferenczi's (1928) "Gulliver fantasies" serving as particularly compelling earlier examples. It was Abraham (1924), however, who first suggested that the mechanism of the body-phallus equation involved the oral incorporation of a bodily part followed by identification of the entire body with that part. Lewin posed the further question: what is the dominant sexual aim in these cases? Following Abraham's formulation that the identification derived from the cannibalistic oral phase is with the bitten-off and devoured penis, Lewin ventured that the unconscious wish and fear expressed at this level of development can only be *to be eaten*. The identification, then, amounts to the passive reversal

---

1. J. Arlow, chair of the Kris Study Group, had simultaneously brought this thinking to bear on the *déjà vu* experience (Arlow, 1959). His work was expanded on by Pacella (1975) and Mahler (1968) in light of Spitz's (1965, pp. 53–149) work on the early nursing face-gestalt configuration.

of the devouring aim, whose object is a parental phallus. Lewin (1950, pp. 102–165) later introduced the idea of the oral triad—the wish to devour, the wish to be devoured, and the wish to go to sleep—all of which originate in the nursing situation. Such ideas often appear in neurosis as *fears,* not only of castration, the oedipal origin of which is regressively defended against by the oral rendering, but also of the sadistic, biting, and devouring wish, defended against and regulated by talion reversal. From this perspective then, we would expect in *all* cases to find the oral triad and its defensive contour lurking beneath the body-phallus equation. In *some* of these cases, we might further anticipate that the body-phallus equation would be central in a prominent defensive regression to the oral phase.

Sandler (1959) demonstrated the protean manifestations of the body-phallus equation in the analysis of a man with a pervasive fear of erection and sexual excitement. Castration anxiety was averted by the displacement of cathexis from the penis to the whole body, which then served the disguised function of exhibiting sexual excitement through rigidity and straightness. Glenn (1971) revisited the body-phallus equation after observing it in conjunction with the Isakower phenomenon. A pregnant woman experienced the Isakower phenomenon on the couch, feeling that her mouth, tongue, hands, and then entire body were swollen and that she was becoming a baby. Identifying with her baby *in utero,* and the baby in turn with a penis, she evinced her own body-phallus equation. As in the oral phase, the head, mouth, and hands are more highly cathected than the genitals, and it is this quality that similarly characterizes the Isakower phenomenon. As vestiges of early self-representation, these regressions can inform exploration of the early formation of the ego's complex representational capacities.

Spitz (1961), working on early prototypes of defense in the infant, distinguished *real* sleep—i.e., the withdrawal of cathexis from the psychic representation of the sensorium, and regression to satiation during nursing—from its prototype, the psychologically null physiological sleep of the neonate. Real sleep is a precursor to all defenses, chief among them regression, the earliest defense mechanism to appear. It also denies the experience of separation and with it the differentiation between the "I" and the "non-I" that Spitz (1957) believed develops out of the repeated experience of loss of the need-gratifying preobject in nursing and early feeding. Easson (1973) applied this thinking to the Isakower phenomenon, seen then as a vestigial manifestation of the earliest awareness of ego boundaries and personhood, most frequently reported in childhood and adolescence, when ego boundaries and the sense of personhood are once again in flux.

Richards (1985) discovered, in light of a ten-year gap in the literature, that there was a dearth of *analytic* material supporting the dynamic formulations of the early work. He invited analysts to make fresh contributions of data. Dann (1992) responded directly, reporting that a patient's perceptual disturbances became a central organizing theme of the analysis. He reiterated Isakower's original understanding but also showed in the case material that revived early sensory memory traces acquire new levels of meaning throughout development. Glenn (1993) was similarly focused in his later study of the Isakower phenomenon as an example of early memories that can undergo developmental transformation. He re-presented, with some additional detail, the case first described in his work on the body-phallus equation (Glenn, 1971). The pregnant woman's identification with the baby *in utero* can also give representation and expression to anal- and phallic-stage psychic conflict. As a matter of historical precision, Abrams (1977) pointed out that the genetic point of view (Hartmann and Kris, 1945; Rapaport and Gill, 1959) rests not only on the principle of antecedent determinism but also on that of epigenetic developmental transformations which occur under sway of both progressive and regressive forces. Glenn emphasized that the Isakower phenomenon *qua* analyzable mental event might be freed of its often singularly oral conceptualization by our greater appreciation of this latter metapsychological assumption.

We would hope, of course, to find this thinking behind our handling of *all* analytic material, but perhaps the drama of the Isakower phenomenon has led to considerable investigation in the literature of some of its facets, with relative inattention to others. We have seen that emphasis in the earlier work was placed on recovered mental contents, their meaning, their place in adult life, and their value in understanding more clearly the experience of both the psychoanalytic and the observable infant, particularly during the oral phase. Later focus on ego functioning helped to demonstrate that regressive perceptual experiences are not infrequent in the analytic situation and can be treated as analyzable. Further investigation revealed that while these experiences are founded in orality and involve regression in the face of anxiety, they can also represent experience and conflict at various levels of organization and development, taking on transformed functions.

CLINICAL MATERIAL

In the following clinical material I will present in some detail the analytic treatment of a man for whom Isakower-like regressive ego phenomena appeared as highly economical representations of his state of mind. They consistently involved *swelling*—swelling of breasts, of hands, and of head. With their changing qualities and precipitants, they became indicators of the advances in ego-building that took place throughout the treatment.

Mr. B. came for analysis in his mid-thirties after moving across the country in pursuit of a woman he hardly knew. He also made the move in part to escape graduate school, which he had all but finished, and in part to escape a female therapist, with whom he had engaged in five years of twice-weekly psychoanalytically oriented work. His chief complaint was a severe inhibition in urinating in public restrooms, requiring him to leave work during the day to use the toilet at home. This was accompanied by the more recent fear that he was homosexual and by a frenetic, handwringing scrutiny of any internal or external occurrences that might be taken as evidence of this. Our initial face-to-face psychotherapy was marked both by his harshly critical attention to my every move and by his frequent near frozen silence in my presence. His difficulty in producing a stream of speech was strongly reminiscent of the urinary inhibition itself. Shortly after beginning therapy with me, Mr. B. reported an episode of the night before in which he wished to be an infant ministered to by an attentive mother. He reported that during that evening's reverie he was lying naked on the bathroom floor of his apartment amid his own urine and excrement fantasizing about being cleaned up and diapered. As time went on and as this account might have foreshadowed, it became clear that in spite of his irascibility, Mr. B. was inclined to form intense, clinging attachments, which he experienced as infantile. We saw over time that any sense of loss, including my so much as shifting my gaze, was met with desperation and rage.

On beginning analysis, he seemed comforted by my physical presence as well as by not having to endure the sight of me, a burden that had in the past stirred him to endless diffuse unfavorable, envious, and loathing comparisons between us. He seemed most comfortable perceiving and imagining me almost solely as an extension of himself. He would become enraged if I made any disturbance in the room such as the sound of adjusting a shirtsleeve or shifting my position in the chair, to say nothing of opening my mouth to speak. He often delighted in describing a recurring dream he had had during his last therapy in which the therapist was an inflatable punching clown that he would hit repeatedly as hard as he could. The clown would immediately rebound to the vertical position with a smile that he took to be mocking his ineffectiveness and yet reassuring him that he was not really as destructive as the strength of his wishes led him to fear.

Over the first six months, he reported a number of episodes of transient perceptual distortion occurring outside of our sessions. He had
had the strange sensation that he was very tall; at another time he had
the feeling that his folded hands belonged to two different people; in
another episode he felt that he was growing breasts. Consonant with his
experience of me as an extension of himself and thus of little interpersonal consequence, these experiences were not initially observable on
the couch. In the seventh month, as Mr. B. was becoming resigned to
my presence as an individual, he offered the following thoughts:

> I feel I started talking right away this morning, but I've missed a chance
> to have a moment of quiet, I was reading about a woman who was in
> analysis for fourteen years with a famous analyst, it took her fourteen
> years to figure out she was depressed, now I just thought if you ever be-
> come famous I'll think, "He was really pretty good and I didn't even
> know it," . . . I think that woman could run circles around that analyst
> **[as *you're* trying to with me, off to a running start]** yeah, now I just had
> the sensation of having breasts, like protective gear, a security blanket,
> but a secret source of power.

In this moment of togetherness, the many threats I posed to him, first
by speaking at all but more specifically by confronting one of his immediate intentions toward me, seemed to call for near-hallucinatory defensive measures. We may retrace his psychic activity in a close reading
of the material by postulating, as is borne out in later productions, that
the moment of quiet he lamented having foregone was, from the perspective of regressive object relatedness, the moment when I was most
nearly completely his own construction, a fantasied person, the em-
bodiment of maternal benevolence and solicitude. This wish for early
oral tranquility with me reflected a retreat from the biting aggression in
his words, the projection of which filled him with a fear of my intrusive
otherness. Over and above his identification with both mother and baby
was Mr. B.'s endopsychic perception—i.e., recognition by his unconscious ego of both his decrement in cathexis of the capacity to evaluate
reality and the resulting ascension of fantasy. Castration anxiety, fear of
loss of love, and terror of disintegration of the self were stirred by my intrusion, and a regressive hallucinatory merger with a powerful and protecting mother was the oral-phase defense up to the task of sustaining
Mr. B.'s ego—for the moment eliminating me from the field.

Our work led to a growing awareness of Mr. B.'s efforts to avoid and
to deny my existence. To do otherwise, he feared, would stimulate a ra-
pacious appetite for emotional nutriment and attachment that could
scarcely be withstood by even the most powerful mother and would certainly consume anyone so incidental and peripherally important as a

man. The following excerpt illustrates the complexity of his struggle, in response to my clarifications, to allow the two of us to share the office. As he contemplates my presence and my potential absence he calls forth a perceptual body image distortion, which again unites him with an ample mother. This reunion is soon threatened, however, by his externalized devouring appetite.

> There's a new man at work . . . I feel the impulse to befriend him . . . I feel all the women at work are powerful, the men aren't . . . working there I'm allying myself with powerful women, being friends with the men is a weak position . . . now I'm feeling as though all this is seductive towards *you* . . . just as I said that I find myself feeling like a buxom woman, with my arms crossed under my breasts like an old peasant woman (*silence*) I'm nervous now, you cleared your throat, maybe it's near the end of the session, I've got to think faster, only a couple of minutes left and then here comes this big hole . . . the weekend . . . like my old shopping-center dream with my mother, the floor opens up in the grocery store and I'm swallowed.

Of the many available themes in that hour, the oral motif of breasts (the buxom woman), food (the grocery store), throats (clearing mine), and swallowing (the floor opens up) pervaded the material in response to his feeling both close to me and seductive. Over many subsequent sessions, Mr. B. continued to elaborate upon what he wished and feared he could do with his mouth.

Further into the analysis, with the development of a slightly greater tolerance for closeness, Mr. B.'s immediate fear of fragmentation had notably diminished. He was somewhat better able to engage with me directly, though primarily by way of fighting, a habit that was readily intensified in response to disruptions of his conflicted attachment to me. In the midst of a protracted rage over my having taken a spring break, he had decided that behavior therapy was going to have to be the solution to some of his inhibitions. Shortly after beginning this "adjunctive" therapy with Dr. D., he began to berate both the therapy and Dr. D. throughout our sessions. He was insulted at the very idea of the therapist's requesting that he close his eyes for imaging purposes. While his familiar fear of manifold regressive dangers had, not unexpectedly, resurfaced in the behavioral therapeutic effort, his dudgeon at feeling told what to do nonetheless remained only halfheartedly displaced from me. Our subsequent interaction led to another transient perceptual distortion in which he felt his right hand enlarging.

> I worry that Dr. D. will get me so relaxed I'll piss and shit all over myself, maybe I *want* that, like a newborn baby, but on the other hand I feel as though I'm saying all this to placate you **[and you feel I *need* pla-**

cating today?], maybe because of my going to see D. yesterday, leaving you and going over to him, all these competing views of reality, like the one I feel you're *bullying* me to accept [**I think perhaps *you're* bullying *me***]. Yeah, I *am* bullying you . . . you know, I actually *do* have some attachment to you, you're not just another doc, nameless and faceless. . . . I felt some *pleasure* just now in your interrupting me, I felt like a runaway train, like you needed to pull the lever to throw the brake on, you usually don't do that . . . *now I feel like my right hand is getting bigger* . . . it upsets me. . . . With my old therapist, who was a woman of course, I'd fear my hands would fill up the whole room . . . actually, it's like the runaway train image, like I'm too big, too powerful.

When asked about "nameless and faceless," he recalled that the names and faces of his past girlfriends tended to run together and to produce *one* woman of great importance. In response to my confrontation about bullying, then, he seemed to do his best to cast me by negation into the nurturant form of the "nameless and faceless" primal woman (breast) of early oral psychic life. This familiar mental refuge from the feared dangers of oral and later aggression derives much of its complexion from the mental functioning characteristic of its developmental origin in early infancy. The perceptual distortion of a swelling hand is consistent with all we have seen in the literature regarding a regression to orality. The predominant bodily cathexes are of the mouth and the hands. Upon regression, cathexis is redistributed along infantile lines, and the sensation is one of swelling of the involved body parts.

In this non-psychotic man, we would further expect to find the Oedipus complex behind his regressive experiences, and it is that component of the process that gained expression through the specific "swelling" of Mr. B.'s dominant hand. As a first pass along these lines, and considering the gender fluidity expectable when regression has relegated oedipal-level functioning to little more than a potentiality, it could be said that Mr. B. felt betrayed that I had gone off on vacation *with someone else*, and that, turning passive to active, he intended to punish me in kind by "going over to" Dr. D. My "interrupting" him in the session not only reassured him but also excited him sexually. The pleasure he expressed in being a runaway train and in ideas of my pulling his lever led to his physical experience of excitation. (He later reported that my interrupting him felt like a potential fight and excited him so much that he "may have started to get an erection.") Here, I was the direct object of his excitement. Great dangers were imminent in his mind, and the regressive oral vortex beckoned. The erection, while still experienced bodily, was displaced from the penis to the hand (a secondary oral characteristic, as it were). This process of displacement, in its entirety, is a manifestation of oral libidinal organization alongside its accompanying narcissistic relatedness.

As Mr. B. became increasingly able to find room for both of us in the office, exhibitionistic and ambitious wishes seemed far less threatening; or, conversely, as his wishes became less threatening, it was easier to find the room for two. As ambitions turned up more straightforwardly in the material, and as we again neared our customary spring break, he reported a dream which involved a new car that he had recently felt emboldened to purchase.

> I had a dream I drove my car into the water, steam was coming out from under the hood . . . a blown valve . . . and water's pouring out like a firehose . . . I woke up last night having to go to the bathroom, but I didn't want to get out of bed.

The regressive oceanic pull continued to seem to offer refuge from the fantasied dangers of adult sexuality and ambition, but, much analytic work having been done, the imagined loss of manhood accompanying his retreat brought into doubt for Mr. B. what, if anything, is actually gained by this maneuver. This burgeoning insight was in evidence several days later when we met in the parking lot as I arrived for the session. The issue was not long in emerging in the transference.

> I had on a baseball cap when you drove up, then I suddenly felt I'd look ridiculous, with a Marlins cap on, maybe I thought I'd have a swelled head, so I took it off, like you might make fun of me, you might be saying, "don't think you're so big," it all makes me anxious.

The allusions to erection and fear of my castrating potential were obvious in the material and supported by Mr. B.'s later associations, but the regressive escape route represented by the water in the preceding dream was more subtle in this material. To be sure, the marlin, named for the marlinespike that its bill brings to mind, had at least as much business in the ocean as the new car in the recent dream, but, in light of what we know, the associative involvement of Mr. B.'s swelled head with this dangerously endowed sea creature nicely betokened his potential for regression to orality in the face of castration anxiety. At this stage of the analysis and under these circumstances, however, the large head (characteristic of an infantile distribution of cathexis) and its swelling (an oceanic manifestation of regression innocently representing erection) were experienced not as regressive perceptual phenomena but rather as ideas, amenable to verbal expression. Perhaps his diminished anxiety was now that of the phallic ariviste, enduring if not prevailing in his effort to share in the world of men.

One day, however, he entered the office thinking about asking to reschedule a session because of a work-related conference he wished to attend, and here verbalization failed him. He felt that speaking with me about rescheduling was risky, and he speculated that it was the potential for not getting things his way and the feelings this stirred that frightened him. His thoughts then went to a "prima donna politician" who felt entitled to do anything he wanted—unlike himself, he hastened to add.

Now I feel maybe I shouldn't have spoken up about rescheduling . . . not take the risk [**which is what?**] not getting my way, and I think it has to do with my *status* here, or maybe I'm concerned about how you'll perceive my *taking* the time off for the conference . . . I feel left out in the cold now, like at home and at work, and now with you, and I'm anticipating you won't be able to reschedule [**but you also *put* yourself out in the cold, it's easy for you to feel that asking me about rescheduling is the bellicose demand of an outsider, it seems safer**]. Yeah, that's true, a fight keeps a distance . . .just now I had a weird feeling of having a big *head,* like my head is *expanding* to fill a space, maybe to push everyone else out, like I say to myself, 'Don't even *listen* to anyone else," . . . "*be* self-sufficient," . . . "I know *everything,*" . . . it's a position of strength . . . I feel my whole head is like a house, and my eyes aren't little openings but plate-glass windows, it's both megalomaniacal and also magnanimous. . . . No, it's *not* that, I think it's also a child's way of bringing myself *down,* after I was just feeling *competitive* about ideas, where I don't want you to get to one before I do. . . .

Speaking of competition, I was joking with E the other day about haircuts, we saw a guy with a Mohawk . . . E said to be competitive I could get my eyebrows pierced, I said, 'If I weren't circumcised I could get my prepuce pierced,' she didn't know the word. . . . In *Ulysses,* Bloom refers to "God, the great collector of prepuces" . . . interesting I went to this after that "big head" feeling [**to genital mutilation?**]. Yeah, I don't know if I have more anxiety about being *big* or being *small,* both. . .

In the days preceding this episode Mr. B. had been troubled by awareness of his intention to ask me about rescheduling a session. It occurred to him that we two busy men might need to negotiate the terms of our work together for that day, but this view entailed in his mind the forfeiture of his investment in my maintaining parental authority. In the course of fearing the impulses that might arise between the two of us as men, he had already covered considerable regressive distance before he actually set foot in my office with rescheduling on his mind.

A simple explanation of some of the session quoted above is that Mr.

B.'s overdetermined fear of what could happen in a direct discussion of rescheduling led to the rationalizations, externalizations, and sense of simultaneous power and safety made available by his regressively communicating to me essentially, "You won't give me what I want, and I hate you for it." To this assertion I replied, as he heard it, "No! it's *your* fault, and *I'm* bigger." And to this perceived attack his humiliated and castrated response was, "Die! I eat you! and I am *biggest* of all!" This exchange stands in precipitate contrast to his civilized manifest announcement, "I fear, sir, that rescheduling may not go my way," and to my response, "That, sir, may be more tolerable than you anticipate," and then to his rejoinder, "Yes, perhaps so." In fact, Mr. B.'s ego was regressively primed by castration anxiety for a struggle, and the anal-sadistic regressive defenses against this anxiety served only to widen the gap between longed-for and felt experience and to amplify the component impulses.

The seized ambivalent opportunity to feel plunged into battle liberated to the brink of behavior, in his mind, impulses that in vivid fantasy dealt a death blow both to me and consequently to his ultimate hope for emotional adulthood. In an instant, his ego "found" that it was only by turning to deep, hallucinatory regressive experience that the situation could be safely represented. Mr. B.'s head was "expanding to fill a space," thus innocently taking the place of an erect penis by way of the regressive redistribution of cathexis. In this instance, the narcissistic object-relatedness, part and parcel of this oral revisitation, was even more clearly demonstrated than in the previous episode. His inflation was pushing "everyone else" out, silencing and devaluating "them." Here again was an unstoppable erectile expansion occurring at the speed of regression. It reflected, among other wishes, that of the dependent or abased subject *already* to be big and powerful, by whatever means available, including the psychic return to an earlier state in which fragile omnipotence was once safeguarded by maternal devotion.

In this state, Mr. B.'s head had become a palace, but noticeable as such only to the monarch's proportionally shrunken ego. All other inhabitants (constituting the "precipitate of abandoned object cathexes") were all but expelled. Object-relatedness itself was thereupon nearly cast out of the house, and for a moment omnipotence was restored. There was a giant infant ruling my consulting room, the magnanimous picture of *noblesse oblige*. But, without mother (her proxy driven out from behind the couch), the regime was tottering, and fragility of the psychic apparatus was the bigger picture in the "plate glass windows" his eyes had become. This imagery reminds us, however, that fusion with mother is integral to this degree of regression and suggests that Mr. B. must also have experienced my comments to him in the session as nurturant and salutary. From this perspective, his regression was an oral expression of both love itself and the desperation to protect it, as seen through the eyes of the symbiont. To all of this Mr. B. declared, "No, it's *not* that," not only affirming by negation the psychic validity of his portrayal but also introducing an additional dimension of the regressive experience—it's regulatory and self-punitive function—"a way of bringing myself down."

Mr. B.'s return to an infantile ego state involves more than simply being drawn away from the fear of loss of love and from castration anxiety by the allure of orality and maternal fusion, which allow innocent expression of the offending aggressive impulses. It also entails being repulsed, by the savagery of the superego's punitive aim, from adulthood and from the mastery of anxiety, and propelled, by the same impulse turned against the self, toward infantile impotence and dependence. In turning punitive, castrating, and infantilizing intentions upon the self, many secondary goals *appear* to be achieved while still gratifying the desires by enacting them against the self. These include reducing the threatening reactions of the original object (withdrawal of love and/or attack) by displacement of aim from the object to the self, by the demonstration of obeisant submission in front of the original object, and by making a preemptive retaliatory strike against the self in response to the original intentions. Further, as in all neurotic compromise, the original aim is in essence achieved, but not without a shift from reality toward fantasy and, accordingly, from active toward passive. In this case, the parent (analyst) is secondarily injured and rendered impotent by the failure to thrive (regression) of the beloved (analyzed) child (analysand).

On emerging from this regressive episode, Mr. B. was then able to work his way back, through further associative links, to a more current representation of the original anxiety. His associations began with the infantile big head of the "guy with a Mohawk" and moved to the piercing mutilation of the eyebrows (not far from nipples and tongues in current piercing culture), thus emphasizing the visual field and the face as forerunners of orality. He then shifted to circumcision and piercing of the prepuce, bringing him closer to the initial castration fears driving so much of the session. At one end of the developmental spectrum from narcissism to relatedness lay orality and maternal fusion; at the other, the castrating father, "God, the great collector of prepuces." The question of "being big or being small," as we shall see, was indeed a salient issue in this analysis, and it involved the narcissistic wish that bigness, in the form of adult ego functioning, be attainable on demand with erectile automaticity, which ensures in turn a position of centrality in the universe of human relations.

The episode of the expanding head represented the themes, fantasies, and defenses in this analysis so economically that it served as an organizing high point. From then on, analysis of the transference was in full swing, and we focused much attention upon the ambivalence so prominent in Mr. B.'s preferred form of relatedness. What he had previously viewed as his angry reactions to my failures of attunement to his attachment were reframed and broadened to reveal the fears that motivated his holding himself at a distance. As the extent to which his attachment to me as a maternal figure defended against aggressive and sadistic impulses, and the extent to which these impulses themselves were amplified by feeling reduced to infantile life, became clearer to him, he became better able to tolerate the awareness of his competitive and ambitious strivings without recourse to mind-altering regression. Following much analysis, Mr. B. married his girlfriend. Several days after his announcement that he and his wife had set a closing date for the purchase of a new house, his thoughts turned as usual toward finances.

> I was going to pay the bill today but realized I need more money for the down payment on the house. . . . I guess I have the feeling it would only be decent of you to let me slide . . . you should want to give me a house-warming gift . . . like you owe it to me . . . but I also feel we're doing something *really* irresponsible buying this house. E says she's envious that I have a lawyer *and* a shrink to help me . . . but of all the people I've spoken to about this, the one I had really wanted to hear from was my *mother.* She finally called last night, and the difference in how I felt was night and day. I got her blessing and I felt very much relieved. . . . I had a dream last night. I was singing *America the Beautiful* in a sort of draconian classroom where you shouldn't misbehave . . . I kept singing in full operatic voice after we were supposed to stop, the rest of the class applauded and I felt good but I feared the punishment that was sure to come. . . . I felt, "Why should we stop singing?" and I wanted to show off, plus sort of tweak the nose of this teacher . . . maybe that's my feeling here in deciding to remain a month in arrears with the bill to help with my down payment, it's like it's kind of "in your face" and I'm going to do it anyway, but it's as though I imagine you're a loan shark. I've paid the principal twenty times over coming here but I have to pay again **[I think you feel you** *need* **the likes of a loan shark to help you uphold your end of the bargain].** Yeah, it does feel that way, plus a set of mothering adult figures **[you mean like the maternal analyst who will give you a housewarming gift].** Yeah, exactly, it's a nice feeling **[and**

much easier for you than to be aware of *taking* the money from me, easy credit where you can get it].

In the past, this was just the sort of moment, a confrontation of his darker plans for me, that might have given rise to a regressive perceptual experience, but in this case the issues so often represented by such experiences were verbalized instead.

> Yeah it's true, the only reason I pay back loans at all is that I'm afraid of what the enforcers will do. . . . I came in here this morning feeling calm . . . a plan to build up the down payment and be in arrears here, like I was pleased that I've found a successful plan, but then I feel I need help [you get nervous enacting your plan with me and then feel you need mothering] (laughs) and lawyering and shrinking, especially the shrinking, like to be made smaller, reminds me of an erect penis shrinking, I feel like I was too big, taking advantage of you, need to be made smaller. . . . Whew, it's been *quite* a week, but there I go again, soliciting your sympathy, when really I'm screwing you.

He began the session with the announcement of his plan to use me for credit but then reverted to the idea of my giving him a gift. With characteristic aggression, he then turned to the feeling of my owing it to him, given the unreasonable demands I've made upon him. Such thinking immediately brought mother to mind, first in the displaced form of his wife and then more explicitly. His relief upon feeling permitted by mother to take this bold step was immediately followed by the report of a dream that began with his participation in a celebration of civilized society, but ended with a narcissistic triumph in which his singing about *the beautiful* in "full operatic voice" resurrected the prima donna, the "first lady" of orality. In this dream, however, castration anxiety (represented by a draconian teacher deserving of a tweaked nose) was plainly evident, as was the triadic life of the classroom and the identification with the phallic mother to which Mr. B. habitually turned for protection. The greater prominence of oedipal dynamics in the dream, as brought into the session and into the transference material, reflected a diminution of both castration anxiety and the related fear of the superego. Mr. B. was now able to verbalize much of his experience. The feelings of becoming big and of "shrinking" once again lost their perceptual quality in favor of ideational representation.

The counterposed themes of being big and being small began to involve increasingly realistic issues of relatedness as time went on, and Mr. B.'s fear of becoming big too fast began to be more available to consciousness as a manifestation of archaic experience, amenable now to verbal expression. The following session, some weeks after the financial one, was also related to his committing himself to buying a house, as well as to whether to apply for a job as the director of a business.

> I don't really feel I'm in a profession, I feel more like a businessman . . . like my father, I suppose. . . . Now I'm thinking of how I left high school to go to college a year early . . . it was partly because F broke up with me and I was humiliated, as we've said, . . . but just now I thought I also had a fear of being a big man, a senior, so I'll go off where I can be the small guy again. I would have been starting goalie on the soccer team as a senior in high school. . . . I did make the team in college, but one kid was a better goalie. . . . I was just as good physically, but he took charge of the defense, yelled at the guys where to go, it was *his* team, he had that kind of presence on the field, I didn't [**you backed away when defense turned to offense?**]. Yeah, I have an anxiety about running things, like I would be in this new job, or even in here, I'd prefer *you* run the analysis, then I can feel pushed around and get offensive, but it's still defensive, it's not *initiative*.

In this particularly free-flowing session, the issues arose spontaneously and constructively.

As similar material made its way more regularly into the work and into the transference, we managed considerable working through, which is not to say that we saw a sea change in character. This was brought into bold relief during the regressive climate of the winter holidays. Mr. B. had decided to go ahead with the purchase of a house and had asked his parents for financial help with the closing costs. His father initially declined to contribute but later softened and sent money. The first night in the new house felt like a mistake, and he "hated" the house. He became even more anxious as he anticipated a holiday visit from his parents, during which he expected disapproving scrutiny from his father, particularly regarding the new house. The session before this visit led to a brief regressive experience on the couch and also to our ability to understand the conflicts even more clearly than in the past. On the previous day, Mr. B. had announced in the last ten seconds of the session that he had had a dream the night before in which his hair had fallen out. I mentioned that it was interesting that this hadn't come up until the end of the session. The next day we encountered the familiar experience.

> I almost forgot to bring your check, I had to stick a glove in the door to keep it open so I could go back to my car to get it. . . . I'm feeling very dependent today, in need of a security blanket . . . with my parents coming. . . . I feel we shouldn't have bought the house, my father was right the first time when he said "no," but my mother had to go and intervene. . . . When my parents arrive I'll feel sad, needy, depressed, and

somehow incapable. . . . (silence) now I'm thinking of the dream coming up at the end of the session yesterday. . . . I feel sad now, low, maybe because we're not meeting the next few days **[but here with me, as with your parents, is it *safer* to feel sad and needy, perhaps you feel there are more dangerous feelings in the background?]**. *Now I have that feeling of my head getting very big,* it seems to go with wanting to hold back a *smile,* somehow putting one over on you, it's the same smile I had to hold back when my first girlfriend told me her former boyfriend had died in a boating accident **[a rival is killed]**. Yeah, it's a triumph, a pleasure, though a guilty one, like getting the money from my father **[and there you feel you and your mother team up against him]**. Yeah, my soft mother who cuts up my brother's meat at the table, who says you don't have to grow up, you don't have to do it on your own, save your own money . . . so I feel with the house that I didn't earn it and don't deserve it . . . **[and your father represents a danger in this regard]**. Yes, I'm actually *afraid* of his visit, like he'll want to know all the details, about the "clothing," I mean *closing* costs. . . . I feel that slip is like a lisp . . . feminine . . . now I feel like you were angry at me yesterday, like I was withholding the dream, maybe that's my anger, at you, feeling criticized . . . which is what I expect from my *father,* or even *want . . . that dream was like a joke,* I mean I really *am* losing my hair, it's no dream, except the bald spot was wider in the dream . . . that same night I had a dream of my old girlfriend G leaving her boyfriend, she was fed up . . . maybe that's like me wanting to leave analysis . . . I wish someone else would pay for it . . . now I just have the feeling that everything has gone too fast, I need to slow down **[mother has let you become too big, too fast?]** yeah, exactly, and I also feel my father *should* have burst my balloon, maybe I feel he still might, I feel I can't *stand* the triumph because I lose him, but I can't stand being a kid either. . . . I enjoyed popping the balloons I got for my fortieth birthday . . . partly to take away H's [his stepson's] pleasure in them . . . now I just thought my parents could watch H for a night so E and I could go out . . . they'd probably be relieved to have the opportunity to be grandparents instead of having to mollycoddle me as though *I'm* the child . . . but that seems a little dull, not so much potential for all that drama; triumphs and dangers. . .

In this example of the regressively swelling head, we are again provided with material that helps to confirm its place within the structure of the mind, including its usefulness as an analyzable element of psychic life. Once again, under sway of external regressive pressures preceding this session, Mr. B. was particularly interested in resisting analysis by keeping me at a distance. A tried and true formula for this involved a generalized regression in which I became a critical parent deserving of his angry and withholding behavior. As he tried not to pay me by leaving the check in the car, he castrated himself in my door and entered my office as a child in search of his security blanket, both castrated and broke (bereft of the fecal column, having paid me). Orality was a wish come true under the circumstances. It is in this state of passively experienced regression that I confronted his defensive *activity*. A surge of aggression once again became his own, and, because of the oral surround, the fantasied consequences of its murderous and sadistic components were extreme, calling for the further regressive step of perceptual involvement.

The malevolent inflatable punching clown so well externalized and feared in his old dreams came to my mind as he described holding back a murderous smile. Earlier in the analysis, his regressive episodes drew attention to the oral sadism in a murderous smile, but at this stage of the analysis, the oedipal incestuous and murderous wishes that were defended against by these phenomena were manifestly evident. Being with mother in the manner of an orally inflated infant, whose phallic intentions are disguised, is to have one's meat cut (as his brother had) in one way by mother and in another by father. The regressively expressed oedipal bond with mother offered Mr. B. oral satisfaction and narcissistic inflation, but at the price of a dedifferentiated relatedness in which attachment by fusion was a requirement; hence object loss would always entail a disintegrating loss of part of the self—castration was built in. Moreover, in his fearful and avoidant relation to father, the only hope of safety lay in becoming feminine, so that Mr. B.'s castration was again the vigorish in this triadic transaction. He then returned in the session to the dream, which he describes as "like a joke," because he is losing his hair in reality. The joke is elusive, however, until we recognize that his wish to lose his hair (to become older and bigger) by becoming younger (an omnipotent infant, also hairless) stood out to him in increasingly absurd contrast to the reality of his position as a man of early middle age. He was ultimately able in the course of the session to allow himself a stint as non-incestuous husband and father, and this paved the way for extensive working through of the Oedipus complex.

As Mr. B. set out freeing his parents, if quickly to recapture them as grandparents, he came to see that he had identified strongly with his mother as a child and had permitted himself to acquire a number of her character traits. These included her habits, under stress, of somatizing psychic conflict, devaluing others with a view to establishing her superiority and centrality, and paying suspicious attention to the details of every "likely story" tendered by Mr. B.'s father and others. Mr. B. found it easy to join his mother in criticizing his father's pretensions, ambitions, and emotional restriction, but he also saw his father as a powerful and effective man. He often felt secretly astonished that his father could have married the inadequate woman his mother some-times seemed to be. This sentiment concealed his belief that he himself could be a better wife to his father than his mother was. Both parents, however, highly valued Mr. B.'s precocious intellectual development, and it was by dint of this approval that he granted himself honorary membership in their generation. This promotion not only reinforced his individual oedipal and negative oedipal victories but also allowed him to broker the parental relationship in ways that each parent un-consciously solicited. This delicate equilibrium of unconscious fantasy seemed both to require and to result in his significant inhibition of phallic aggression, and it was in this environment that his oral-narcis-sistic / anal-sadistic character had been tempered.

DISCUSSION

Mr. B. presented for analysis with pervasive symptoms demonstrably linked to separation anxiety and dysfunctional attachment. Indeed, his adult relational patterns during the early analytic work exhibited a frozen vigilance, resistance to comfort, and ambivalent mixture of ap-proach and avoidance reminiscent of the more pathologically inhib-ited attachment disorders of infancy and early childhood. In addition, as we have seen, Mr. B.'s inclination toward ego functioning that is re-gressive to the point of perceptual disturbance yielded phenomena firmly rooted in orality, as described by Isakower and substantiated by a wealth of subsequent contributors. In this case, the hallucinatory prominence of the *head and hands* that occurs as infantile libidinal cathexes are revived was also a magnification, in every sense, of the ef-fectors of the earliest form of extrauterine attachment to an object. It is the breast, in its function as the physical anchor of object attachment and as the source of nourishment, that anaclitically acquired libidinal stature as the first part-object in the structuralization of the mind. As such, it became both the source of narcissistic vitality and the benefi-ciary of love. In this neurotic illness, the rapid regression of specific early ego functions, such as proprioceptive integration and mainte-nance of body image, marked earliest orality as a fixation point. The fixation was stabilized both by the capacity of the oral mentality to pro-vide comfort and by its ability to give less troublesome regressive rep-resentation to higher order conflicts. It is not surprising, then, that we find a parallel tendency toward regression of the more *complex* ego function of object relatedness, so that narcissistic attachment to a ma-ternal part-object characterized much of the analysand's adult rela-tional functioning.

These issues, spanning a range of psychoanalytic concepts, raise familiar questions regarding such ideas as the natural history of narcissism, the development of the self and concurrent threats to its integrity, the instincts as object-seeking versus pleasure-seeking, and the place of object-relations theories in understanding disturbances of attachment. Succinctly, this is the discourse of character analysis. More specifically, in an analyzable case in which orally determined ego functioning plays a major role—i.e., in which ordinarily autonomous ego functions become transiently disrupted and thus point to a locus of derangement in earliest orality, the crucible from within which ego nuclei are forged—it is character analysis that will elucidate pathology and stimulate growth. Throughout an idealized analysis, there is a migration from the complex to the simple, from the outside to the inside, from the displaced to the immediate, and from the defense to the impulse. Interpretations early in an analysis can reveal how far down this path of defense-relaxation the analysand will comfortably go, and these initial exchanges identify the psychic venue of the beginning work. As in all development, disturbances in the early stages decrease the stability of later structures, some of which must be supported if the reworking at the foundation is to succeed. As our theory evolves, it is not this model that is called into question so much as our understanding of the *process* of moving toward it and the effect that various ways of doing so or not doing so has upon clients, patients, and analysands.

In the case of Mr. B., developmental fixation and regression have left higher-order structures enfeebled by castration anxiety, but he has been spared the ravages of developmental arrest in which they might seem absent altogether. Mr. B.'s regressive symptoms reflected the state of the ongoing character analysis and thus helped to sharpen the focus of the work. For example, very early in the analysis we saw that Mr. B. functioned in a narcissistic miasma out of which emanated extensive vituperation at moments when I displayed even a trace of autonomy. When he complained in one session of missing his potential moment of quiet, and then thought of a woman running circles around an analyst, I might have interpreted any number of the distortions, confusions, reversals, externalizations, and fantasies that accompanied the episode, but I chose to highlight the one agenda item common to every other mental operation in that and preceding sessions: the effort to stay as far away from me as possible. That this resulted in a near-hallucinatory experience speaks to the magnitude of the threat posed by my presence and my analyzing, but the phenomenon itself also provided a window in to the specifically activated unconscious conflict with which the patient was immediately concerned. His near-hallucinatory experience of having breasts, as we have seen, gave clear representation to his narcissistic isolation and level of relatedness in the transference and otherwise. Had I focused on a more differentiated specific element of his initial productions, such as his need to see himself as a woman in relation to me, I would have been treated to a flood of intellectualized commentary which would have served nicely in turn to maintain the barrier that Mr. B. felt to be so necessary. Instead, he became quite interested in the *apparent* contradiction inherent in his fantasied avidity for attachment and his actual behavior, which was dedicated to holding onto me by being sure that I was there to push away.

Continuing attention to the ambivalence of his relatedness led to our awareness of both his desire for and his fear of merger with me as a defense against standing on his own and being responsible for his thoughts and words. This led slowly to our further understanding that such wishes and fears, and their many derivatives, were themselves warded off and yet expressed through his intense orally aggressive fixation. We had moved from addressing the superordinate issue of his ambivalent attachment to me toward identifying not only the specific fears and pleasures in oral aggression but also its defensive role as a whole. This work, having helped to clarify some of the difficulties beneath his ambivalence, led to an additional shift from the experience of attachment as it finds expression in loss, longing, and a sense of thwarted opportunity toward the experience of attachment as it involves affinity, concern, and fulfillment. Mr. B.'s increasingly important and close relationship with me then allowed for an even more vivid view of his development, particularly in the management of both attachment and power. Our relationship began to reveal more clearly the ways in which he expressed complex adult aims regressively, in infantile modalities.

As we have seen, this well trodden regressive pathway became most evident after the vacation that had led Mr. B. to turn his attention toward Dr. D., the behavior therapist. It was during this exchange that Mr. B. experienced the feeling that his hand was swelling and then reported accompanying fantasies of omnipotence and megalomania. The infantile hand is both an end organ of clinging attachment and a gavel of narcissistic sovereignty. A demand for both attachment and independence is expressed in this response to his experience of my leaving him and going off with another.

The perceived swelling of the hand takes place, however, with the fulminant automaticity and separateness that can be attributed by men to their erections through a partial externalization of the sexual drive. The penis, expanding in this manner, as though by its own intention, leaves the man in the passive position of shrinking in relation to it and thus of feeling at once diminished by the very power of which he is otherwise possessed—a fitting description of the status of his ego under these circumstances. When conflict is more deeply threatening and displacement of the drives is achieved by a wholesale regression, available through fixation, to earliest orality, then the swelling penis of sexual excitation is replaced by the swelling hand of appetitive urgency. Here the swelling itself represents inversely the velocity and force of the regressive undertow that effects the replacement of the wishes and fears of adult sexual life with those of infantile oral life. Being big and powerful becomes a matter of oral incorporation, accomplished in actual eating by the physical experience of adding to what is inside by consuming and thus reducing what is outside, and in loving by the more conflicted psychological fantasy of the same in relation to a loved object. Narcissistic omnipotence at the price of annihilation of the loved and needed woman is clearly expressed in Mr. B.'s fear that his "hands would fill up the *whole* room," which, to put it benignly, would leave room for no one else. We might add that in this case, the atavistic conversion of phallic experience to oral experience was achieved by displacement, regression, and neurotic compromise without clear evidence for fantasies of oral incorporation of the penis as seen in more primitive instances of the body-phallus equation. For Mr. B., the threat of loss and the shrinking of his body and ego relative to his hand served regulatory purposes; that is, they were cautionary threats, every bit as important in the equilibrium of the overall process of compromise as the gratifications they addressed.

Mr. B.'s earlier feeling of having breasts, a source of protection and power, reflected a walled-off, narcissistic level of regressive relatedness. Fusion with mother was paramount, and the minimal differentiation of self from the dyadic unity was displaced in the maternal direction—i.e., away from the face and mouth, away from the hand, and toward the breast. This regressive fixation was held in place by a boundary of oral aggression, attacking and repelling the external world while maintaining the repression of higher-order conflict. The episode of the swelling *hand* came after much working through and reflected, in oral terms, an increased differentiation between inner and outer and, hence, between self and other. Mr. B.'s less ambivalent attachment to me followed on our mutual survival of his aggression, and it reduced his fear of fragmentation sufficiently to allow a dim awareness of potential adult gratifications, though again expressed in the oral-narcissistic mode of perceptual alteration.

As the analysis continued, the next spell of regressive ego functioning involved the feeling of the swelling *head* in response to Mr. B.'s crossing my path with a highly instinctually laden wish to reschedule a session for business reasons. By this time, his relationship with me had been firmly enough established and rendered safe enough from annihilation that a symbiotic merger with me no longer seemed a vital necessity. Significant differentiation of self from object could be said to have occurred. This progression was demonstrated in the latest regressive *swelling head* episode by the prominence of the head and face, the psychic loci of the self. The self, having previously been one with the breast (a buxom woman) and subsequently an appendage of the breast (the clinging hand and suckling mouth), was now in apposition to the breast, to me, and hence to "the other." In this psychoanalytic work, where regression involved primarily specific, well circumscribed ego functions, this change not only reflected considerable diminution in vulnerability to regression but also revealed the development of sufficient emotional flexibility (independence) to allow the regressive ideation to give even clearer representation to the oedipal future, albeit in the seemingly innocent ways that Isakower described. At this point in analysis Mr. B. had begun to find his psychic bearings in three dimensions, and the oedipal scaffolding could be seen to arise from the preoedipal psychic foundation.

That Oedipus, a name that means "Swollen Foot," brings us the condensation of human psychological truths, affirms the enormous penetrance of the epistemological legacy of classical antiquity. Rudnytsky (1987) points out that the name Oedipus suggests not only *oidos* (swollen) but also *oida* (I saw, I know), and he cites Thass-Thienemann's (1957) elaboration of the idea that the prehistory of words can reveal, under psychoanalytically informed scrutiny, latent meaning which is far older than the written record. Thass-Thienemann offers the following discourse on Oedipus:

> The attribute "swollen-footed," however, should not be understood simply as referring to the physiological "tumescence" or "erectibility." It is symbolically expressive of the very core of Oedipus' personality. The Greek verb *oidaō*, "to swell, to become swollen," denotes the physiological tumescence but refers also to the specific character trait "to be inflated," "to ferment," "to be troublesome." . . . To "swell" or "to be swollen" is the bodily expression of "boasting" or "bragging" in all our languages. The braggart whose pride has no objective foundation appears to be inflated. Oedipus, the solver of riddles, is inflated and infatuated by his "knowledge," but such knowledge "puffeth up," Paul said (I Cor. 8:1–3). The logical consequence of such infatuation is stumbling and error.

Mr. B.'s "getting a swelled head" constituted, among other representations, a regressive resurgence of his own archaic introduction to the knowledge that he had a powerful rival for the primary object of his love and to the fantasy that this rival could be vanquished. Oedipal victory, consequent upon the dangerous and conflicted elimination of the father, constitutes a denial and a deflection of the "ionizing" force which acts upon primal attachment and stimulates further psychic structuralization. Rudnytsky tells us that Oedipus renders himself contemporaneous with three generations (beyond being the son of his parents, he is the husband of his mother and the brother of his offspring) and thus encounters the transcendent curse to which he is heir. The psychic equivalent of Oedipus at Thebes involves the individual's failure to resolve and relinquish the external oedipal relationships in such a way that they might then function internally as the agency of futurity (Loewald, 1962)—as the superego. It is the superego, heir of the Oedipus complex, through which the ego presents its own future. (Loewald would have us "verb the noun" *present* to fully appreciate *presentation.*) Without a workable future the management of the present by the ego falls prey to the unopposed inherited past of the id, the ego's dissolution becomes inescapable, temporal boundaries dissipate, and hierarchical structure is eliminated. It is the father, when development is unimpeded, in his position orthogonal to the mother-son axis, who so readily catalyzes the emergence of this structure. The unconscious, evolutionarily inherited curse of Oedipus—i.e., the "knowledge," by now embedded in biological structure, that psychic differentiation must take place for adaptation to be served, sets the stage for the internal representation of this organizing triadic force to unfold. This developmental imperative in turn gains its proscriptive psychic expression in the dread of maternal assimilation (Loewald, 1949) under the threat of prevailing castration anxiety and its nomothetic power in the wish for freedom from primitive attachment under the promise of both a conduit for constructive aggression and a means to enhanced libidinal gratification.

Mr. B.'s "expanding head," the leading edge of self as distinct from object, was now able to alert him to the presence of the quintessential oedipal polarity of tumescence versus growth. In all apparent psychic polarities, of course, the kinship of extremity in the unconscious can bring the poles toward unity and the midpoint to the extreme, as we are fond of pointing out about love, hate, and indifference. In biology, there is no growth without tumescence, and in the libidinally structured psychoanalytic mind, no knowledge without affect. There is no identification without incorporation and no superego without id. Reality evaluation involves an alternating current of projection and introjection such that objective reality without psychic reality would be meaningless. These dialectic traversals emphasize not polar opposi-tions but rather the emergent epigenetic differentiation of higher lev-els of psychic organization, which, adult development already having been approximated, appear to function in counterpoise to their re-gressive precursors. It should come as no surprise, then, that the psy-chic apparatus is particularly well able to represent in the idiom of low-level organization a glimmer of the high-level organization toward which it strives and away from which it regresses. Specifically, earliest orality, the seat of narcissistic object-relatedness and the medium for unrestrained drive gratification, bears every resemblance to phallic mastery, except for its degree of adaptive potential. In phallic mastery, narcissism has evolved into non-incestuous object love, and drive dis-charge is channeled, not only out of disillusionment with the old ways, but also out of a new-found ease, which, while resembling that of ear-lier and simpler times, has been hard won through the anabolic process of structuralization.

In accordance with the laws of the primary process, these discom-forts may be sidestepped in fantasy by the regressive substitution of undifferentiated primitive experience for newly imagined psychic achievement. In a conflicted situation for Mr. B., which invites and pos-sibly demands phallic mastery, the head expands, becoming engorged by the flow of libidinal cathexis in the direction of early infancy, and this in turn reawakens an aggressive sense of sovereignty while provid-ing the protective extenuation of helplessness. This is the economy of "*having* an inch and taking a mile." It is allowed to become *analytically* useful by the regressive dialectic, in which the past is substituted for the present but the present is then brought uniquely to bear on the past. The swelling infantile head at first seems merely an anatomical and temporal displacement from the penis, regression filling in for erec-tion; but it is, on further thought, a representation of the ego whose growth, dependent upon libido, is wishfully fantasied to be of an erec-tile nature. In truth, however, ego erection proceeds in alternating in-crements, advance followed by advancement, enlargement followed by evolution, expansion followed by maturation. Mr. B.'s regressive per-ceptual experiences were followed by associations and fleshed out by words. Affective surges took place within a progressively elaborated verbal and historical context, and repeating gave way to remembering. The analytic situation provided Mr. B. not only the safety and freedom to swell up, but also the time and the structure to grow into the part.

In these ways, Mr. B.'s regressive ego experiences of perceptual dis-turbance and body-image distortion can be seen to conform to the principles outlined by Isakower. All of Mr. B.'s "swelling" episodes were rooted firmly in orality, all occurred as defenses in response to anxiety, and as such all served to give representation to the higher-level fantasies from which conflict and anxiety stemmed. Occurring on the couch and thus in the atmosphere of the transference, these episodes corroborated the earlier findings and also demonstrated that such experiences are amenable to the same extensive analytic work generally afforded other evidentiary specimens of unconscious activity, such as dreams and parapraxes. Of further importance are observations about the nature of the regressive behavior of specific, usually autonomous, ego capacities. Such functioning reflects a return to states integral to the early formation of the ego, and an ideal analysis in which they are prominent will entail extensive character analysis. Orality and its mechanical cousin, attachment, hold in their primitivity the pluripotent capacity to represent the spectrum of psychic development. Physical attachment gives rise to narcissistic psychic attachment, and the lifelong struggle of making and breaking bonds gives rise to libidinal structure, which by turns bespeaks independence, admits of solitude, and engenders the fertile peace of mind that subtends enduring adult attachment.

In the course of Mr. B.'s analysis, episodes of regressive ego functioning provided, by way of their extraordinary representational capacity, an index of this development of the capacity for attachment. As development was reawakened and as the inclination toward regression receded, so went the tendency toward episodes of ego deformation. Human character is, of course, individual history, and what is now will always bear the stamp of what came before. Even after words had become the predominant currency of our interaction, Mr. B. would often refer to my bill as "the check," a condensation of developmental phases (a dinner check, a bank check, and a hockey maneuver to keep him in check) that never lost the prominent oral backdrop against which I had been cast as the source of sustenance. Late in the analysis, as Mr. B. was preparing to seek a promotion at work after having just married, he described his new determination to "step up to the plate and get into the game." This resolve was followed shortly by, "As soon as I said 'plate' I thought of the dinner table." Here, Mr. B. demonstrates not only his newly permissible ambition but also his deeply held preference for the fantasied safety and gratification of framing his strivings within the spectrum of the oral phase, only this time in associative imagery and words, open to interpretation and choice. Indeed, the elevation of sensory history to the status of conscious ideation reflects "ego erection" of consequence.

BIBLIOGRAPHY

ABRAHAM, K. (1924). A short study of the development of the libido, viewed in the light of mental disorders. In *Selected Papers of Karl Abraham.* New York: Basic Books, 1953, pp. 418–501.

ABRAMS, S. (1977). The genetic point of view: Antecedents and transformations. *J. Amer. Psychoanal. Assn.,* 25:417–425.

ALMANSI, R. J. (1958). A hypnogogic phenomenon. *Psychoanal. Q.,* 27:539–546.

ARLOW, J. A. (1959). The structure of the déjà vu experience. *J. Amer. Psychoanal. Assn.,* 7:611–631.

DANN, O. T. (1992). The Isakower phenomenon revisited: a case study. *Int. J. Psychoanal.,* 73:481–491.

DEUTSCH, F. (1953). Instinctual drives and intersensory perceptions. In *Drives, Affects, Behavior,* ed. R. M. Loewenstein. New York: Int. Univ. Press, pp. 216–228.

EASSON, W. M. (1973). The earliest ego development, primitive memory traces, and the Isakower phenomenon. *Psychoanal. Q.,* 42:60–72.

FERENCZI, S. (1928). Gulliver phantasies. *Int. J. Psychoanal.,* 9:283–300.

FINK, G. (1967). Analysis of the Isakower phenomenon. *J. Amer. Psychoanal. Assn.,* 15:281–293.

FINN, M. H. P. (1955). A note on a waking "blank stage" analogous to Isakower's phenomena, the dream screen, and blank dreams. *Psychoanal. Rev.,* 42:99–103.

FREUD, S. (1900). The interpretation of dreams. *S.E.,* 4 & 5.

GLENN, J. (1971). Regression and displacement in the development of the body-phallus equation. In *The Unconscious Today,* ed. M. Kanzer. New York: Int. Univ. Press, pp. 274–287.

——— (1993). Developmental transformation: The Isakower phenomenon as an example. *J. Amer. Psychoanal. Assn.,* 41:1113–1134.

HARTMANN, H. AND KRIS, E. (1945). The genetic approach to psychoanalysis. In *The Psychoanalytic Study of the Child.* New York: Int. Univ Press, pp. 11–30.

ISAKOWER, O. (1938). A contribution to the patho-psychology of phenomena associated with falling asleep. *Int. J. Psychoanal.,* 19:331–345.

JOSEPH, E. D. (1965). Regressive ego phenomena in psychoanalysis. In *Kris Study Group, Monogr. 1.* New York: Int. Univ. Press, pp. 68–103.

KEPECS, J. G. (1952). A waking screen analogous to the dream screen. *Psychoanal. Q.,* 21:167–171.

LEWIN, B. D. (1933). The body as phallus. *Psychoanal. Q.,* 2:24–47.

——— (1946). Sleep, the mouth, and the dream screen. *Psychoanal. Q.,* 15:419–434.

——— (1948). Inferences from the dream screen. *Int. J. Psychoanal.,* 29:224–231.

——— (1950). *The Psychoanalysis of Elation.* New York: W. W. Norton and Co., Inc.

——— (1953). Reconsideration of the dream screen. *Psychoanal. Q.,* 22:174–199.

LEWY, E. (1954). On Micropsia. *Int. J. Psychoanal.*, 35:13–19.

LOEWALD, H. W. (1949). Ego and reality. In *Papers on Psychoanalysis*. New Haven: Yale University Press, 1980, pp. 13–17.

———— (1962). Superego and time. In *Papers on Psychoanalysis*. New Haven: Yale University Press, 1980, pp. 43–52.

MAHLER, M. S. (1968). *On Human Symbiosis and the Vicissitudes of Individuation. Vol. 1. Infantile Psychosis*. New York: Int. Univ. Press.

MURPHY, W. F. (1958). Character, trauma, and sensory perception. *Int. J. Psychoanal.*, 39:555–568.

PACELLA, B. L. (1975). Early ego development and the déjà vu. *J. Amer. Psychoanal. Assn.*, 23:300–318.

RAPAPORT, D., & GILL, M. M. (1959). The points of view and assumptions of metapsychology. In *The Collected Papers of David Rapaport*, ed. M. M. Gill. New York: Basic Books, 1967, pp. 795–811.

RICHARDS, A. D. (1985). Isakower-like experience on the couch: a contribution to the psychoanalytic understanding of regressive ego phenomena. *Psychoanal. Q.*, 54:415–434.

RUDNYTSKY, P. L. (1987). Freud and Oedipus. New York: Columbia University Press, pp. 266–267.

RYCROFT, C. (1951). A contribution to the study of the dream screen. *Int. J. Psychoanal.*, 32:178–184.

SANDLER, J. (1959). The body as phallus: a patient's fear of erection. *Int. J. Psychoanal.*, 40:191–198.

SPERLING, O. E. (1957). A psychoanalytic study of hypnagogic hallucinations. *J. Amer. Psychoanal. Assn.*, 5:115–123.

———— (1961). Variety and analyzability of hypnagogic hallucinations and dreams. *Int. J. Psychoanal.*, 42:216–223.

SPITZ, R. A. (1955). The primal cavity. *Psychoanal. Study Child*, 10:215–240.

———— (1957). *No and Yes: On the Beginnings of Human Communication*. New York: Int. Univ. Press.

———— (1961). Some early prototypes of ego defenses. *J. Amer. Psychoanal. Assn.*, 9:626–651.

———— (1965). *The First Year of Life*. New York: Int. Univ. Press.

STERN, M. M. (1953). Trauma and symptom formation. *Int. J. Psychoanal.*, 34:202–218.

———— (1961). Blank hallucinations: Remarks about trauma and perceptual disturbances. *Int. J. Psychoanal.*, 42:205–215.

TAUSK, V. (1919). On the origin of the "Influencing Machine" in schizophrenia. In *The Psychoanalytic Reader*, ed. R. Fliess. New York: Int. Univ. Press, pp. 52–85.

THASS-THIENEMANN, T. (1957). Oedipus and the Sphinx: The linguistic approach to unconscious fantasies. *Psychoanal. Rev.*, 44:10–33.

The Dread of Integration

Integrative Processes in a Chronically Ill Borderline Patient

M. A. TALLANDINI

Integration of the patient's mental organization is an important part of all psychotherapeutic experiences. Generally, it is welcomed and thought well worth the effort needed to achieve it. However, there are some patients who feel terrified by this process. They seem to think that integration involves a loss of the self: they feel it is dangerous and even resist it with psychotic-type defenses. This was certainly the case for the patient described in this paper, who was affected from an early age by brittle diabetes. For her, this reaction was always activated by separation, and it also appeared prior to any developmental step she needed to take—e.g., in recognizing self-boundaries, sexual identity, and facing the oedipal conflict. On all these occasions her reaction was to run away from treatment in a state of deep regression, feeling suicidal, and liable to seriously harm herself through the mistreatment of her diabetes. The issue of integration, seen to arise with the concomitant loss of omnipotence, presents itself at different levels of development of the self and of the drives.

Associate professor of genetic epistemology, University of Trieste; senior lecturer, University College, London; associate member of the British Psycho-Analytical Society and of the Italian Psycho-Analytical Society; member of the Anna Freud Young Adult Group for Research in Psychoanalytic Processes.

I am greatly indebted to Dr. Clifford Yorke for his continuous help in the treatment of this patient and for the extensive and very fruitful discussions of the ideas presented in this paper. I gratefully acknowledge the intellectual support and stimulation of A. M. Sandler (chair) and the other members of the Young Adult Research Group at the Anna Freud Centre. The Young Adults Project has been funded through the generous support of Mr. Philip Granville.

The Psychoanalytic Study of the Child 54, ed. Albert J. Solnit, Peter B. Neubauer, Samuel Abrams, and A. Scott Dowling (Yale University Press, copyright © 1999 by Albert J. Solnit, Peter B. Neubauer, Samuel Abrams, and A. Scott Dowling).

INTEGRATIVE PROCESSES HAVE BEEN UNDER SCRUTINY IN PSYCHOANA-
lytic theory for a long time. They are at the core of construction and
reconstruction within the analytic process. Whereas anxiety linked to
the fear of disintegration has been repeatedly investigated and discussed theoretically, little attention has been paid to the analysis of the
fear of integration, except by Gaddini (1981). Yet it seems to be a common phenomenon, particularly in young borderline patients. In this
paper I discuss a borderline patient, Miss T., who seriously endangered
her body by her long-standing mistreatment of brittle diabetes, and in
whom the fear of integration was a cardinal concern. This fear was not
so much of disintegration, as in many other patients, but of integrating the parts of the self at different levels of libidinal development. In
particular this anxiety appeared to be aroused by any separation when
the object seemed at risk of disappearing; this aroused and exacerbated the emotional intensity of libidinal and aggressive wishes. My
contention is that such patients are unable to deal with integrative processes because their early object relationships did not provide them
with the initial capacity for binding together aggressive and libidinal
energies. Moreover, an absence of adequate physical care makes them
unable to provide safety for their own bodies.

In this paper I will discuss the repeated catastrophic experiences in
the treatment of Miss T. every time an integrative process was in danger of coming to the fore. Each catastrophic experience presented two
correlated aspects: one psychological, with a total loss of the self; one
physical—that is, the inability of providing her body with the care it
needed. Facing the integration process requires that the aggressive
and libidinal drives to be bound together through an introjective
process, leading to identification with the parental figures. Such a
process can be impaired if the negative aspects of parental figures over-
whelmingly prevail. In such a situation the introjection of parental imagos is seen as a danger, and the patient cannot form a true identification. Identification is seen and feared as negative, and the patient
therefore withdraws from it. Certain consequences follow: it becomes
impossible to accept separation because not having internalized an object makes it impossible to separate from it; and the absence of an internalized object makes it impossible to find internal resources to cope
with separation.

I would argue that for many patients with borderline characteristics,
the task of facing separation is, at different levels, extremely difficult.
However, their extreme vulnerability to such a painful event and often
inability to face it is due not primarily to separation per se but rather
to the difficulty in integration that results (Gaddini, 1981). In less

damaged patients it is quite common to observe disintegration anxiety which, even though it results in fear of loss of the self, aims ultimately at reaching integration. By contrast integration anxiety brings all the forces of the mental apparatus into the service of non-integration: the outcome can be a permanent psychotic state. Such patients generally lack an adequate degree of bound drive energies and therefore cannot afford to internalize separation, which would require bringing libido and aggression together in order to give way to the process of grief. At any level they fear that this will be death-inducing and that any integrative process will require the total use of the little bound energy they have or, even worse, would install a new integrative process, making them fear catastrophe, going to pieces, and going mad.

INTEGRATIVE PROCESSES

The problem of explaining the coterminous presence of libidinal and aggressive forces has long given rise to dispute. Freud (1920) stated that the pleasure principle comes into operation only after the energy, the excitatory processes, has been bound, in this way enabling freely flowing energy to change into a state of quiescence. From this perspective, binding means mastery or integration of stimuli. Subsequently Freud (1923) added the concept of defusion and established that maturational instinctual progression is associated with increasing drive fusion and drive regression with drive defusion.

In line with this interpretation, Anna Freud (1949, 1966) noted deficiencies in emotional development when "the aggressive urges are not brought into fusion and thereby bound and partially neutralized, but remain free and seek expression in life in the form of pure, unadulterated, independent destructiveness" (p. 496). As Furman (1985) points out, illness or injury and their attendant treatments can seriously affect the balance between the drives, significantly increase the stimulation of both drives, and, at the same time, damage the synthetic function of the ego. She adds that this is especially true with children who have experienced overwhelming trauma from whatever cause especially when the body has been involved. This is the case for the patient I will be discussing. She emphasizes the importance of the environment, particularly the role played by caring adults. The overstimulated or traumatized child experiences difficulty with fusion because his or her integrative capacities cannot bind the excess of stimuli and/or, in the case of overwhelming trauma, because the synthetic function is damaged (Furman, 1985). Only the presence of a mother who, acting as an auxiliary ego, shields the child from excesses of libidinal and aggressive stimulation can provide the necessary balance to the realization of such integrative processes. A relative preponderance of aggression impedes fusion altogether or allows only developmentally primitive forms of fusion to occur, as in sadomasochism. Furman and Furman (1984) and Rosenfeld and Sprince (1963) note a lack of fusion, integration, and neutralization as major characteristics of borderline children, and they point to "excessive aggression characteristic of the prephallic stage." It seems, therefore, that fusion depends not only on the quantity of available libido but also on its quality. By this I mean that the libido must be bound so that it comes securely under the sway of the pleasure principle and is capable of being absorbed and contained by the available forces of the ego. When the excitatory processes cannot be bound and mastered, they lead to overwhelming trauma or to very intense, uncontrollable sexual excitement. In these conditions, fusion appears not to take place or to take place only to a limited extent, as in the form of primitive sadomasochism.

From a different theoretical perspective, Winnicott (1962) described what he called "the non-integration phase," which is identified with a stage of infantile mental development. In this stage Winnicott foresaw the contemporaneous presence of different aspects of the mind that stay together as if by magic. Only later will the child start to integrate them, because she will need an "integrated" unity to enable her to deal with the internal and external world. Gaddini (1981) distinguishes his position from Winnicott's, linking the fear of integration phenomena to acting out. He gives two different meanings to acting out: the first is progressive and at the service of development; the second, when acting out aims to eliminate tensions and therefore tends to retain a state of non-integration and makes the integration processes impossible. He underlines the fact that in a situation of loss of the self the patient can face either non-integration anxiety or integration anxiety and that the latter "represents the true pathological aspect." It is stronger than non-integration anxiety, impedes the natural developmental processes, and contributes substantially to retaining the non-integration state as an extreme defense.

ACTING OUT AS CONSEQUENCE OF INTEGRATION ANXIETY

I will put forward a different viewpoint from which acting out can be seen as resulting from a fear of integration, which can present itself at different levels of development. I will present clinical material from a patient who revealed these characteristics. The appearance of these phenomena in the clinical situation could easily be attributed to the negative therapeutic reaction, but what I have in mind can be distinguished from this reaction, for two reasons. First, the negative therapeutic reaction usually presents itself after an important insight, whereas with Miss T. the phenomena appeared before any insight was reached; it was a sort of aura that silently but steadily came into the analytic setting. It appeared to me that a shock, instead of suddenly appearing, was anticipated and its development observed until there was a terrifying loss of control over external and internal reality (Eidelberg, 1959). At first, indications of this were almost imperceptible: for example, the sessions would start to become too intellectualized, then the material would become indecipherable. Later, the content was blurred, with Miss T. speaking so quickly that I could not understand the point she was making; I did not have time to elaborate her meaning in my mind. Subsequently the sessions continued to have these characteristics but, in addition, I was actively stopped from interpreting; at the same time Miss T. began to miss sessions, and it was difficult to foresee when she would come, irrespective of the quality and intensity of prior session's contents (that is, not coming to the session just after a very intense and, in my view, productive session and/or from a flatly non-productive one). Invariably this situation was accompanied by acting out, sometimes reaching the point where I feared an interruption of the analytic treatment or her putting herself at risk through abusing her body by binging, making herself sick, or, even worse, injecting an overdose of insulin. I invariably felt disappointed, bored, hopeless, persecuted, useless, irritated, revengeful, fed up, cross—the recipient of the kind of feeling that Weintrobe and Harrison (1994) describe in patients as "too-muchness," except that in this instance it was the analyst who was having the experience of engulfment and intolerance.

The second feature that seems to distinguish this situation from the negative therapeutic reaction is that it presented itself *before* a developmental step occurred in the patient's psychological organization and/or her external life (for example, when her periods returned, when she first had sexual intercourse, when she finished her degree). The feeling she induced in me was of something that seriously threatened the psychoanalytic situation. Each time the analytic couple found themselves in this situation of panic and despair, it was invariably linked to the prospect of major improvement and understanding, both psychologically and in the practical management of Miss T.'s diabetes. Each push toward development (any process of integration) was halted by her pathological anxiety of a loss of the self that would make "any change in a precarious situation a total catastrophe" (Gaddini, 1985, p. 740).

But these events happened *before* any insight took place. It seems to me that there are two essential aspects to this fear: one is of growing up and is triggered by any movement toward autonomy, and activated at the level of the ego. A second aspect of this fear is placed at the level of the id and refers to the integration of repressed and sexualized material every time a new issue of development in the area of the drives occurs.

In clinical practice it often happens that, over a period of time, an aspect of the patient's mental life becomes familiar to both members of the therapeutic couple. When this happens the repetition of all behavioral schemata linked to it reactivates a kind of ineluctable process.

It felt as if the psychoanalytic situation was seriously threatened, and this usually began *in sordini*, becoming increasingly dangerous. Each time before recovery set in, Miss T. and I reached the point where we believed that the analysis was going to be interrupted. Even after years of analysis, having experienced this situation many times previously, it was still impossible to prevent it from resurfacing. Interpreting the fact that it would lead us to repeat the usual scenario did not help: each time the tension and danger were real. I did not know whether the analysis would continue. What, in retrospect, is also clear was Miss T.'s terrible fear that she would lose me.

With my patient the acting out always followed and never preceded the fear of integration. Acting out was interfering with the treatment whenever material requiring integration came near the surface. The issue of integration arises together with separation and the loss of omnipotence, and it presents itself at different levels of development that can be considered from the viewpoint of the self and of the drives. It seems to me that in our society, this issue presents itself when a person is expected to make a definitive step toward autonomy but has failed to reach a level of developmental organization that makes self-support and independence from the parents possible. From this perspective, it is not surprising that our more seriously ill patients live on Social Security and find it unbearable even to think of supporting themselves.

I will present clinical material from four periods of Miss T.'s analysis. In the first we can observe the annihilation of any distinction between mind and body, giving her body the task of expressing her thoughts; in the second the state of confusion between self and non-self and her fear of a more integrated self appear; the third phase illustrates her difficulty in integrating her sexual characteristics at a point where her psychological resources allow integration only at a homosexual level; the fourth session is built around her conflictual wish to define herself as an adult. Chronologically, the first session dates from the beginning of the analysis, the second relates to the second Christmas break, the third to the following summer break, and the fourth excerpt is from the fifth year of analysis, when the topic of termination began to be discussed.

CLINICAL MATERIAL

Miss T.'s clinical material is often rich and compelling. I greatly respect her for her efforts to deal with painful material and am grateful to her for giving me the opportunity of understanding ways of functioning that are difficult to discover in less ill patients or in patients who are just as ill, if not more so, but who do not dare to go as deeply inside themselves as she did.

Miss T. was referred by the consultant of a casualty department that she had often attended in a serious state of ketosis. She had been in and out of the hospital whenever her life was in serious danger. After her last recovery, she realized that she would die if she failed to manage her diabetes more effectively. Her diabetes is of the brittle type[1] and was diagnosed when she was seven years old. She is the youngest in a family of four, with two older sisters and one brother. Hers is a long and intricate story of painful illnesses. Mother is a chronic schizophrenic, and father, unable to cope with the situation, left home when Miss T. was between 8 and 9, rarely reappearing. Miss T. and her brother were left with the mother while her sisters were taken in by relatives until they could live independently. When T. was 13 years old mother was married again, to another schizophrenic. The family situation became even more unbearable. During her early adolescence, when the issue of her genital sexuality came to the fore, Miss T. had to face the presence of this second husband, who would threaten mother and daughter when he was in a crisis.

Miss T. stayed at home until she was 18, unable to leave her mother, whom she thought she had to look after, but at the same time finding

---

1. Juvenile (brittle) diabetes is a chronic metabolic disease in which there is a relative or absolute lack of insulin produced by the pancreas. The onset of the illness is characterized by a breakdown in the child's physical conditions that include weight loss, fatigue, inordinate thirst, and frequent urination. These symptoms reflect the abnormal elevation of food glucose levels, a condition which, if untreated, will eventually result in ketoacidosis. High blood sugar, unmitigated by insulin injections, will eventually also lead to coma and death. Secondary complications include blindness, cardiovascular diseases, and shortened life expectancy. Poor diabetic control increases the likelihood of secondary complications (Hockaday, 1985).

her mother the only person who could look after her. Her adolescence was characterized by various kinds of self-abuse: drinking alcohol, taking drugs, binging and making herself sick. Insulin was used to keep herself together rather than to control diabetes; in this way, she could exert control, master her body and her mind, be ideally slim, and avoid feeling sad or depressed (Yorke, 1985). It was a way of splitting off her illness, one of many aspects of her lack of integration.

Both parents colluded with Miss T. in externalizing and denying her diabetic identity. Miss T.'s father, astonishingly, used the same procedure described by Fonagy et al. (1993), of injecting her with insulin while she was asleep. Mother colluded in a perverse and psychotic way in denying her daughter's illness: she used to make an alliance with Miss T., agreeing to lie to the doctor about Miss T.'s diet. In this way both parents contributed to bypassing "the confrontation with reality necessary for normal adaptation to the disease" (Fonagy et al., 1993, p. 476) and avoiding the necessary integration. Miss T. expressed her fear of the sensation of annihilation and falling to pieces when a hypoglycemic crisis occurs. In medical practice, when diabetes has been recognized, the child and his family are told that there must be drastic changes in the child's daily routine, and family life undergoes these changes revolving around the ill child (Baum and Kinmonth, 1985). Miss T.'s family reacted in a contradictory way: her diabetic identity was denied as an illness but enhanced and praised as the way by which she could be considered a special and privileged child. Father, described by the patient as violent and aggressive with her siblings, was careful and attentive toward her. She remembers the whole family's helplessness in dealing with her ketotic crisis, her experience of zooptic hallucinations, of falling into a never-ending dark space and dying. It is interesting to note that the diabetes was a central theme at the beginning of Miss T.'s analysis, and later, even though a recurrent theme, became a less important issue as her control improved.

After she left mother Miss T. went to college and became even more self-damaging, behaving as if her mother, despite her limitations, could provide an auxiliary self. When I first saw her for assessment she was detached and withdrawn. Her speech was blurred and distant. To keep her mind on the present I had to put questions to her, which she answered as if she was returning from somewhere far away. She expressed her sense of detached despair: she had no friends, no interests, no sex life. Petite, dressed in black, she gave the impression of being clean yet untidy. Curiously, she appeared to me to be potentially pretty. The beginning of her analysis was characterized by extreme uncertainty, due not primarily to explicit conflict but in large part to her incapacity to manage her everyday life well enough to arrive at my office at the right time and on the right days. She was obsessed with painful and overwhelming suicidal thoughts that she could communicate to me only occasionally.

What she recounted was very difficult to put together into a picture. She could not allow herself to recognize her body: she was completely covered in black, and once, when she noticed her white skin through a hole in her tights, she was surprised and disgusted. She could not acknowledge her genitals. She did not menstruate.

The whole of the first year of analysis was concerned with the patient's emergence from a sense of chaos and confusion.

BODILY ILLNESS AS A WAY OF AVOIDING MENTAL INTEGRATION

The beginning of the analysis was characterized by her continuously daunting and death-carrying mismanagement of her diabetes. She binged in order to fill her mind and silence her thoughts. Then she made herself sick so as not to become fat and in order to feel the pain in her body rather than leave mental space for her desperation. Insulin was used at random in order to tell me the danger she was in without having to face her aggression or her wish to attack me violently and my mind inside the session, as a place where she could integrate her thoughts. She sometimes came to her sessions hours before they started, and sometimes just in time to catch the last few minutes. Analysis, like insulin, could not be taken at fixed times. She would come bearing a heavy weight: a huge briefcase, a huge handbag, and also at least a couple of shopping bags full of food. In fact, each day before the session she went to a nearby supermarket, often binging while in the waiting room and coming to the session with a full stomach and no insulin at all. Of course the alternative behavior was to keep her bags around her and, not having eaten all day, to be on the verge of collapse. Interpreting that she was showing me she could provide for herself and did not want what I could give her met with a clear rejection: the only reason she could see for her behavior was that the supermarket was very handy. No integration was allowed at that time between action and thoughts. This situation reached its apex when she started to bring aggressive contents, that emerged particularly after the weekends, under the influence of a separation, as in the following clinical material.

Her flatmate complained that my patient had left bread crumbs on the table. Miss T. thought that for this reason her friend would leave and she would be left completely alone. When her fear was interpreted that if she made some minimal disruption with me I would take it as a reason to get rid of her, she replied, "You are fed up with me." During the following part of the session it was nevertheless possible to work on her aggressive wishes toward me-mother, unable to provide for her needs and to look after her. The surfacing of aggressive content and its interpretation were apparently accepted but not internalized. In fact, in the following session she complained that the day before she had had the impression that her head was blowing up. She continued to blame analysis for her physical and mental state, at the same time disparagingly attacking the analytic work. She claimed that, like her parents, I was unable to provide any sense of safety or to make her diabetes disappear; the only choice she had was to turn her anger against herself by taking laxatives and making herself sick. I interpreted her difficulty in confronting her anger toward her parents and my lack of omnipotence to the fact that she would prefer to leave and not continue analysis, to which she exclaimed, "If I am angry towards my parents they go blank." After this sentence her speech became a flood of words, sometimes lacking coherence. She was evidently having a hypoglycemic crisis during the session. She asked me to help her by providing something to eat. At that time she went around without any provisions, such as glucose or something similar, for any emergency. She wanted me to be concretely her caring parent, because, at the time, physical and psychological aspects were indistinguishable.

Anxiety related to aggressive impulses is intensified by the fear of death, deriving from the real danger inherent in the illness (Moran and Kennedy, 1984). What was striking in this material was the immediate correspondence between bodily expression and mental components, where the anger that could not be contained by the mind was immediately translated into aggression against her own body and displayed together with the need for dependence on the loved-hated parents-analyst. This aggression was linked to the unbearable discovery of their lack of omnipotence, made evident by the fact that they could not make the diabetes disappear. When facing such a painful discovery, Miss T. resorted to her bodily needs that were indistinguishable from her psychological needs. These needs could only be expressed through enactment because the mental components were too heavy, difficult, and dangerous to hold. The use of her diabetes to express her feelings and to obtain concrete fulfillment of her needs was making her understanding of her internal world even more difficult because she was ascribing her emotions to the diabetic state.

THE FEAR/INABILITY TO RECOGNIZE THE BOUNDARIES OF THE SELF

About a month before the Christmas break, in the second year of analysis, I was feeling worried about the possible development of this analysis and uncertain about what was the main problem to be addressed. The patient was missing sessions, and I had the impression that something important was going on without knowing what it was. At this time I felt I was taking part in something disastrous, but this was variable and the situation did not feel altogether familiar. Yet I was certain that the analysis would not survive. Nothing I said seemed able to reach her. My own feelings echoed my patient's feelings of impending catastrophe; but while she was convinced that she would not survive, at the same time she felt that the analytic relationship was still alive. Survivors of a catastrophe have had the terrible experience of the certainty of dying within the catastrophe itself, and this was the sensation that Miss T. was conveying to me. Certainly the Christmas break, with the inevitable separation, was an important element in all this, but I had no idea what it could be linked to.

After a more balanced period, Miss T. was again in a state of complete and despairing disorganization, binging and vomiting, thinking of suicide. She suddenly decided to move into a new flat that she had not even seen. She ran away from the previous one, where an intrusive landlady had suddenly became a persecutory and an unbearable "concretization" of her negative transference (Sandler & Sandler, 1978). When I drew attention to her moving toward something unknown, turning away from feelings that had become so unbearable that she felt it preferable to throw herself into something completely dark, and unknown, she answered, using concrete thinking devoid of metaphor, that she did not like the flat where she was living and found it completely natural not to see her new flat before moving in. As for her work, a productive period was followed by a cessation of all activity at college. She was terrified by a change in her view of herself that derived from the awakening of her sexual interest. Her body, her feelings, herself— all had to be reorganized because she was now aware of the sexual parts of her body.

She always said she was afraid of traveling, especially by herself, but she suddenly decided to visit the best friend of her childhood and adolescence, who lives in California. Her decision was unexpected and compulsive: she ordered her ticket even before checking to make sure her friend would be at home at Christmas or whether it was appropriate for her to stay with her friend's family.

At the time my countertransference alerted me to a fear that she was on the verge of a terrifying danger and might go mad. I could see in her panic the same fear she had transmitted to me. In order to avoid it she was running away. Her attendance at sessions again became erratic. I had no idea when she would keep her appointments. Even so, the sessions were often dramatic, with important issues that could not be properly analyzed because she would interrupt interpretations that she saw as dangerous and unbearable.

The following material comes after a session missed without notice:

She arrived on time. She appeared distant, aloof, estranged, disoriented. She immediately apologized for her absence the previous day and recounted what happened. The day before yesterday she went to bed late and slept deeply. When she finally awoke she went around her flat doing little domestic chores. She was feeling strange and blurred, as if she was having an hypoglycemic episode. With some difficulty, she checked her blood-sugar level and found it normal. Then she felt very hungry, she thought because the day before she had had only vegetables for dinner. The day felt weird: it was very dark. She had an appointment with the hairdresser at 10:30 a.m. It was already after 10:00 and, fearing that she would miss her appointment, she telephoned for a cab. When the cab came she told the driver where to go, asking him to hurry because she was late for her appointment: to have her hair cut. The driver looked surprised, saying that it was a very strange time to go to the hairdresser. At that point Miss T. realized that it was very dark. Greatly confused, she rang up a friend who confirmed that it was 10 in the evening and not in the morning. Terrified by her own disorientation, she went to see a friend and stayed with her because she was too scared to go back home and stay alone.

Miss T. described this event with a mixture of surprise, fear, and protest. She was still very confused and frightened by it and was convinced that the episode was linked to her fear of becoming blind. She also said that during the night she had awakened and wanted to use the toilet, but instead of going upstairs to the women's toilet she went downstairs to the men's one (she was living in a shared house where there were two toilets, one for men and one for women). She thought she knew the meaning of this mistake: she thought she was driven by her sexual needs, which she had only recently discovered and of which she was ashamed. She was also ashamed of the fact that she had told me she loved me. Suddenly she changed the topic, complaining that she had lost the whole of the day before when she meant to do a lot of things to be ready for her journey: she had to collect her ticket, to have her passport photographs taken, to have them signed, to have her hair cut. She said she was scared because she wanted to withdraw from reality into a fantasy world. In particular, she said, almost casually, that she felt unsafe without me. She went on to say that, to feel safe, she was going to see her friend, getting her to take my place. I pointed out that she was going to the edge of another ocean, putting a great distance between her love and her hate for me, since it seems impossible to keep them together. Miss T. reacted with surprise: "To go to the edge of another ocean? What are you saying?" From the following sentences I gathered that she had no idea where she was going except that it was far away, nor did she know how long the journey would take. She nevertheless explicitly told me that she was planning to stay there to start a new life.

This session shows features characteristic of this patient. There is abundant clinical material from different levels of development, not even minimally contained in a hierarchical organization. In my interpretations I had to choose the elements that seemed closest to the possibility, not of her *understanding*, but of her *integrating*. I said that to feel her link to me at the same time as a separation was unbearable, and that it also seemed to her cruel for me to persist in my decision to have a break. I added: "You are telling me you would like me to go with you up in the sky where we could be together, in the dark, in space. A place where nobody and nothing else could interfere with us. It is as if you are trying to unify the two of us by traveling around the world to a place where maybe one could dream of staying forever." I added: "This separation is bringing into *our* session the terrible reality that we are not a whole person. That each of us has our own boundaries is so hard for you to bear that you feel the world is upside down, and night and day are confused." (I chose *not* to interpret the transference—that is, not to bring this material into historical perspective. I thought she needed to have her *actual* need recognized.)

She responded by protesting vigorously against analysis and against me, asking in a disparaging voice "what is it for," commenting widely on the uselessness of her coming, not allowing any space for me to speak. I had to force myself into this flood. I told her that she found this situation overwhelming and felt there were too many things that needed to be kept together: her new knowledge about sexuality, her fear of becoming blind, the separation over Christmas. I added that she felt unable to contain all this by herself; that it was as if she might fall to pieces if I was not there to help her to keep it all together. I empathized, saying it was particularly painful to be so dependent, like a child who is breast-fed and suddenly deprived of her source of support. I said I could understand how, for this reason, she felt discarded and her survival threatened. Miss T. said that she had been blind about her sexuality until now, and now she was "obsessed" with her body.

The following session she was in a much improved state. She told me she had thought about my interpretation and understood that she was sucking from my breast and felt very dependent. She said she had talked about her mother with a friend and would like to make a link with her (mother) but finds it very difficult to do so. I told her that she was expressing her wish to have contact with her mother and me but also her fear of receiving something from me or her mother that could endanger her. At the same time she was asking me if I could bear to give her what she needed. Miss T. replied that she had spoken with a friend the day before about the high rate of suicide among analysts.

Miss T.'s account had the quality of a lack of boundaries between events. It seemed more like a dream that had a vivid sense of reality than the other way round. Some of the latent meanings, such as the urgency of going to see the hairdresser to reshape her hair, were immediate and accounted for her need to see me, to try to reshape her thoughts and prevent her from acting out against such awareness. Her diabetes is represented by her fear of going blind, fear that in turn represents her wish to be blind to her newly discovered needs. Different levels of development were simultaneously present and made the psychological situation intense and unbearable: they did not appear to be hierarchically organized but, on the contrary, were contiguous. It was possible for her to bear the coexistence of these levels because they were contained by the omnipotent couple and needed no clarification. To recognize the existence of a distinct and separated object meant having simultaneously to contain libidinal and destructive forces; if she did not she would have ended, as she said, "in pieces." Thus the necessity to re-enact the omnipotent unified object through using, as a substitute, the friend who represented, for her, the best experience of her childhood. The extremely regressed state the patient showed in this session bore witness to Miss T.'s great difficulty enduring even an initial state of integration, the regression triggered by the event of separation; the developmental failure that made it impossible for her to integrate her love and her aggression beyond the initial infantile omnipotence, in which nothing was distinguished but in which, for the same reason, nothing could face the test of reality. As Gaddini (1981) says, "The fragments are the pieces of self which have survived the catastrophe, immersed in a dark and infinite space in which they can be absorbed and scattered for ever. There now appears the dominant urge to hold the residual fragments of self together, to maintain and protect the state of survival" (p. 169).

THE DENIAL OF SEXUAL IDENTITY THROUGH NOT INTEGRATING
THE EXISTENCE OF THE OPPOSITE SEX

Her first experience of intercourse was very important; she enjoyed it, but the young man did not continue their relationship. Miss T. felt abandoned and rejected. Her feelings were so strong that she tried to keep them at a distance. When, one evening, this man knocked at her door she did not open it. She could not bear the hostility she was experiencing in contrast to her feelings of dependence and neediness. She again entered a phase of her analysis in which I felt impotent in the face of an emerging destructiveness. She lost control over her diabetes, as if *only* in her self-abusive and self-destructive behavior was she able to manage her feelings. Her sessions were full of rage: she shouted at me, she swore, she derided me, and she told me, with evident pleasure, about different ways in which she mismanaged her diet and made herself sick. All her previous progress was endangered; the precariously recovered balance started to disappear, and, at that time, her periods stopped. The atmosphere was again characterized by a crescendo of mismanagement and a stream of talk that left no space for interpretation. Miss T. was evidently terrified by the upcoming summer break.

In the session that follows she reported how much she had been shocked by a book she read. It is the story of an only child, a boy who was in fact a girl. The parents had told her that she had lost her genitalia in an accident, being bitten by a dog. This child was really uncertain about whether he was a girl or a boy. He/she used to go to the men's toilet and was really uncertain about her/his gender. I ask Miss T., "What about you?" She says she saw herself with her parents and thought that for her the terrible event was the discovery of her diabetes when her mother told her that from now on she would be a very "special" child. She remembers herself as an adolescent when, having no periods and no sexual relationship, her sexual identity was uncertain. At the time she wanted to be slim so as to avoid any evidence of her feminine identity. She was binging and vomiting and was very ill. At this point in the session she was overcome by shame and said she saw me on a table: she wanted to make pieces of me and eat me. I took this up indirectly, saying it was a way of making what happened to the child in the story happen to me. I said she was surprised, threatened, and excited by her wish to eat me. It was as if she could find how exciting the food in her mouth might be and how powerful she could feel in cutting me into pieces and swallowing me. Eating instead of having sex. Miss T. said, "All that is crap" and immediately added, "it is crap but it is true."

Miss T. was clearly involved in this story. After the session her self-destructive behavior increased: she was evidently aiming to kill herself. In the following sessions she repeatedly expressed the wish to become so ill that she would have to be hospitalized. My interpretations about separation had no effect. Her pain and desperation became unbearable: the session had a sense of death and impending catastrophe. The emotional conviction that she was not endowed with both male and female genitalia resulted in a total loss of omnipotence and the feeling of being powerless and dead. Interpretations of this were rejected. She protested against what she called "the Freudian model," accusing me of constraining her in a prefabricated theory. To ward off any possible effect from my interpretation she joined a class in women's studies in which she prepared a seminar contrasting Freudian theory with others. Miss T. was repeatedly angry when confronted with the task of recognizing her own sexual identity. This was inextricably linked with her father's abandonment, reactivated by her boyfriend's disappearance, as she pointed out in a later session.

Session after session, Miss T.'s appearance was increasingly androgenous. She decided to spend her summer holiday in a lesbian camp. She was now thinking of making love with a woman. She said she knew she liked men but wanted to feel liberated from them. The obvious fear of castration shown in the previous material was warded off by Miss T. before I could even allude to it. My interpretation, that she was very scared by her feelings of loneliness, desperation, and the wish to destroy me, because she cannot keep me with her as she could not keep her father, who went away with another woman, was quickly dismissed. Miss T. commented bitterly that this woman was nothing special, and at the time her father left she did not feel any distress.

Miss T. went to the lesbian camp, which she very much enjoyed. She found herself at ease in this environment and told me that she wanted to keep her father and all other men out of her mind and thoughts. Immediately after returning, she started a brief homosexual relationship in which she assumed the male role. The subject of men was avoided for many months. When, occasionally, the subject was raised, perhaps in a reference to some men who were part of her group, she would react by not coming to the following sessions.

At that time she seemed completely oblivious to her previous sexual experience. I think her need to stay within a homosexual environment corresponded to the maximal integration of her sexual drives she could achieve. It was too much for her to keep together the love and hate linked to both separation and her sexual needs. She could recognize them only at a preoedipal level, in which she was afraid she would disappear without the presence of the caregiver's support. The sadness, anger, and jealousy of her father's abandonment, at the oedipal level, with the discovery of her need for a male partner, needed to be warded off. Furthermore, the wound to her omnipotence when she could not fulfill all her mother's needs made her exclude men's presence and feel permanently aggressive toward them. But, at the same time, she assumed an unnatural caricature of a male manner: she spoke loudly and swore heavily in a strong and deep voice, showing a kind of supremacy over "inept women," as she described me and her mother. She was in fact terrified of discovering her sexual needs and denied them by assuming the aggressor's characteristics (A. Freud, 1966). The theatricality of this aggression brought into the session with great obstinacy was impervious to any attempt at understanding. Miss T. was very carefully protecting the degree of drive integration she had achieved, again avoiding touching anything that could threaten this. The homosexual constellation was the maximum integration she managed at that moment. She could not allow herself to integrate both her wishes toward and her anger against her father, facing at the same time the abandonment of her casual boyfriend. One could speculate about what might have developed if her occasional relationship with her boyfriend had continued or if the analyst was a male instead of a female (Rafael-Leff & Perelberg, 1997). For this kind of patient the impact of concrete events is especially strong because they can scarcely rely on metaphorical thinking (Kernberg, 1967); their containment depends in larger proportion than any other pathology on the external and concrete situation.

AVOIDING THE INTEGRATION OF LIBIDINAL AND AGGRESSIVE DRIVES
TOWARD THE PATERNAL FIGURE

While often failing to attend, Miss T. continued with her analysis: very fruitful sessions were followed by absences. She could bear neither continuity nor the idea that the analysis might end. We had discussed termination over the previous years, and she became aware, unwillingly, that analysis could not go on forever.

She made some important modifications in her external life: she moved from a shared house to a flat by herself; she finally decided to enter a teachers' training course. She was having a good social life visiting with friends and vice-versa. Each of these steps was taken with extreme difficulty and reported to me with evident ambivalence, as if I would intrude into her external life. She repeatedly complained about her inability/unwillingness to look after herself. It was as if there were a stowaway (Gaddini, 1981) in the session and the real Miss T. stayed outside. For her, I was not a supportive parent: on the contrary, her caution in speaking about the events of her life, of hiding her intentions, made me realize that for her I was a jealous competitor who would destroy her achievements. She had to be wary. When I interpreted this she told me that her father was always competing with her and would not accept being second.

She pointed to another reason for being guarded: that if she were better I would "chuck her out." In fact I had the impression that there was a planned, clandestine, if semi-conscious, project to induce a situation where the analysis would end without either of us being aware of it. Another unconscious goal was to make me "give up on her." This was a clear reference to her father, who, the last time he saw her, had told her that he had given up on her. The sessions assumed the characteristic of a long monologue of rationalization, though she missed many sessions without warning. Her absences became so numerous that I decided to raise the issue and speak abut her fear that even analysis could reach an end. She was in her fifth year of treatment, and the Christmas break was coming in four weeks. Miss T.'s reaction was one of panic. She did not come to her sessions for a whole week and I felt deeply worried, to the point that I asked the receptionist if Miss T. had telephoned.

When she returned she appeared to be in reasonable shape although she asserted that it was useless to come. After the session when I had raised the issue of termination, she had gone as usual to the Buddhist center to meditate and had been terrified by the realization that all her meditation was about planning her suicide. At the end of the meditation she had been unable even to deal with the final rite that the meditation required. She planned her farewell letters. She held a mental image of her parents, toward whom she felt very angry, then bought a bottle of Paracetamol (aspirin). After her meditation she could no longer bear to feel like 'a shit' and decided to kill herself. She kept the pills in her pocket, even though she knew very well that she could kill herself far more quickly with an overdose of insulin. She told no one of her decision. She went to see many of her friends, and stayed quietly with them. She found it particularly bizarre that one of them said to her that she (T.) was very strong. Miss T. said she gave that impression but it wasn't true. She felt deeply damaged inside, as if the analysis had had no effect. She said she wondered if this was the right therapy for her. I said she felt abandoned, and the fear resulting from talking about the end of her analysis put her into a terrible state. She wanted to tell me how very fragile she felt. Perhaps the anger was also hard to bear because it was like the anger she had felt toward her parents in meditation. She felt I would give up on her, as her parents had done: her mother because of her illness, her father because he left home. For this reason it was terrifying even to speak about ending the analysis. Miss T. insisted that if she still felt that she went to pieces in the face of any separation, it meant that the work we had done together was useless and this wasn't the right therapy for her. I told her she wanted to run away from it because she found the pain it evoked too difficult and almost preferred to kill herself. Miss T. said she has always faced a tragedy with every separation. She thinks this is because her mother was completely absent when she was little. She recognizes that it is her habit to run away from problems instead of dealing with them, but she had hoped to be able to leave analysis without these frightening feelings. She wanted to know how her analysis was going and pursued this train of thoughts for the rest of the session.

The content of the session and, even more, the emotions associated with it left me worried and dissatisfied; there was something bizarre about it: she presented herself as a relatively well-adjusted person who brought into the session someone suffering deeply, without integrating the two. After the session I discovered that Miss T. had called the center's receptionist asking for an assessment of her analysis by the psychiatrist who saw her when she initially applied for treatment. She told him on the telephone that she wanted to find out whether psychoanalysis was the right treatment for her, even though she had no reason to criticize me as an analyst and did not want me to be informed of her inquiry. The consultant took a very pragmatic, realistic, and, from my point of view, supportive stance. He told her that he would have to tell me what was happening since no one knew more about the analytic situation than analyst and patient and that, if she needed an appointment, he would see her.

The following day she did not come to her session, and just as the time for the session had run out, she called and left a message asking for an extra session! As it was a Friday I told her she could come at the usual time on Monday. When she did so she spoke of her terror of being deserted by me over the weekend. If the analysis came to an end, she said, she wanted to have another one. I said she seemed terrified even by the *idea* of speaking of termination. But before I could complete my interpretation Miss T. agreed with it and started a long and, to me, surprising list of complaints. She felt she couldn't express her anger inside the analytic setting. She didn't know what she could say and how far she could express herself. Could she cry? How loud might she speak? How much and how vigorously could she shout? Finally, she said she had to find someone who would lay down rules. She came to the conclusion that as I couldn't give her rules because of my role as her analyst, she could go to see the consultant to find out what the rules were.

Miss T.'s request was double-edged. She was asking me to assume the role of the father and at the same time telling me that this was too much for her. She had to keep it outside the session, identifying the father in the person of the consultant. I chose to interpret her feelings without reference to the transference. I told her that sometimes we feel in danger because we don't know our limits, even if having limits can make us angry. I went on to say that this could also happen inside a family, where one parent usually had more of a duty to set limits than the other. Miss T. immediately became alert and tense. She said, "Nobody in my family did it" and after a while, in an undertone, "My father did it." Then, speaking aloud again, she continued in a challenging and deprecating tone of voice: "That was because my mother was hopelessly weak." Only in the following session did she give me the opportunity to tell her that maybe the reason for her anger was the threat of thinking of me like a father, like her father who sets the rules, and it was safer for her to envisage somebody else, like Dr. X, doing so. She responded by quickly and loudly criticizing me. She finished by saying that she didn't want to "freak out." I told her that she feared loving me and hating me, and was frightened of feeling alone, of desperation, regret, and of her wish for revenge. She feared I couldn't be with her *and* stand these feelings without retaliating and menacing her. In one of those sudden revelations that she is unexpectedly able to make, Miss T. said that one of her fears was that I would return her hostility.

Miss T. clearly expressed her inability to face her feelings toward her father. She was terrified because she could see me in this way. She wanted to see me as a fragile and inept mother, unable to manage her upbringing. Later in the session she painfully reminded me of how, as young as nine years old, she used to look after her mother and deal with the household when her mother was ill. She tried to exclude her father from her thoughts in the session, as he had excluded himself from the family. At the same time she made it clear how many strong emotions she had at the time when, dealing with her deluded mother, she felt forced to assume the paternal role as provider for the family. The integration of the experienced internal relationship with feelings that had been denied for such a long time was an enormously crushing effort. She could imitate her father but she couldn't deal with her fear and fury for having been left without the protection she desperately longed for. What was very clear in this session was her inability to introject her father as a figure of authority with superego characteristics.

Miss T. needed to end analysis silently, without taking notice of what was happening, because she could not cope with integrating her aggression and her love for her father, nor could she direct toward me the feelings she had for him. Faced with this emerging theme, she saw the end of the analysis as a withdrawal from a situation of emergency. To avoid taxing her ego with any further emotion, she needed to reach the end silently because she thought that in this way she could avoid the excruciating pain of a final separation.

DISCUSSION

The fear of integration in the clinical material just presented has two correlates. The first is the loss of omnipotence and is an internal psychological experience. The second is separation and relates to an external fact that also carries with it complex internal psychological factors. The second seems to trigger the first in each of the situations depicted: both find an appropriate stage inside her diabetes. The occasion for all four episodes was provided by the separation that is inevitable in the analytic setting, as it is in life, which reactivated previous experiences of loss and the impossibility of coping with intense feelings of love and hate. In all four situations there is, at different levels, the issue of loss of omnipotence. The narcissistic components and therefore the impossibility of having an object separate from herself make her feel an extreme loneliness. In Miss T., the narcissistic withdrawal is defensive; yet it prevents her from attachment to a libidinal object. In any case, the object is so damaged and negative, and she is so resentful toward it, that she cannot tolerate its presence. Closing her mind to metaphorical meanings and instead using concrete thinking and her ill body meant excluding any space for the existence of others' minds. Recognizing the boundaries of the self means realizing that there are others, and the self is only a small part of the world; to accept one's sexual identity again indicates a limit to omnipotence; to accept the existence of rules and to introject the superego is another wound to omnipotence. All these aspects are triggered by the issue of separation because at different developmental levels separation brings with it a sense of impotence, together with love and hate toward the person who is leaving.

Separation is a very powerful psychological experience, but it is also inevitable, which makes its acceptance indispensable for reality testing. Miss T. was impaired in her capacity to deal with reality and specifically with the reality of her physical illness by growing up with traumatized parental figures who denied their own traumatic experiences. She repeatedly said that her mother became schizophrenic because she did not want to face reality. On the other hand, to overcome separation it is necessary to bind together the libidinal and aggressive drives.

As to whether fusion occurs within the ego or the id, there are different opinions. Freud (1920) and A. Freud (1949) relate it to the id. A. Freud (1966) pointed out the need to take into account "intrasystemic contradictions within the id" when excessive amounts of aggression are turned inward against the self and the individual becomes torn within himself and develops a preference for inner strife as opposed to striving for inner harmony" (p. 246). Nunberg (1930), on the other hand, attributes fusion to the synthetic function of the ego. According to him, it is the synthetic function of the ego that unites, binds, and brings coherence to the personality and its functioning. Hartmann (1939) utilizes Nunberg's concept of the synthetic function in his framework of adaptational processes. Furman (1985) considers ego and id equally involved in the fusion process, noting that clinically, synthetic function is not linked to any specific ego apparatus but affects all of them. In Miss T.'s analysis, the collapse of her capacity for integration presented itself with issues of aggressive and libidinal drive development in the presence of ego and id components.

It is interesting to consider the different levels of achievement to which such a capacity needs to be applied (to use metaphorical meanings, to define self-boundaries and sexual identity, and to training for work). The capacity to carry out these processes reflects the individual's id and ego endowment but is also related to such factors as variations in the strength of drives and the intactness of the ego apparatus (Weil, 1970). For Miss T., the presence of an infantile illness affected the balance of the drives because of the bodily experiences linked to her illness. The experience of falling to pieces when in hypoglycemic or ketotic crisis could significantly increase the stimulation of both drives and damage the synthetic function.

The effects of impairment of the ego apparatus have been widely documented (Burlingham, 1972; Sandler & Edgecumbe, 1974) but it is open to question how much such (physical) defects actually interfere with the development of integration. As Moran and Kennedy (1984) point out, analytic work with diabetic patients exposes the nature and quality of reciprocal interaction between psyche and soma in a way that other forms of psychological treatment cannot.

Miss T. often speaks of her fear of falling to pieces both physically and mentally. These, or similar expressions, are familiar to psychoanalysts but for Miss T. the correlate is not the non-integrative process; the real danger is that integration carries with it the necessity of recognizing her diabetes as a bodily illness and not as a way of controlling herself and others. If the patient has a sufficiently solid self, the most common anxiety will be of non-integration, which makes possible a much more solid therapeutic alliance. However, if the self as a separate entity is very fragile, there will be much greater integration anxiety, and therefore resistance to the unfolding of the analytic process will be stronger and sometimes insurmountable because the anxiety will act against any improvement effected by the analytic process itself. As a consequence of her lack of integration Miss T. is using imitation much more than identification, which requires integration of different aspects of the psychic apparatus. But the acquisitions deriving from imitation are, by their very nature, fragile and unstable. Anxiety about losing control, linked to her experiences of ketotic and hypoglycemic states, may reinforce the wish to fuse with the analyst, a wish that further intensifies anxiety at the possibility of loss of control.

From a developmental point of view this anxiety has its roots in the first object formation and in this way it is widely influenced by the environment (Greenacre, 1967), specifically by the role of caring adults in which the mother and her relationship with her child play an important part. I do not know what was the "material" truth (Freud, 1939) of this relationship for Miss T., but one can infer how difficult it might be to relate to a mother so deeply damaged that she used her daughter to contain her own immense anxiety. Miss T. repeatedly told me how mother was emotionally distant; such painful unavailability could be linked to an inability to integrate aggressive and libidinal forces in her own mind. Therefore it would have been impossible for the mother to support and develop her infant's integrative capacity by reflecting them in her own mind. The main task for the analyst in Miss T.'s treatment was to be the auxiliary ego and the id mediator, the place where fusion could be realized and contained, and only later to transfer this function to the patient. This task was not always successful with Miss T. because of her fragility and the need to calibrate interventions with the level of the patient's tolerance. This was often the result of striking a very difficult balance between the different components as the analyst understood them.

Furman (1985) points out that a mother's difficulty with fusion and integration in her own personality and in her investment in her baby interferes with her role as the child's auxiliary ego, as would a discontinuity in the relationship due to physical separation or emotional unavailability. Miss T. experienced both kinds of absence, due to mother's mental illness and to her repeated hospitalization. A. Freud (1956) indicates that the mother as auxiliary ego and id-ego mediator must gradually transfer her function to the child. This was not possible for Miss T.'s mother. On the contrary, Miss T. had to develop precocious ego functions in order to care for her mother and for her body in the way prescribed for diabetics (A. Freud, 1975). Hartmann (1939) has pointed out that precocious development of ego functions is related to a retarded development of the synthetic function.

If we envisage the analytic situation as a repetition of the process of growth, we can see how hard it is to help patients with this kind of difficulty to structure autonomous capacities, which require the ability to integrate. Integration is described as a process that fuels itself throughout its own functioning. As the autonomous capacities develop, every step in the process of fusion aids integration and, in turn, increases the capacity for fusion. But for Miss T. the fused energy with which she was endowed was scarce. When she had to face the task of a new integrative process, she had to use all the integrated forces she possessed; therefore she felt completely at the mercy of contradictory unbound emotions. A situation of panic ensued, in which Miss T. aimed to avoid, at any price, getting into contact with her catastrophic experience. It is in this context that, at the beginning of her analysis (see the Christmas trip), her defensive behavior was so chaotic and disorganized that it was difficult to compare it with structured defensive mechanisms. Rather, it should be likened to Tustin's (1981) "protective maneuvers."

One of the techniques I found useful with my patient was to help her hold together memories from previous sessions, building up a sense of continuity that I offered to her from my own mind. I have recently noticed that she has started to remember analytic events from previous sessions as if she had internalized them. I discovered that with this patient I did not need to vocalize what I understood, even if the material was uncontroversial. What I really needed to understand was how much she could tolerate of what *I* understood, and this was difficult and delicate because if I disappointed her by not saying enough she felt abandoned and empty, as if not fed well enough. She would run away (since unfulfilled needs would make her feel disoriented and empty, betrayed in her exploratory steps). But if I said too much, she found this even more threatening, would fear imminent catastrophe, and would run away. In an apparently contradictory manner, any progress she made was used against the psychoanalytic process. In fact, as she became better able to deal with herself and apparently more structured, it became more difficult to intervene because her defenses were stronger: she had to defend what she had achieved, and this new status was more organized than the previous one, as were her defenses. On the other hand, she was much more aware of her internal world and recognized that she was generally much better.

The definitive step toward adulthood ideally requires a final integration of aggressive and libidinal drives directed toward parental figures and the related mourning for the ideal parents one never had. When there have been difficulties in internalizing parental imagos and this resulted in very unstable internal objects, the mourning process cannot take place because of the fear of a total loss of the object. The integration between aggressive and libidinal wishes, present in the mourning process, cannot take place because, given the scarcity of libidinal components, the patient fears complete loss of the object. The definitive step toward adulthood also means, ideally, considering the parents no longer as providers and caregivers but as peers. Patients like Miss T., whose parental figures were inadequate carers, must renounce the dream of receiving the protection and care they never had but need so much, in order to build up a good enough internal object. To abandon this hope for good is particularly difficult because these patients have to re-experience their hate and despair and to recognize that they were full of these negative feelings, at the same time dealing with the emptiness in which they are left without them.

In this paper I have presented only one aspect of this patient's functioning. From my point of view, it is one of the most compelling and challenging features, on which many other analytic themes are based, and which may be the "kernel of truth" (Freud, 1939). In this patient the historical truth is at the point in Miss T.'s development where she has to go back to try to bring together her seemingly irreconcilable experiences.

BIBLIOGRAPHY

BAUM, J.D., AND KINMONTH, A. L. (eds) (1985). *Care of the child with diabetes.* New York: Churchill Livingstone.

BURLINGHAM, D. T. (1972). *Psychoanalytic studies of the sighted and the blind.* New York: Int. Univ. Press.

EIDELBERG, L. (1959). Humiliation in masochism, *J. Am. Psychoan. Assoc.,* 7, 2, pp. 274–283.

FONAGY, P., MORAN, G., & TARGET, M. (1993). Aggression and the psychological self. *Int. J. Psycho-Anal.,* 74:471–485.

FRANKL, L. (1961). Some observations on the development and disturbances of integration in childhood. *Psychoanal. Study of the Child,* 16, 146–163.

FREUD, A. (1949). Aggression in relation to emotional development: Normal and pathological. In *The Writings of Anna Freud,* New York: International Universities Press, 1968, 4:489–497.

—— (1952). The mutual influences on the development of ego and id. *Psychoanal. Study of the Child*, 3:42–50.

—— (1956). Psychoanalytic knowledge applied to the rearing of children. In *The Writings of Anna Freud*, New York: Int. Univ. Press, 1969, 5:265–280.

——. (1966). *The ego and the mechanisms of defense*, Int. Univ. Press, New York.

—— (1975a). Psychoanalytic psychology of normal development, Int. Univ. Press, New York, 8, (1970–80).

—— (1975b). Psychopathology seen against the background of normal development. Int. Univ. Press, New York, 8, (1970–80).

FREUD, S. (1920). Beyond the pleasure principle. The *Standard Edition of the Complete Psychological Works of Sigmund Freud* [S.E.], ed. and trans. J. Strachey. London: Hogarth. 18:7–66.

—— (1923). The ego and the id. S.E., 19:12–68.

—— (1939). Moses and monotheism. S.E., 23:7–140.

FURMAN, E. (1985). On fusion, integration and feeling good. *Psychoanal. Study of the Child*, 40, 81–110.

—— (1982). Mothers have to be there to be left. *Psychoanal. Study of the Child*, 37, 15–28.

FURMAN, R. A., & FURMAN, E. (1984). Intermittent decathexis, *Int. J. Psycho-Anal.*, 65, 423–433.

GADDINI, E. (1981). Sulla imitazione. In Gaddini, *Scritti (1953–1985)*, Milan: Cortina, 1989, 159–182.

—— Acting out nella situazione analitica. In Gaddini, *Scritti (1953–1985)*, Cortina, Milan: 1989, pp. 535–546.

—— (1985). La maschera e il cerchio. In Gaddini, E., *Scritti (1953–1985)*, Milan: Cortina, 1989, 735–742.

GREENACRE, P. (1967). The influence of infantile trauma on genetic patterns. *Psychic trauma*. Ed. S. S. Ferst, New York: Basic Books.

HARRISON, A., & WEINTROBE, S. (1994). Psychoanalytic treatment and understanding of violence in children and young adult. *Seventh International Scientific Colloquium*, London: Anna Freud Centre. (Unpublished paper).

HARTMANN, H. (1939). Comments on the psychoanalytic theory of the ego. *Psychoanal. Study of the Child*, 5, 74–96.

HOCKADAY, T. D. R. (1985). Pathogenesis and natural history of the treated disorder. In: *Care of the child with diabetes* eds. J. D. Baum & A. L. Kinmonth. New York: Churchill Livingstone, pp. 12–28.

KENNEDY, H., & MORAN, G. S. (1984). The developmental roots of self-injury and response to pain in a 4-year-old boy. *Psychoanal. Study of the Child*, 39, 1, pp. 195–212.

KERNBERG, O. (1967). Borderline personality organization, *J. Amer. Psychoanal Ass.*, 15, 3, pp. 641–685.

KOGAN, I. (1992). From acting out to words and meanings, *Int. J. Psychoanal.* 3, pp. 455–465.

NUNBERG, H. (1930). The synthetic function of the ego. In *Practice and theory of psychoanalysis*. New York: Int. Univ. Press, 1, pp. 120–135.

RAFAEL-LEFF, J., AND PERELBERG, R. (eds.) (1997). *Female experience.* London: Routledge.

ROSENFELD, S. K., AND SPRINCE, M. P. (1963). An attempt to formulate the meaning of the concept "borderline." *Psychoanal. Study of the Child,* 18, 603–635.

SANDLER, J., AND EDGECUMBE, R. (1974). Varieties of aggression turned against the self. In *From safety to superego,* ed. J. Sandler. New York: Guilford, 1987.

SANDLER, J., AND SANDLER, A.-M. (1978). On the development of objects relationships and affects. *Int. J. Psycho-Anal.,* 59, 285–296.

TUSTIN, F. (1981). *Autistic States in Children.* London: Routledge & Kegan Paul.

WEIL, A. P. (1970). The basic core. *Psychoanal. Study of the Child,* 25, 442–460.

WINNICOTT, D. W. (1962). Ego integration in child development. In *The maturational processes and the facilitating environment.* New York: Int. Univ. Press, pp. 56–63.

YORKE, C. (1980). Some comments on the psychoanalytical treatment of patients with physical disabilities. *Int. J. Psychoanal.,* 61, 187–193.

——— (1985). Fantasy and the body-mind problem. *Psychoanal. Study of the Child,* 40, 319–328.

ADOLESCENCE

Adolescents and Popular Culture

A Psychodynamic Overview

DEBRA S. ROSENBLUM, M.D.,
PETER DANIOLOS, M.D., NEAL KASS, M.D.,
and ANDRES MARTIN, M.D.

Adolescents occupy a difficult and seemingly elusive developmental space, which makes them enigmas to most adults, including psychotherapists. Building upon dynamic theory such as that formulated by Winnicott or Erikson, this paper explores the relationship between adolescents and material elements of popular culture within a psychodynamic and developmental framework. Theoretical perspectives are integrated with case material to illustrate some of the roles of popular music and fashion in the lives of teenagers as a means of expression and in potential ther-

Debra S. Rosenblum, M.D., is clinical instructor, Harvard Medical School, staff psychiatrist, Cambridge Hospital, Division of Child and Adolescent Psychiatry. Peter Daniolos, M.D., is consulting associate in the Department of Psychiatry and Behavioral Sciences, Duke University Medical Center; Medical Director, Chapel Hill Pediatric Psychology; staff psychiatrist, The Durham Center, Durham, N.C. Neal Kass, M.D., is clinical instructor in Psychiatry, Harvard Medical School, Concord, Mass. Andres Martin, M.D., is assistant professor of Child Psychiatry, Yale University Child Study Center.

Some material in this paper was presented by the authors at the Annual Meeting of the American Association of Child and Adolescent Psychiatry, October 1996, Philadelphia, and the Annual Meeting of the American Psychiatric Association, June 1998, Toronto, Canada. (The names of the patients described in the case studies have been changed to protect their privacy.)

The authors would like to extend their appreciation to Dr. Lawrence Hartmann for his editorial suggestions on an earlier draft of this paper. They would also like to acknowledge the contributions of Dr. Leston Havens, Victoria Kass, Rebecca Martin, Bradley Rosenblum, Dr. Lenore Terr, and Ray Williams.

The Psychoanalytic Study of the Child 54, ed. Albert J. Solnit, Peter B. Neubauer, Samuel Abrams, and A. Scott Dowling (Yale University Press, copyright © 1999 by Albert J. Solnit, Peter B. Neubauer, Samuel Abrams, and A. Scott Dowling).

apeutic alliance formation, dynamic understanding, and working through developmental conflicts in displacement.

ADOLESCENTS OFTEN PRESENT A UNIQUE CHALLENGE TO DEDICATED AND empathic psychotherapists. Unlike younger children, who express themselves in play, or adults, who frequently seek treatment on their own, teenagers sometimes demonstrate substantial resistance to the therapeutic process. This reluctance to engage results not only from the reality that most adolescents in therapy find themselves there at the behest of authority figures, usually their parents, but also from characteristic developmental phenomena, such as the defense mechanism of denial, as well as the conflict between the wish for autonomy and the regressive pull of dependence. "I don't know why I'm here, there's nothing wrong with me," is a familiar opening line in therapy with this population. One means around this resistance is to address issues in displacement, as in play therapy with the younger child. Whereas teenagers may be hesitant to reveal vulnerability by discussing their feelings, they may be more comfortable talking about popular music or clothing styles, areas in which they enjoy some sense of mastery. The exploration of such topics, including tattoos and piercings, not only facilitates alliance formation but also emphasizes integral concerns in adolescent development, such as body image, sexuality, and the search for identity.

Popular Music within a Developmental Framework

A good deal of psychoanalytic literature has focused on the role of fairy tales and nursery rhymes in realizing the developmental needs of the preschool child. According to Bettelheim, fairy tales aid in the mastery of the psychological tasks of growing up by providing symbolic expression for these rites of passage. These tasks include: (1) overcoming narcissistic disappointments and the oedipal dilemma, (2) relinquishing childhood dependency and escaping from separation anxiety, (3) organizing the chaotic pressures of the unconscious, and (4) gaining a feeling of selfhood and self-worth (Bettelheim, 1976). Fairy tales legitimize inner experience by providing vehicles for working through unconscious pressures in fantasy and play. As children grow into adolescence, their developmental needs are no longer met by fairy tales or imaginary play games. For many teenagers in contemporary Western culture, popular music serves as the agent of expression for age-specific conflicts and defenses.

Popular music has a dynamic attraction for many adolescents. In one survey, 81 percent of students described music as a "very important" part of their lives (Reston, 1984). Between the seventh and twelfth grades, the average teenager listens to 12,500 hours of music (Avery, 1979). Since its inception in the early 1950s, rock and roll music has presented itself as the medium for the outsider, the lonely, the alienated. It purports to supply a voice for the rebel who dares to stand apart from mainstream or adult culture. This dissonance comes across not only in the thematic content of the songs but also in the way the music performer presents him- or herself in contrast to mainstream adult society. Even the sound of rock and roll or rap music—often loud, rhythmic, and agitated—proclaims the underlying sense of "difference."

Children enter adolescence with the mandate to grow toward adulthood, an obligation that inspires ambivalence. One developmental challenge is to decathect from early object ties in order to achieve an autonomous and consolidated sense of self. A sense of loss, grief, and perceived abandonment emerges related to a sense of parental loss and disappointment. This process is characterized by an oscillation between progression and regression; autonomy and dependence. The resurrection of pre- and post-oedipal identifications that led to superego formation can become a source of anxiety in the context of emerging sexual impulses that need to be controlled. As the teenager rejects the external controls of latency as vehicles of dependency, the ego has less support, leading to a greater sense of isolation and perceived abandonment (Blos, 1962).

"I hurt myself today / to see if I still feel / I focus on the pain / the only thing that's real" (Reznor, 1994). These themes of loneliness and marginalization are evoked in popular music, from "I can't get no satisfaction" (Jagger/Richards, 1964) to "I'm a loser, baby, so why don't you kill me" (Beck, 1994). Adolescents listening to these songs hear some of their most powerful thoughts and feelings echoed and expressed. In this music, they feel that their internal turmoil has been matched and understood. Through its romanticization of the antihero, popular music rearticulates the perceived powerlessness of youth as a source of identity: "Hope I die before I get old—talking about my generation" (Townshend, 1966). The listener is able to transcend self-doubts in the realization that he or she does not suffer alone and is not "crazy" for having these feelings. Like fairy tales for younger children, popular music provides settings for the adolescent imagination through which unconscious conflicts may be played out and resolved in displacement. Listening to music can provide a source of guidance and comfort. An adolescent girl wrote to *Rolling Stone* magazine after the suicide of Kurt Cobain, lead singer of the "grunge" group

Nirvana: "I could be feeling like total shit and hear a Nirvana song and end up feeling renewed afterward. Maybe that's not supposed to happen. Maybe someone singing about anger and pain and confusion and loss and the shallowness of it all isn't supposed to make you feel better. But it always made me feel happy and alive afterwards" (*Rolling Stone,* 1994).

As adolescents pull away from their parents and look to others as ego-ideals, the popular music star can become healer, teacher, shaman. Performers appear to reveal and articulate emotions that the listener feels but does not know how to express. Adolescents often view these performers as their confidants, the only ones who understand how they suffer. As internet message boards testify (America Online, 1998), many teenagers were devastated by Kurt Cobain's suicide. Some felt as if they had lost their best friend, and a number of copycat attempts have been reported anecdotally (Goldberg, 1997). Through outrageous dress or behavior, many rock and rap stars present themselves as a "different" kind of adult or a bridge between the kids' world of fun and the grown-up world of responsibility. These artists serve as projections for the adolescents' fears and fantasies on a number of metapsychic levels, including sexual awareness, primal release, and emotional identification. A teenage music fan may play the Rolling Stones' song "Sympathy for the Devil" and imagine him- or herself as Satan, the narrator of the song, or as Mick Jagger, the superstar performer who sings it.

Musical affiliation also plays a role in adolescent peer relations. Musical preference as a means of communication becomes a nexus for group identity, extending to clothing style and expressed beliefs as well as, on occasion, drug use and other risk-taking behavior. With music, teenagers form their own distinct subcultures—hip hop, Deadheads, Goth, Heavy Metal—as a challenge to the parent culture, in part as a resistance to growing up but also, paradoxically, as a way of staking out their own territory upon which to grow. An exile assumed voluntarily, this space becomes, in Winnicott's term, a new holding environment to replace the one that the family can no longer provide. This space, comprised of shared fantasies that speak to the adolescents' inner reality and impacts on how they perceive external reality, resembles a transitional phenomenon: an "intermediate area between what is subjectively and objectively perceived" (Winnicott, 1958). External experience is encountered in this transitional space so as to coincide with the subject's perception or illusion of having created it and thus perpetuating a sense of omnipotence or mastery through the shared medium of music.

ELEMENTS OF MUSIC

Why does music, rather than some other expressive art form such as poetry or visual arts, appeal so strongly to most adolescents? One factor is the great availability of music through radio, recordings, and music videos. Another is the ability to share music in a peer setting. Music can be "owned": a song can be played again and again, sung along with and danced to in interactions perhaps not possible with fine arts or literature.

Music induces a regression to preverbal ways of experiencing. With the exception of some musicians who process music in the left hemisphere, like a native language, most people process music in the right hemisphere, which also governs the emotional nonverbal aspects of speech, such as facial expression and prosody (Feder, 1993). Verbal exchanges between infant and caregiver are organized around affective intonational features more than actual syntax or words. Many popular music songs use the call-and-response pattern, an echoing of phrases between the lead singer and the rest of the band, which also is evocative of early communication attempts between infant and mother. With the inherent pressure to achieve distance from the family, the adolescent seeks out music, a medium that recapitulates the early dyadic interchange and recaptures a version of the early holding environment.

Most popular music songs possess a verse-chord structure that quickly oscillates between tension and release. Rock and roll and rap are organized around rhythm to a greater extent than other musical styles such as classical. The most dominant sound apparent to the developing fetus in utero is the maternal heartbeat. Rhythm and a repetitive tempo anchor many contemporary songs, notably rap, which has no melody but is spoken or chanted to an insistent, repetitive beat. These structural elements make popular music unconsciously recognizable and more accessible than other forms of music in which longer periods of time elapse before a return to the familiar (the tonic chord, or "home," in classical music). Many rock songs are predictable both within themselves and also because adolescents will play the same song or album over and over, just as a younger child will beg to hear the same nursery rhyme or fairy tale "one more time." The ability to anticipate and master a piece of popular music creates a sense of safety and order for teenagers, who often feel that they have little to keep them—or some of their thoughts and impulses—contained.

Popular music, by virtue of its emphasis on the backbeat, which accentuates the second and fourth quarter beats, encourages movement and participation. Teenagers, more than younger children, are aware of having a body and often are ashamed of or confused by sensations within the body. Emerging sexuality accounts for some of the appeal of popular music both thematically, in its implied rebelliousness, and structurally, through its embrace of rhythm. Sexuality is enacted in displacement through dancing or "losing oneself" in the music; these can be safe ways of coming to terms with problematic issues such as the acceptance of a new adult body and the sexuality this maturity presupposes.

MUSIC IN THERAPY: THEORY AND CASE STUDIES

Clinical work with adolescents requires a capacity in the therapist to join the experience of the patient without participating in the actual behaviors that led the teenager into treatment. Music can allow the willing therapist immediate and visceral collaboration with the adolescent patient. Listening to and discussing music with the adolescent patient resemble play. According to Winnicott (1958), "Psychotherapy takes place in the overlap of two areas of playing, that of the patient and that of the therapist. Psychotherapy has to do with two people playing." When a therapist joins the semi-hypnotic reverie of a younger child playing, the greatest therapeutic results can arise. A shared engagement with music allows for this interplay with an older child.

Clinical Case I: Robin

Robin, age 14, came to treatment by parental order because he was doing poorly in school and had begun to spend time with a "bad crowd." He appeared disengaged and depressed to school staff and demonstrated oppositional and disrespectful behavior toward his mother. He had adamantly refused prior treatment attempts and had spoken in virtual monosyllables to the counselors at school and the HMO psychiatrist who had referred him. His father was a hard-working, well-meaning construction worker who was often out of the home because of a busy work schedule. Mother was a small Italian-American woman who had her hands full with five children, of whom Robin was the oldest. Although she always had enjoyed a close relationship with her son, he had dramatically distanced himself in the year after the youngest sibling was born, coinciding with his beginning middle school. The black clothing Robin wore constantly was of particular concern to his parents.

When Robin walked into his first therapy session with one of the authors (N.K.), the therapist was struck by the meticulous attention that had obviously been paid to his outfit, which bore the trademarks of the rock icon Marilyn Manson. The therapist began the interview by expressing admiration for Robin's manner of dress and found him quite willing to explain the details of color, slogans, rings, hair, and related musical interests. Most of this first interview was spent discussing these details. Robin, visibly more engaged with the therapist, was able to explain his attraction to Marilyn Manson, saying that he had a Marilyn Monroe side as well as a Charles Manson side. Despite his apparent disinterest and difficulty in school, he was reading Marilyn Manson's autobiography and was fascinated by it. The interview ended with patient and therapist agreeing that one of Robin's biggest troubles was getting his parents to tolerate his choices. Both parents were surprised when Robin and the therapist emerged from the session laughing and planning future sessions.

The work has not been confined to this sphere, but the encounter provided the therapist with a solid backing to enter more intricate negotiations between Robin and his parents. He spent time with the parents discussing their relations to music, their reactions to the music Robin was listening to, and the healthful aspects of this form of play. Robin's father was able to pick up on this point remarkably and joined his son not only in listening to music but also in reading and discussing the Manson book; the two had rarely spent time together previously in these pursuits. It may have been through the transitional phenomenon of music that Robin was able to discuss in therapy the parallel issue of his anger and hurt that his mother (he ignored his father in this) had borne so many children and left him feeling neglected.

The consolidation of group identity, forged out of a personal identity, is a critical adolescent developmental task that is accessed well by clinical attention to music. The adolescent's "crowd" often alarms adults but sometimes is organized around musical and cultural themes. In the case of Robin, he had an interest in Gothic dress, music, and movies. The film *The Crow,* a Gothic parable, involves the eventual triumph of good over evil, a theme that provided substantial relief to Robin's parents. In contrast, yet in service to these needs for group and personal identity formation, is the fact that music also provides equally well for the adolescent's need for privacy and private thoughts.

Clinical Case II: Chris

Chris is a male with 40-percent renal function, the result of a birth anomaly that required more than ten hospitalizations and surgeries before he was eight. He was referred for psychiatric consultation at age 16 for explosive behavior and possible psychosis. He had been attending a therapeutic day school because of his outbursts and had little commitment to academics. Most of his behavior and affect seemed to revolve around his mother, who was described as enmeshed with Chris, erratic, child-like, self-preoccupied, and volatile. The therapist, who had known the family since Chris was twelve, described the mother as having a severe borderline personality disorder. She had left the family suddenly, just before Chris's thirteenth birthday. (She was still in touch with Chris during her absence from the home.) His father, who worked as a deliveryman for a biotech company, had been surprised by his ex-wife's action, which rendered him emotionally limited in the parenting of his son. The treatment had broken down: Chris would refuse to attend most sessions and when he did attend, with his father, would present as silent or obtuse and occasionally would fly into a rage and bang at the walls.

At the first meeting between Chris and N.K., the boy reported, with some delight, that he was seeing images or "scenes" in his head from multiple visual perspectives simultaneously and without needing to move his body. He described MTV videos playing all the time in his mind. He and this therapist discussed the details of the music videos: the bands involved, the colors, speed, technical quality, and sound. He clearly presented as intelligent, creative, imaginative, and interested in talking about these details. The therapist asked him, since this was a psychopharmacological consultation, whether there was any aspect of these images, thoughts, or sounds that he would like to eliminate if a medication were able to perform such a function. By this point, Chris was more interested in talking about music and said that he would not like to change any of these perceptions. He said that there were advantages of these perspectives, his "gift," for becoming a filmmaker, to which he aspired. The rest of the hour was spent discussing music: his tastes, his therapist's tastes, and the group tastes at school. His father and the referring therapist were told that meetings with N.K. would occur for a while before it could be determined whether medication was appropriate; for now, Chris just wanted to come and talk and commit to weekly meetings.

Over the first few weeks of treatment with N.K., Chris found it difficult to speak about his history, relationships, parents, or peers. He stated that he did not want to talk about his mother but would "kill" anyone who badmouthed her. He said he loved his father but did not feel understood by him. He elaborated that he did not feel understood in any context, that he had been born in the wrong century, and that his values and intelligence were mismatched to those of people today.

Chris was an overweight boy who wore a tattered leather jacket during all sessions, with a dark baseball cap pulled low over his face. Most of every early session turned to the discussion of music, the subject in which he was clearly most at ease. The therapist struggled with the worry that he was not accomplishing enough. After playing with ideas about music and lyrics, Chris announced that there were some songs he wanted his therapist to hear.

The therapist brought a portable compact disc player to the sessions, and Chris supplied the CDs; they listened together, and the therapy shifted. The music deepened the therapist's understanding of this timid boy, who could seem so fierce in moments of outburst but felt small and vulnerable. Chris's favorite bands were heavy metal: huge musical structures with firm background bass and drum-work guitar textures. Chris claimed that he did not pay attention to the lyrics, yet he mouthed them to all his favorite songs. With the therapist, he studied album covers, and eventually the therapy settled into a session of listening, the way teenagers do by themselves or with their friends. He announced one day that he had brought the "mama of them all," referring to a 1991 album by the heavy-metal band Metallica which contained the song "The Unforgiven." The sound seemed enormous and medieval. The lyrics spoke: "New blood joins the earth./And quickly he's subdued/Through constant pained disgrace/The young boy learns the rules/With time the child draws in/The whipping boy done wrong/Deprived of all his thoughts/The young man struggles on and on . . . What I've felt/What I've known/Never shined through in what I've shown/Never free/Never me/So I dub thee Unforgiven" (Metallica, 1991). At the song's end, the therapist stated, sadly and awkwardly, "It's you and your mother." Chris, who prior to this time had refused to assign any meaning to the songs, quietly nodded, and asked, "Would you like to hear it again?"

For Chris, listening to this song with the therapist signified a turning point in their relationship. The song was played often, and Chris became much freer and more articulate in expressing his feelings about his body and his fear of dying young from renal failure. He spoke of his rage at his mother for being overprotective and smothering when he was a young boy, yet he sensed that she loved him no matter what he did. He described his anger that he never could join the military (the family had a long and distinguished history of military participation) and his despair that he would not, could not, amount to anything. Apart from these dynamic issues, the music conjured a fantasied personality that he and the therapist were able to play with as he made his way in society. The character was a strong, principled figure with the qualities of a knight in shining armor whose task was to protect and fight for the underprivileged. The character had exaggerated qualities: a bellowing voice, the capacity to intimidate, anger that would make others tremble, and a heart of gold. This character was invoked as Chris navigated the adolescent difficulties of failed love relationships, low self-esteem, chronic feelings of abandonment, and, at times, behavior intolerable to his father or the therapeutic school.

Ultimately, Chris's behavior became less of a problem, although he continued to struggle with his father over cleaning his room or participating in their small household. He had experienced a core narcissistic injury but could barely acknowledge his entitlement and pleas to be taken care of. He continued to meet with the therapist, to listen to tunes on the radio and "surf the waves" to pick up on songs and themes at random while discussing everyday aspects of life or playing at darts. Chris's decision to join his mother, a considerable distance from the therapist's office, has currently disrupted his treatment, but he keeps in frequent contact. The work together remains rooted in the mutual experiencing and playing with musical themes, sounds, and lyrics. The music paradigm afforded a basic trust.

FASHIONING IDENTITY

Much thought, creativity, imagination, feelings, fears, hopes, conflicts, and desires fuel an adolescent's clothing choices and the way he or she presents the self to the world. Fashion is a complex expression of identity for the adolescent, the end result of intrapsychic and external forces. It is worthwhile for the therapist to notice and understand the way an adolescent presents as an expression of inner life and an adaptation to external reality. Questioning adolescents about style is a powerful clinical tool to gain access to their emotional lives and also creates a connection so that therapeutic work may occur in a safe space.

CASE STUDY: ZEV

Zev, now aged 16, first presented at age eleven for severe panic disorder with agoraphobia. For the next two years he received cognitive-behavioral treatment combined with paroxetine, which decreased his anxiety. He entered treatment with P.D. at age thirteen, at a time when he was being home-schooled because of severe anxiety as well as a language-based learning disability.

Zev is the youngest child and only son of a university professor and an educator, who reside in a medium-sized city in the Southeast. His father comes from a working-class background and acquired an Ivy League education. He works out regularly and values his appearance.

He has been very accepting of Zev's anxiety and has never pushed him to re-enter public school. Zev's relationship with his father has been one of awe, respect, and some fear—his father has an unpredictable and forceful temper. As Zev entered adolescence, his father attempted a closer relationship with him, revealing much about his own youth and current life to his son in an attempt to bridge the distance between them. At times, he disclosed intimate aspects of his sexual behavior, which made Zev uncomfortable.

Zev's mother was psychiatrically hospitalized for psychosis and depression when he was three, following the miscarriage of what would have been his younger sister. She was diagnosed as bipolar and has been maintained on lithium since that time. Trained as an educator, she readily took on the complicated role of becoming his teacher for grades seven through ten, with part-time home schooling for his junior year. Zev always has been close to his mother and privately worries about her happiness and whether his parents enjoy much intimacy between them.

Zev described his parents as "too good" because he felt he owed them so much for their sacrifices resulting from his panic disorder and that he had "very little room to mess up." He feels he has been a disappointment to his father: prior to his birth, a faulty amniocentesis identified him as a female. "Then I had a penis and he was so excited." He believes he has not lived up to his father's expectations of a son but has been a burden because of his panic disorder and has "no room for normal teen things."

In the initial sessions, Zev's style of dress changed frequently: "I like to have a variety of styles, not just one. I collect them and think about what I'm going to wear each day. I try not to be influenced by styles but I am influenced by music groups. I like the Beastie Boys: they wear classy clothes with something different. I definitely care about my clothes but I don't want to look like everyone else." Soon after making this comment, he took to wearing ski caps in the hot, Southern fall and old-fashioned thrift-store clothing.

After these early sessions, Zev plunged into massive alcohol use, a new behavior for him, leading to a conjoint session between him and his father. As he began to restabilize, he said: "A lot of my feelings never have been expressed to [my father] . . . he doesn't understand teen culture." He stated that the thought-blocking skill he had learned in his previous cognitive-behavioral therapy now was impeding his ability to tolerate or understand his dissonant thoughts and feelings: "I block all my feelings . . . it is easier . . . they build up, and alcohol provides a vent to clear temporarily." Later, he tearfully revealed: "I feel that regular feelings have been muted by my learning thought-blocking techniques, I'm struggling to maintain a sense of myself . . . a desperate attempt to form an identity."

During this phase, Zev informed his mother that he was contemplating getting a nipple pierced. He disagreed with her view that this was self-mutilation. "It is something that I want to do on my own . . . not really an answer . . . a private thing that not a lot of people see." Although he never had his body pierced, the day he talked about it he also brought in a drawing entitled "Christianity": "People lose themselves looking to one guy—Christ—for answers. They become weak—like when I had panic disorder. It is like looking to parents and God for answers. They become copies." At this time, Zev described himself as an atheist, and the world as meaningless and malevolent. His father is a devout Catholic. When asked if he saw any similarities between himself and his father, he replied, "I will be like him in some ways. If he had grown up like me, he would be me."

Zev formulated his own theory of development: "By the age of ten, you are pretty much a hard mold of what you will be. You can be cracked with something bad. At my stage it is pretty much glazing. Once you get glazed over, you are not untouchable. You have formed a protective shell—it keeps you from being easily changed except for tragedies." Zev believes he developed a tough shell because of his feeling that he did not fit in with others. He thinks that, with the exception of his mother, his therapist, and, sometimes, his father, most people see only his shell. "My parents reminded me that I need to be aware of the image I project. People jump to conclusions . . . they need to separate the shell from the real person . . . I appear to be tall but am a very short person inside." He described himself as a snail with "parts sticking out . . . so I jumped in and puffed out the shell with bright colors, to keep away the bad guys. But it's temporary—when I grow up I will not need it."

Although his parents appeared to be supportive, his father became enraged when Zev came home with a mohawk hair cut: "My Dad went crazy, shouting at me." Frightened by the intensity of his father's response, Zev decided to remove the mohawk. At age thirteen he tried on make-up: "I was sitting on the can and bored and I wondered what my lips would look like if they were a little more red." His parents and sister reacted intensely, telling him that he could not wear make-up. "It was just my creativity, just paint, but it set a bomb off in the household." He added, "People are uncomfortable with the feminine in males. It threatens them."

Eight months into therapy, Zev commented: "Clothing style reflects the way a person lives. Some people really in trouble wear stuff that no one thinks looks good—not trying to make a statement. That is different from the kid with boots, chains, and dyed hair because they cared enough to fit a look they like. It takes a lot of work. Like a mohawk: kids spend 15 minutes at least on their hair. And a lot of gel!"

Zev's mother reported overall improvement: he seemed happier, able to tolerate long road trips with outings to shopping malls and other locales. He remained involved with friends although he decided not to rejoin them in public school but to enter a newly formed charter school. He became tearful when talking about punk music: "The complete outcasts come into this punk community and find refuge . . . those who were fat, tortured, not many prom queens. Punk music originated from nerds in plaid pants and messy hair. It's a nonjudgmental place held together with common interest." He asked his therapist to listen to an album by the hardcore group Minor Threat. "I've learned more from these lyrics—'Nothing is fair . . . go ahead and try'—than from all my therapy. It has been a bible to me—inspired me to make the best of myself and sink or swim . . . I get emotional about it and wish I had an outlet . . . I feel a lot of feelings are trapped and it can be destructive."

Zev explored the meaning of music in his life, connecting it to his sense of style. After going to a Kiss concert, he stated: "I wore an old plaid suit so as not to be dressed like everyone else. I don't have a single friend who likes Kiss, so I wanted to go. Huge concert but I didn't have much anxiety. I didn't know people were still feathering their hair back."

Zev described feeling drawn to a peer, Sally. One rainy day, she made a dress from an old shower curtain and wore it to school "so that she would not have to use an umbrella." Zev liked her "extreme form of self—a form of innocence. We are two people who do not exactly fit the teen stereotype." Zev also identifies with his pet rat, Ollie: "Rat. My pet has that label, and it is not fair. I have this teenage label, and that is not fair . . . I am so much more. I relate to Ollie: metal bars that can't be broken."

Zev took pride in carefully blending different clothing styles. Once he entered the therapy office attired in a mechanic's canvas jacket with a faux leopard collar. When asked about the jacket, he described not only the evolution of his current style but also his personal path of identity consolidation: "At first I wore clothes at the edge, but I got sick of it. Two years ago, I was trying to be different when I was a freshman in home schooling. It was a rush for identity; random and chaotic. I lost so many years being a kid and was not happy. I had been dressed by others until then. Then, this winter in charter school, I wanted more traditional stuff, like 50s suits, relaxing 50s kind of things. I also got into work pants. I didn't want to put no thought into it, but also not be the fashion statement I was earlier. Now I have more balance. I put more thought into it, am more careful and less random. I'm using things I like from different groups or cultures and wear what I like even if it is not cool. I respect the working class culture." The therapist asked Zev to elaborate about his mechanic's jacket and he replied: "I like the idea of a mechanic wearing leopard print—silk and a hammer."

At this point, Zev had successfully integrated into a chaotic charter school for his junior year. Conversations with his teacher revealed that he was an excellent student who contributed to class and was a talented writer despite his learning disability. He was well liked and respected by his peers. Zev went on to public high school for his senior year, fulfilling his dream of having at least one year in "regular" high school. He also tolerated a decrease in his paroxetine and began to work out regularly in a gym with his peers. He described feeling less preoccupied with how others viewed him and, for the first time, comfortable with being a teenager. His father bought a motor scooter for him, resulting in enhanced mobility and freedom. Zev successfully navigated through traffic without a single panic attack. He also took on a part-time job as a mechanic's assistant, and he now arrives for therapy attired in an auto-worker's uniform.

The study of Zev illustrates how fashion serves as a window into the adolescent's internal world. By asking him about his clothing choices, the authors therapist learned about the anxiety that has plagued him for much of his life and better understood his identity conflicts and adaptive coping patterns. Conversations about clothing led to deeper, affect-laden insights into his role in his family and with his peers. Themes of alienation and resilience emerged, and shifts in style clearly reflected shifts in his mind, serving as a marker of growth. Zev's clothes reflect the struggle described in Erik Erikson's developmental stage of identity versus role confusion. Erikson (1950) suggested that adolescents form groups based on petty aspects such as dress as a defense against role confusion. In Zev's case, he worked hard to create a look that both defined himself and expressed his sense of difference from his peers.

This case illustrates the powerful understanding that may emerge from noticing and asking adolescent patients about their clothing choices. As Havens (1986) has written, therapy is much more powerful if the patient believes the therapist is seeing the world from his or her perspective. Changes in Zev's clothing and musical interests reflected his identity consolidation, including improvement in self-esteem and lessening of anxiety. Zev moved from being overwhelmed by anxious and aggressive feelings, in part projected onto a world that had become meaningless, hostile, and dangerous. As he began to tolerate these feelings and block them less, the world became a more "Buddhist" place, with meaning, purpose, and kindness. His armor for the former world was "on the edge," with much energy invested in wearing attention-getting clothes and shaving his head to "scare the enemies," as he invoked in the metaphor of the snail that pulls in its soft parts and puffs out its shell. He felt vulnerable, defective, and weak. For the later, gentler world, his suit was a synthesis of different cultures and times, including the 1950s of his parents. He proudly declared his individuality and belonging, experiencing himself as stronger and less frightened. He comfortably joined his peers, asserting that he was really a teenager after all. In *Adaptation to Life*, George Vaillant (1977) describes growth as adaptive shifts in defenses—for example, evolving from acting out and projection to reaction formation and intellectualization, to sublimation and humor—to reflect increasing maturity. He likened this process to a hermit crab shedding an old shell and finding a more suitable one. Zev would fully agree with this conclusion.

TATTOOS AND PIERCINGS

> Those two bastards got us nice and early and made us into freaks with freakish standards, that's all. We're the Tattooed Lady, and we're never going to have a moment's peace, the rest of our lives, 'till everybody else is tattooed too. J. D. Salinger, *Franny and Zooey*.

Tattoos have rarely been seen under a gentle medical light or studied from a kind psychological perspective. The psychiatric and psychoanalytic literature have been particularly harsh on them, typically associating tattoos with severe disturbance because of their correlation with assaultiveness and sociopathy (Newman, 1982), "deviant behavior, self-destructive tendencies and satanic activities" (Farrow, 1991), and the more radical "bizarre sexual practices" (Caplan, 1996), such as "sadomasochism, fetishism, and bondage" (Buhrich, 1983). The medical and dermatologic literature has not been any more sympathetic, usually focusing on their infective potential, on techniques for their removal, or on the lasting regrets reported by many of their recipients (Hall-Smith, 1991). These views stand in sharp contrast to anthropologic and sociologic perspectives (as well summarized in Brain, 1979), which have typically been more developmentally based; more sensitive to the role of tattoos and other body decorations in the individual's life and to the function they serve in the individual's community at large.

The demonization of tattoos not only results from cultural and professional tradition; it also serves defensive purposes, distancing viewer from subject and offering means of dealing with the disturbing reactions they arouse. Tattoos evoke powerful feelings in the observer. Many of us stare dumbfounded and tantalized, with a mixture of awe, repulsion, interest, and visual attraction. It is difficult to disregard them or to become oblivious to their presence. No longer confined to seamen or prisoners, tattoos have beome a ubiquitous part of the everyday landscape. They have entered the mainstream of fashion and have become increasingly common among American youth, in some settings as common as earrings, make-up, or baggy jeans. A therapist who demonstrates not only tolerance but actual interest in an adolescent's tattoos or wish to be tattooed reveals a willingness to get to know teens and delve beneath the surface. It is a way of making contact, on their terms and in their language, as well as quite literally on their turf: on the territory of their skins.

What have come to be known as the bodily arts—tattoos, piercings, scarification, and branding—can be construed as non-verbal communication. They reveal more than meets the eye and serve as windows to experiential truth that is more than "skin deep." By their very natures, such arts may be described as playful: an elaborate exercise in the creative transformation and embellishment of the body and the self. Like play and music, the skin and its decorations can be seen as a transitional area where inner and outer realities converge.

Just as tattoos can demarcate inner from outer experience so as to establish boundaries between the two, they also unambiguously demarcate the bearer from others (Grumet, 1983). In using radical and extreme attire, adolescents set the limits of their persona, not only differentiating themselves from their families and the mainstream but also erecting boundaries around a nascent and diffuse sense of self. The prevalence of tattoos among adolescents points to the normative developmental crises in identity consolidation, for which tattoos may offer a concrete and readily available solution. Furthermore, feeling vulnerable to a rapidly evolving body over which they have no say, adolescents may find that self-made and openly visible decorations restore a sense of normalcy and control, turning a passive experience into an active entity. By indelibly marking their bodies, they can lay claim to their growing and increasingly unfamiliar physiques or strive to reclaim their bearings in an environment experienced as alien, uncomfortable, or suffocating. In either case, the final outcome can be a resolution to unwelcome impositions: internal and hormonal in one case, familial or societal in the other. In the words of a sixteen-year-old facially pierced girl who could have been referring to her body as easily as to her family: "If I don't fit in, it is because *I* say so." This statement embodies one meaning of many teenage styles and enthusiasms that offends adults: conscious and unconscious awkwardness and insecurities are masked by purposeful flouting of adult or mainstream standards.

> Abby, a sixteen-year-old, had what at first appeared to be the Roman numeral "XX" tattooed on her arms and chest. The tattoo actually represented the female sex chromosome pair, not a number or random letters. "I have a say on my sex and my gender," she explained; "even if my chromosomes determine this is the way it is, they do so under my say." Through her tattoos, she transformed the passive sense of being a female at the mercy of her chromosomes into an active identity through which her feminine self emerged only through her discretion.

Tattoos and other self-made designs are commonly seen not only among gang members and in juvenile correctional facilities, but also in regular and boarding school settings (Thomson, 1983). At times fabricated with materials as rudimentary as paper clips, eraser heads, or even sheets of plain paper, such markings can spread rapidly in an epidemic fashion, outwitting and puzzling supervising staff. In these settings, adolescents may use the designs to assert a sense of bonding, affiliation, and allegiance to a group. They can attest to shared experiences, to adolescence itself, lived and survived together. They may bear witness to life's vicissitudes: adolescent excitement and exhilaration interspersed with growing pains, shared misfortune, or even incarceration, actual or imagined.

Imagery along religious, skeletal, or morbid lines, the likenesses of fierce animals or imagined creatures, and the simple inscription of names historically comprise the favored themes of many tattoos. These marks not only signify ideograms for dearly held persons or concepts; they also serve dually as magnets and repellents, incorporators and exorcisers. Images and abstract symbols gain substance on becoming a permanent part of an individual's skin. They may originate as testimony to an ongoing relationship and afterwards become the only evidence that the relationship ever existed, literally becoming the relationship itself.

> Bob, a thirteen-year-old, proudly showed A.M. his tattooed deltoid. The tattoo depicted a roll of the dice marking the month and day of his birth. He then revealed his unmarked back and drew the "great piece" he envisioned for it: a menacing figure displaying a hand of play-

ing cards: two aces, two eights, and two sets of dates. His father had belonged to "Dead Man's Hand," a motorcycle gang named after the set of cards (aces and eights) held by the legendary Wild Bill Hickock in the 1890s when he was shot dead over a poker table in Deadwood, South Dakota. The boy had only the vaguest memory and sketchiest information on his father but knew he had died in a motorcycle accident: the fifth card marked the dates of his birth and death.

Sailors and adventurers were the first to import tattoos from the Far East and make them popular in Western culture. For a long time, tattoos were the mark of the nomad: yet the popularity of the anchor motif may have had less to do with guild membership than with an intense longing for rootedness and stability. The resurgence of tattooing in our increasingly mobile, almost virtual society hardly seems a coincidence, for tattoos are loud statements of existential permanence: unchanging bearings on a fleeting body. Like photographs, tattoos serve as testimonial keepsakes which endure despite the passage of time. A sense of permanence and constancy may arise from permanent marks that can be carried on the body no matter what physical, temporal, or geographical vicissitudes may occur. Tattoos remain the same when all else changes.

> A seventeen-year-old, self-described as a "professional drifter," Cody reported having started scattered self-made tattoos before he turned ten. At age 15, after running away for the first time, he started to have tattoos applied professionally. He especially cherished a compass of winds tattooed on his chest and the abstract representations of the planet Saturn scattered along his arms. These images seemed to orient him within earthly and cosmic dimensions. In his words, they were the "coordinates" he carried with him on his unpredictable wanderings.

> A proud father at seventeen, Don had the smiling face of his three-month-old daughter tattooed on his chest. Displaying the image proudly, he explained that he would "always know where she is, no matter what happens," when years hence he saw her semblance etched on himself.

Their very immutability on the evanescent canvas of flesh renders tattoos mesmerizing conduits to a lasting sense of permanence. Irreversibility sets these bodily arts apart from other modifications such as attire, cosmetics, or hairstyle. Irreversibility, however, is a relative concept. Most piercings can be removed without a trace, and even tattoos can be modified, painted, or surgically removed. This potential "undoability" of piercings and tattoos may explain why the more radical practices of branding and scarification have become popular in recent years. A gradation of body alterations can be hypothesized, with bell-bottom pants at one end of the spectrum and whole-body branding and scarfication at the other. The greater the need to establish permanent and immutable referents, the more loudly an identity, boundary, or commitment needs to be expressed, the more likely it is that extreme body alterations will be employed.

Adolescents' bodily decorations, no matter how radical and dramatic in their presentation, can be perceived in terms of figuration rather than disfigurement (Brain, 1979). These demarcations become adjuncts that sculpt and define the self by means of external manipulations. They can be understood as self-constructive acts rather than mutilatory or destructive ones, transforming the natural body into a personalized and therefore self-made and self-owned body. Therapists' awareness of these issues will allow them to become sensitized through an adolescent's skin to another level of internal reality.

CONCLUSION

This article attempts to provide an overview as to how certain facets of popular culture intersect with adolescents' developmental needs. Rather than dismissing these elements as "superficial," practitioners should be sensitive to this material when it arises in therapy, as a means of exploring identity issues in displacement. Encouraging the teenager to talk about what is important to him or her about music or clothes can strengthen alliance formation and increase the patient's comfort within the therapeutic space. The capacity of the therapist to communicate to parents about music, style, and their relation to transitional and developmental phenomena can play a critical role in deflecting their anxiety about what they perceive as aberrant and frightening behavior. Although the songs and styles change with time, teenagers will continue to stake out territory they define as their own, as separate, and to adapt the available cultural material to satisfy and express their internal developmental needs and longings. Recognizing the influence of popular culture on the adolescent is one way in which therapists can attempt to explore and understand the wonders and paradoxes of this often difficult population.

BIBLIOGRAPHY

AMERICA ON LINE (1994–98). *Nirvana Message Board.*
AVERY, R. (1979). Adolescents' Use of Mass Media. *American Behavioral Scientist,* 23: 53–70.

BECK. (1994). "Loser." *Beck: Mellow Gold:* Geffen Records.

BETTELHEIM, BRUNO. (1976). *The Uses of Enchantment.* New York: Knopf.

BLOS, PETER. (1962). *On Adolescence: A Psychoanalytic Interpretation.* New York: The Free Press.

BRAIN, R. (1979). *The Decorated Body.* New York: Harper & Row.

BUHRICH, N. (1983). The Association of Erotic Piercing with Homosexuality, Sadomasochism, Bondage, Fetishism and Tattoos. *Archives of Sexual Behavior* 12 (2): 167–171.

CAPLAN, R., KOMAROMI, J., AND RHODES, M. (1996). Obsessive-Compulsive Disorder, Tattooing and Bizarre Sexual Practices. *Br J Psychiatry* 168: 379–380.

ERIKSON, ERIK. (1950). *Childhood and Society.* New York: W. W. Norton.

FARROW, J. A., SCHWARTZ, R. H., AND VANDERLEEUW, J. (1991). Tattooing Behavior in Adolescence. *Am J Dis Child* 145: 184–187.

FEDER, STUART, ET AL. (1993). *Psychoanalytic Explorations in Music.* Madison, Conn.: International Universities Press.

GOLDBERG, R. (1997). Teens Commit Cobain Copycat Suicide. *Music News of the World:* 3.

GRUMET, G. W. (1983). Psychodynamic Implications of Tattoos. *Am J Orthopsychiatry* 53 (3): 482–492.

HALL-SMITH, P., AND BENNETT, J. (1991). Tattoos: A Lasting Regret. *Br Med J* 303: 397.

HAVENS, LESTON. (1986). *Making Contact: Uses of Language in Psychotherapy.* Cambridge, Mass.: Harvard University Press.

JAGGER, M., AND RICHARDS, K. (1964). "Satisfaction." *The Rolling Stones.* Decca Records.

KLEINMAN, ARTHUR. (1988). *The Illness Narratives.* New York: Basic Books.

METALLICA. (1991). "The Unforgiven." *Metallica: Metallica.* Elektra Records.

NEWMAN, G. (1982). The Implications of Tattooing in Prisoners. *J Clin Psychiatry* 43: 231–234.

RESTON, V. A. (1984). The Mood of American Youth. *National Association of Secondary School Principals.*

REZNOR, TRENT. (1994). "Hurt." *Nine Inch Nails: The Downward Spiral.* Nothing/Interscope Records.

ROLLING STONE. (1994). "Correspondence Column." *Rolling Stone Magazine* 683: 11.

SALINGER, J. D. (1961). *Franny and Zooey.* New York: Mass Market Paperbacks.

THOMSON, W., AND MCDONALD, J. C. H. (1983). Self-Tattooing by Schoolchildren. *Lancet* 26 (2): 1234–1244.

TOWNSHEND, PETER. (1966). "My Generation." *The Who: My Generation.* Fabulous Music LTD/BMI.

VAILLANT, GEORGE. (1977). *Adaptation to Life.* Boston: Little, Brown.

WINNICOTT, D. W. (1958). *Through Paediatrics to Psycho-Analysis: Collected Papers.* New York: Basic Books.

—— (1971). *Playing and Reality.* London: Routledge, Kegan Paul.

Use of Insight in Child Analysis

ANITA G. SCHMUKLER

The role of insight in working with a preadolescent girl, who was en-
gaged in a seven-year analysis, is examined from the perspective of ther-
apeutic action. The patient's use of insight, within the context of a trans-
ference neurosis, contributed substantively to changes in the depth of
object relations, modulation of affect, return of development to its an-
ticipated pathways, marked reduction of obsessive-compulsive sympto-
matology, and profound flowering of intellectual development.

THE CENTRAL ROLE OF INSIGHT IN CHILD DEVELOPMENT AND PSYCHO-
analytic treatment was explored during the course of the 1978 Symposium,[1] a meeting at which Anna Freud, during a summary statement,
raised the salient question: "Has psychoanalysis moved away from the
original conviction that it is knowledge of the unknown inner life that
cures?" Further, Miss Freud declared, "Without wishing to devalue the
importance of transference, I think we have to keep in mind that it is
the insight produced by the transference that is the central idea: insight for the analyst and insight for the patient." With respect to child
treatment, Anna Freud spoke of analysis as offering the possibility for
"increase in insight that is not generally achieved in normal develop-

Training and supervising analyst at the Institute of the Philadelphia Association for
psychoanalysis; clinical assistant professor of psychiatry at the University of Pennsylvania Medical Center and practitioner of child and adult analysis.

This paper is an expanded version of a presentation at the Twentieth Annual Colloquium sponsored by The Anna Freud Centre on November 6, 1998, at the Royal College of Physicians, London.

1. A Colloquium has been sponsored by the Anna Freud Centre, in London, each
year since 1978. (This paper was presented at the 20th Annual Colloquium.) The first
few meetings were referred to as "Symposia."

The Psychoanalytic Study of the Child 54, ed. Albert J. Solnit, Peter B. Neubauer, Samuel
Abrams, and A. Scott Dowling (Yale University Press, copyright © 1999 by Albert J.
Solnit, Peter B. Neubauer, Samuel Abrams, and A. Scott Dowling).

mental processes." She referred to the fact that some older children, following psychoanalytic treatment, might potentially feel more isolated, experiencing their peers as less insightful than they.

At the first Symposium, Hansi Kennedy presented a pivotal paper in which she traced the developmental line of insight. With respect to adolescents, she took the position that they have the potential for "gaining objective insight into unconscious motivation and conflict resolution." Lampl-de-Groot recalled that Sigmund Freud viewed insight as a talent or gift. The examination of that which is constitutional does not seem to have become fully integrated into current thinking about children in analysis (with the notable exception of the seminal work of Mayes and Cohen, 1995), yet I think it is worthy of further study. If insight indeed represents a "gift," one must address the question of what provides opportunities for it to flourish. Is its emergence phase-specific—that is, more accessible at particular phases of development and less accessible if there is a lack of the requisite liberty and encouragement to acknowledge inner states and to travel within the mind between past and present, preconscious and conscious? What is the fate of this gift during the massive repression of infantile amnesia? How are matrices established so that the capacity for insight may be integrated into emerging structures as development proceeds? Does the development of insight parallel the emergence of metaphor, which demonstrates a distinct forward movement during the phallic-oedipal phase and then recedes during latency?

As a working definition, I'll quote from Peter Neubauer's paper at that Symposium: "Insight during psychoanalysis comprises the expansion of the ego by self-observation, memory recovery, cognitive participation, and reconstruction in the context of affective reliving." At the first Symposium, Anne-Marie Sandler also underscored the essential affective component for any insight that moves treatment forward. From my point of view, imagination is another crucial component of mutative insight. Of course the responsible use of insight requires particular strengths: the capacity for self-observation, the ability to tolerate unpleasant affects, regression that is limited to the analytic situation, superego function (or its precursors in children under five), the capacity for synthesis, and a degree of creativity and playfulness that enables the individual to entertain new ways of thinking and experiencing.

CASE PRESENTATION

Dee was a lively eleven-year-old girl who presented with an acute onset of severe compulsive symptoms, abiding hysterical traits, and a suggestion of possible learning disability on psychological testing. For two months she had been telling her parents of persistent and distressing obsessional and compulsive symptoms. She felt the urge to rewrite her school assignments at least five times, a major interference in completing school assignments. She also exerted considerable energy each evening in rearranging the clothing in her closets and drawers, an activity that she imagined would "protect" her and her family from intruders.

Dee's compulsive symptoms, present but relatively unobtrusive from about age seven, had intensified dramatically within weeks following the death of her favorite aunt, who had died suddenly at age thirty-five following a cerebral hemorrhage. Dee had responded to her aunt's death with denial, quickly followed by compulsive symptomatology.

A few weeks after Aunt Kathy's death, Dee suffered a second blow. A girl who took much pride in her intelligence, Dee was rejected from the prestigious private school that her mother, Aunt Kathy, and two oldest siblings had attended. Her performance in the verbal-aptitude admission test had been dramatically low.

Dee was the fourth of five children. The two oldest were away at college. Ted was twenty months older than Dee and Ruth, two years younger. Dee's mother, a secretary, remained at home until Dee was eight. A live-in, Portuguese-speaking housekeeper, who had entered the household before Ted's birth, assumed substantial responsibility for the care of the three youngest children. She remained Dee's (ambivalently) trusted companion even at the time that treatment began.

Dee was toilet-trained by her housekeeper at age two and, with the exception of several week-long episodes of constipation, both before and after her sister's birth, she reportedly demonstrated no regressive symptoms at that time. Dee's constipation was treated vigorously by her housekeeper, who administered a kind of triple therapy—enemas, suppositories, and laxatives. Dee's persistent thoughts and feelings (reconstructed during the analysis) once her sister was born were notable: she felt "not really in charge of anything any more." At two-years, nine-months she had told her parents that "sometimes the only thing [she] feel[s] the boss of in this family are [her] poopies." Self-observation was in progress.

Dee attended nursery school from age three, separated easily, was perceived as very quiet and obedient, and had close girlfriends by the conclusion of the school year. When Dee was six, her almost eight-year-old brother was a soccer star and her youngest sibling, Ruth, then four, was an unusually gifted musician, attracting considerable attention from the family and the community. Dee became increasingly passive and angry. It appeared to her that her efforts to engage her father's interest were thwarted by his interest in her siblings and his deep involvement with his professional obligations as a senior partner in a law practice. When Dee confessed to her first-grade teacher that she sometimes preferred her housekeeper's company to her mother's, the teacher reprimanded her and delivered a "loyalty lecture." Dee recalled that her earliest response was fury, which, suppressed by intense shame and guilt, was supplanted by compliance. As we spoke, Dee recalled that eventually she yearned for total control over her feelings and was distressed that she didn't feel able to "just shut 'em off, like a faucet."

When Dee was seven, her housekeeper took an extended leave to return to her home in Brazil. Dee's parents found a "short-term replacement," and, while they acknowledged the likelihood of the housekeeper's return, they tried to suppress conversation about her, since at that point her return was uncertain and they wanted Dee to avoid suffering. The parents had heard that children should not be given promises about the distant future, since they lack an adequate conception of time. The housekeeper returned after one year, but during her absence, Dee first experienced compulsive symptoms and became a "picky eater." She repeatedly returned to affectively charged memories of the housekeeper's departure, to which her initial articulated response was "I can't believe she did this to me." We also returned to the experience when, prior to the second summer break, Dee felt urgently that she needed to know where I would be. While able to tolerate the lack of gratification of actually knowing my destination, she expressed most cogently her wish to "see it on a map."

Psychological testing performed immediately prior to the treatment showed significant disparity between Dee's verbal abilities and her visual-motor skills. The psychologist's impressions included "compulsive defense mechanisms"; although acknowledging that the evidence was limited, he felt that Dee's scores "might be suggestive of a learning disability specifically in the visual perceptual area." Impressed by a very strong emotional component to Dee's difficulties, he recommended psychotherapy and tutoring.

Dee appeared very sad when we met, and she described her problem of "fixing and checking things." Dropping a book, for example, might bring harm to some member of her immediate family. She spoke of her oversolicitous posture with her unappreciative peers and siblings. As she continued to describe her feelings and experiences, anger replaced sadness, particularly when she spoke of her envy of her siblings who were living at home and her anger at the siblings who had "abandoned" her to live away at college. She longed to discover a way in which she might surpass her siblings and win her father's admiration.

Dee reported a dream from prior to our meeting in which a "mean" woman confined prisoners in a room that was about to collapse. Mother was aware of the danger and, as Father was about to step into the room, asked someone to trade places with him, not because she wanted to *hurt* anyone, but to try to save Father.

Dee had awakened terrified. She referred to a recent house fire in her neighborhood in which several members of a family lost their lives and arson was suspected. The event, occurring in a affluent suburb, was described by investigators as "the work of a hate group," and Dee's perception was that the violence was a natural response to the existence of "different belief systems" in the world. Dee tried her best to suppress her impulse to "like one person more than another," and she experienced similar pressure within her own family, in which she tried to love everyone exactly equally, a formidable task.

My recommendation for analysis was based on an interference with development that appeared to be related to Dee's unresolved oedipal conflicts, which were encumbered by both developmental issues and a possible neurophysiological component. Considering the interplay of conflict, development, maturation, object relations, and possible neurophysiological issues, I felt that analysis was likely to provide Dee with the widest opportunity to resolve her problems.

Dee began by complaining about "unfairness" in her family, among her peers, and in the world in general. For extended periods, most notably during the first year, we worked almost entirely on displacement, trying to understand the presumed motives of "mean girlfriends," "cruel teachers," and "heartless" parents and siblings. In this context, we delineated feelings, conflicts, and defenses and began to explore the world of associating thoughts to feelings and memories. Dee worried that her friends in her very bright peer group would not respect her when her academic performance failed to meet their standards. Academics were important to her father, and Dee spoke of her longing for her father's respect. With some difficulty, she expressed feelings of marked denigration toward her mother and, tentatively at first, she expressed curiosity about me. I commented on her difficulty tolerating conflictual feelings. Twirling her curly blonde hair and smiling, she asserted, "Knowledge is power." Then I interpreted her wish to discover facts about me as one way to feel more powerful. In associating to power over the other, she reported an impulse that had begun several months before treatment began: to kiss her mother "a certain number of times, like seven," an action that she knew her mother found particularly distressing. While Dee "hated violence," even becoming distressed if her father did not slow his car for a bird that "might land in the middle of the road," she adopted a form of "bothering people, like Mom," by her "habits," which she experienced as unavoidable.

When Dee's parents attempted to share household tasks, she became angry that her father sometimes engaged in "motherly" tasks like "cooking." Dee had clear notions of what was permissible in terms of gender-associated activities. Toward the close of the first year of our work, Dee referred to the breast development of her classmates and wondered aloud, "Which are better? Big breasts that make the woman seem powerful or small ones, like models, with another kind of power?" Her recognition of concerns over her own breast development led to her expression of an acute sense of shame, particularly with respect to her worries that "one breast seems to grow faster" and her fantasy that asymmetry was a sign of weakness and inferiority.

When I commented on Dee's conflicted feelings about being a girl, she asserted that "girls who are feminine are interested in boys and makeup. They are dumb, whiny, and immature. Girls are smart until they are about twelve and then they become inferior." She wanted to become an adult with "total control."

As Dee railed against her emerging femininity, she linked this to her widely variable academic performance, insisting that men and boys "have it" and that women must try harder to achieve academically. She began to show an interest in counting my books and assessing their contents, and concluded that one of her aunts and I had academic interests because we were "part-male."

A repetitive behavior appeared in which Dee presented her mother with average or below-average exam scores at a crucial moment, just as her mother was hurriedly leaving the house for an "important appointment at the beauty salon or day-spa." When I pointed out how disappointed Dee became when her school failures did not bring anticipated help from mother, she responded with tears, followed by efforts to engage my attention. She would empty her book bag on the floor at the start of a session, scattering dozens of papers, and she would proclaim that I would "organize" her if I really cared. At this point, "caring," "controlling," and "protecting" were intertwined inextricably.

I underscored Dee's longing to feel loved by forcing people to "organize" her and, in a way, control her. She expressed the fantasy that she could never do well on her own. Dee was puzzled about the fact that she had always been friendly with only the brightest girls, felt "just as smart" as they were, but had difficulty "showing it" in school. "It's like a hidden smartness," she lamented, "and most of the time even I can't find it." In this context, there were indirect references to penis envy, but they were not yet available for interpretation.

As Dee's conflicts were engaged within the transference, her parents reported that she was "less volatile" and that she was performing school assignments in a more independent and attentive manner than previously. She appeared to get along with her siblings more easily and was beginning to engage in relationships with girlfriends who appeared "more reliable" than her previous friends. Her parents also observed a marked decrease in compulsive symptomatology. At this juncture, Dee's parents complied with her request to discontinue the tutoring. This followed several episodes in which she was very anxious in an exam and unable to recall information that she "knew." Identifying with our work, she asked herself during the exam, "Now, why would I forget that now?" When correct answers emerged "from nowhere," Dee decided that "our thinking together" was a preferred method for dealing with school performance.

During the winter break of our second year, Dee accompanied her father on a week-long business trip to Tokyo. On the evening of her return, she asked her mother to kiss her goodnight. Then Dee began to complete an overdue school assignment on the Revolutionary War. She awakened, terrified, from a dream in which many innocent people were being hanged. A man, her father's age, was seated, and a woman, who seemed extraordinarily friendly to Dee, gratified his final wish by bringing him a glass of mineral water.

In her associations, Dee spoke of the pleasure of kissing her mother the previous evening. She loved to touch Mom's soft, fresh-smelling hair. At once she demanded to know what hair conditioner I used. I observed that she wanted to know all about me and find out what we share, which sometimes might feel safer to express than some of her further thoughts. She replied: "We're different. I hope you are not offended by this, but sometimes I think I am really pretty. Prettier than my mom, too."

In the dream, she recalled later, she had been a princess, yet she wasn't certain if she'd be killed. A series of associations led to conflicted wishes for closeness with various girlfriends, her oldest sister, then a senior at college, Mother, and me. This appeared to represent both longing for the preoedipal mother, reasserting itself in early adolescence, and a defense against oedipal wishes and attendant retaliation.

Dee's initial response to her menarche at age twelve and a half was pride, followed by a litany of complaints. She dealt with feelings, frequently surprising to her, of profound similarities between vagina and anus. It was in this context that I recalled reading Freud's "hurried" note in the *New Introductory Lectures* that interest in the vagina is essentially of anal-erotic origin. In a footnote (added 1920) to the *Three Essays,* Freud quoted Salome's 1916 paper in which she discusses the history of the prohibition of anal pleasures. Freud added: "From the time of prohibition [of anal pleasures] what is 'anal' remains the symbol of everything that is to be repudiated and excluded from life." He sought the origins of obsessional neurosis in the anal phase, and his focus was on male patients. What of the earliest links, historically, between the anal and the genital in the female? We can begin by examining the Book of Leviticus, in which God asks Moses to instruct the people that "if a woman conceives and bears a male child, then she shall be unclean seven days . . . but if she bears a female child, then she shall be unclean two weeks." What are the implications of these deeply rooted notions for female development, particularly for girls whose perceptions of their genitals is encumbered by anal conflicts and defenses? While current literature examines female genital anxieties, the interest in anal influences remains on the back burner, so to speak.

Dee's anality had a profound effect on her obsessional illness and on her adolescence, particularly on her defenses, modes of thinking, and affective relatedness. When she soiled furniture in my office by accidentally spilling paint that she had brought along from her after-school art class, she attempted to use denial and explained her behavior as accidental; yet she was capable of using my interpretations to gain insight that permitted her to acknowledge her envy and hatred of me, wishes for revenge, and humiliation for feeling "less than perfect." In this context, she shared her disappointment at my "imperfection" and therefore my presumed inability to help her. Perfection, in her estimation, was the characteristic of the men in her family. This material gave us an opportunity to begin to understand her envy of men.

My interpretation of Dee's ambivalence toward her mother led to her anger over her mother's preoccupation with her appearance and her frequent appointments at the beauty salon. Dee's mother spent hours organizing closets at home, and Dee responded by presenting herself as particularly "disorganized." She took refuge in her own disorganization to enlist Mother's help, punish her for unavailability, deny responsibility for her own actions, assert her "femininity," and force her parents to "organize" her, while hoping that I would do the same. Disappointed by my insistence on "just talking," Dee associated to potential harm that might befall me. I pointed out that her worry about my having an accident while on vacation appeared to be linked, in her associations, to similar thoughts about her mother, particularly when she was angry with Mother. Dee was silent, yet moments later she burst into tears and said that at the time she first came to treatment, she wished, fleetingly, that her mother instead of her aunt had died of a cerebral hemorrhage. She had entirely forgotten that thought!

As Dee became increasingly tolerant of her destructive fantasies and freer in expressing them directly in our work, there was a further diminution of her compulsive symptoms. She appeared able to use insight not only for the purpose of affecting current pressures but to re-examine earlier perceptions and experiences in the light of newly acquired understanding.

Following this piece of analytic work, Dee's grades rose in an unprecedented manner. By then, most of her assignments were completed in a timely fashion, and her earlier forgetting of assignments was replaced by a conscientiousness of which she felt proud. In the previous months, Dee had examined a multitude of affectively charged fantasies related to impaired mental capacity, experiences of "the intact" and "the injured," her feelings about her own injury and its sequelae in relation to her aunt's illness, and her notions of the origin of her compulsive symptoms. Dee was a keen observer, and one direction of her aggression was that of intellectual curiosity. Earlier, her head (thoughts) had been one locus of her dangerous impulses. While hatred and rage were so prominent and her conflicts so intense, an adaptive use of sublimation had been difficult for her to achieve. As the treatment proceded, Dee became much freer in her ability to use her intellectual energy.

During the third year of our work, Dee, at 14, exhibited further movement toward socialization. New girlfriends appeared, and Dee described "crushes" on a series of boys. In tandem with this, we observed an episodic recrudescence of anal conflicts. Her parents were distraught about the mess in her bedroom, and Dee thought that she sometimes unwittingly "messed up" her relationships with girlfriends, by whom she frequently felt "overlooked." Some of this may have been developmentally expectable, yet the intensity of Dee's struggles with girlfriends became a subject for analytic scrutiny. My interpretations permitted Dee to view her provocations of her girlfriends, and me, as part of her efforts to maintain connection, as, earlier in her life, messing was part of an effort to get attention (love) from her mother and her housekeeper, whose attention to "spotlessness" was, even then, a source of frequent struggle.

One day I opened the waiting-room door and saw Dee busily engaged in doing homework. I told her that we could begin as soon as she was ready. Dee heard this as "not caring," for which she expressed intense anger and disappointment, similar to her experiences with her mother. This permitted us to examine in greater detail her comparing my perceived behavior with that of her mother, as well as her expectation and wish that we behave and respond "the same." She began to reassess her mother's responses, acknowledged her mother's love for her, and began to speculate on her importance to me, expressing her disappointment that our relationship was not "real enough."

At 15, Dee returned from a summer vacation reporting that she had "missed [me] so much." She was delighted that she had gotten along well with her family. She was also aware of a marked diminution of her compulsive symptoms and asserted that, for the first time since age seven, she felt free to eat a wide variety of foods. She announced proudly that she finally had a boyfriend. Her adolescent development was marked by increasingly successful efforts at independence, and a new sense of relatedness appeared as anal defenses and conflicts over femininity were analyzed.

This material coincided with her work on keeping and revealing secrets, partly a developmental issue of adolescence, intensified in Dee's case because of family issues. While on the trip she overheard a family secret, which she had suspected, about the violent death of two uncles prior to her birth. Her associations led us to examine a major defense in the analysis, her avoidance of seeing and knowing. Earlier she had adopted the stance taken by her parents, that "knowing" would impose too great a burden on this already anxious girl. Dee referred to her (then) diminishing compulsive symptoms and her learning problem as her "hidden secrets," linked associatively with being "dirty" and "out of control." For the first time, Dee acknowledged that this led to her feeling "special." Her problem of compulsive actions was a fact that her parents had tried to conceal, even from close relatives, and she had categorized that secret along with others, including her work with me, as issues that involved excitement and intrigue. Earlier, when her siblings were commended for their talents, Dee had imagined that her only notable behavior was, and would be, that of pathological content. Exploring this, Dee said that once she had imagined that her parents' keeping her problems secret indicated a "caring" for which she had been willing to pay dearly in the past. "But now I am becoming my own person, and I can own my strengths and even my weaknesses, which, by the way, aren't nearly as bad as I used to imagine," she observed. Dee's increased synthetic function appeared to be a pivotal factor in her expanding capacity for insight. Insight and synthetic ability appeared to be mutually dependent, enhancing development.

During the fifth year of treatment, Dee tried to engage her younger sister in playing music together informally; she came to a session complaining of a severe headache and spoke of her fury with her sister, whose occasional boasting over the attention gained by her performances Dee considered "cruel." On the previous day, Dee had acknowledged her own "gloating" over a less fortunate classmate. I underscored Dee's externalization, and this intervention appeared to permit Dee the freedom to begin to examine some of her sadistic impulses in detail. When I failed to give opinions or to tell her of my vacation plans, Dee sometimes became furious, entertaining fantasies of destroying my office or harming me physically. As she reflected on these feelings and fantasies, for which her tolerance had expanded significantly, she related them to anxiety over early losses, in response to which she had felt overwhelmed, unable to master the experience.

Following an analysis of Dee's "certainty" that she would be more attractive than I was to my "husband or boyfriend," her relations with her father, previously burdened by frequent heated discussions, improved substantially. She enjoyed his appreciation of her and their interests in common, some of which she had suppressed previously.

Dee enjoyed a succession of boyfriends. While she was distressed over "breaking up," she was always optimistic about her next encounter. When she met James, whom she "adored," she was uncharacteristically "shy." James was the first boy who wasn't "just a jock" but had "a real brain too." Dee struggled with her impulses to compete with him and "be the best" and feelings that she "just wanted to be a good friend and a girlfriend." She said thoughtfully, "I used to think I could get James's attention if something terrible happened like if my mom died suddenly, just like my aunt did, but I don't want to be a person who always looks for pity. I guess now I just want him to like me for me. And now I know that when I used to imagine Mom sick or dead so much, it was partly because I was so mad at her and wished it. Whew! Long ago I used to be afraid to even say that," she observed with satisfaction.

When the death of Dee's grandfather was linked to a medical error, Dee struggled with her notion that "you can never trust a doctor." I linked this material to Dee's worries about trusting me. Dee spoke of friends whose physician parents discussed patients at dinner, and she questioned my loyalty to her. Sometimes she had felt closer to me than to anyone else. Feeling so trusting was still a little scary, but mainly she was glad of it. Dee felt that the experience of analysis had helped her to trust herself, a state that she found most helpful in working with earlier concerns about being alert, aware, and able to learn. "I always used to avoid guessing answers because I was so sure I would be wrong," she said; "my brain didn't seem trustworthy, controllable. You know what? Now I don't even think of it as 'my brain' but just as 'me.'"

Following this piece of analytic work, Dee announced that she would most certainly outdo me professionally. She would become an architect whose buildings would be identified by her name, while my work is accomplished in relative anonymity. "Your favorite aunt doesn't even know that you have an analyst, let alone her name," she observed.

At 16, Dee reported a dream involving intimate contact with her boyfriend, with whom she had spent the previous evening. Shortly after this episode, she had had an intense argument with her mother, whom Dee described as disrespectful to a neighbor. I interpreted Dee's finding a reason to fight with her mother immediately following a pleasurable episode with her boyfriend as a response to her guilt over intimacy and sexual excitement. Dee's many affectively laden associations led to the recovery of an early memory of her babysitter's severely reprimanding her for genital touching. Her next association was at about age four; she felt that she "had it all" when her parents each held one of her hands and lifted her above a puddle as they walked. "I guess that in some ways I still want to be the little girl who's lifted over puddles, you know, like feeling powerful because I'm connected to someone who seems powerful, but I also want to be a regular teenager and, sooner or later, probably later, have intercourse. My Mom wouldn't agree, but I don't care." Dee's recognition that intimacy with a boyfriend coincided with distancing from her parents stirred anxiety and was linked to early separation difficulties and to notions that independence and autonomy were related to isolation.

Dee worked a good deal at differentiating her views of gender in relation to perceptions of control and mastery, with emphasis on the differentiation of vaginal and anal. Following this work, Dee approached her schoolwork with renewed vigor and was rewarded with prizes for academic excellence. At once she was beset by anxieties. She wanted "perfection." She elaborated a fantasy that when I was a high school student I had only "perfect" scores. She felt disappointed that, in view of her fantasy, she could not "beat" me. The analysis of a dream led to Dee's notion of punishment for early scoptophilic impulses, and this afforded us extended opportunities to explore her problem of "missing details" in academic efforts and to continue to work on the idealizing transference.

Dee's emerging academic success also led her into direct and conflicted competition with boys who were her peers. Her successes were punctuated by episodes of "forgetting," behaving as if she "knew nothing." Ultimately she wrestled with her conflicts so that she felt confident that she could be successful academically without relinquishing the femininity she was beginning to enjoy. A more balanced view of gender issues emerged. "I used to think men had a right to be furious and show it, but women who behaved that way were not really women. What a restrictive thought!" she said with a satisfied smile.

During the seventh year of treatment, Dee received a prize for outstanding work in a subject that required considerable visual perceptual skill. In the context of the transference, she re-examined her fears of competition in surpassing her mother and her analyst and she renewed her exploration of her identification with her father and brother Ted. As Dee reworked her idealization of parents and analyst, she was able to conclude that each had strengths that had contributed to her development. At the same time, each had weaknesses that were now tolerable rather than frightening.

Termination work involved revisiting disruptive (affective) separations early in life. Dee also re-engaged her struggle over the narcissistic injury she suffered when, in a family of many extraordinarily talented academics, she had felt unable to compete with siblings who were very close in age. Early in treatment, Dee's obsessional illness had resulted in constricted thought, difficulties with affect modulation, limited affective engagement with peers, immaturity, and excessive dependence on parents and friends, and had markedly interfered with her use of sublimation. At termination, Dee exhibited a greater synthetic capacity and a more durable superego. Her demands on herself and others had become more flexible. When Dee began to feel capable of taking care of herself and increasingly independent of parents, the requirement for "perfection" in a boyfriend subsided, and she was comfortable with the ordinary strengths of a peer. With respect to her (then) most recent boyfriend, Dee mused, "We can both be winners."

DISCUSSION

The case of a preadolescent girl with compulsive symptoms and hysterical traits served to illustrate the use of insight for deepening material, integrating past and present experiences, affects, memories, conflicts, and defenses, and facilitating synthetic function and development in general. As pathways for insight were established and re-established, primitive defenses, previously an encumbrance to her development, had yielded to greater use of sublimation and permitted her creative capacities, previously bound in conflict, to flourish. As her superego became more flexible and she exhibited greater tolerance of fantasies and impulses, obsessional and compulsive symptoms receded, object relations demonstrated striking improvement, and intellectual development flourished.

An early insight was the patient's recognition of fantasied links between knowledge and power and her fear of her own destructive capacities. Her early theory that girls experience loss of potential power as they reach puberty was associated to her notion that only then was gender determined irrevocably. Ultimately, she linked the "dumb and whiny" posture that she had attributed to pubertal girls to her view of herself as a prelatency girl with a brother whose gifts appeared to be unbounded and a toddler sister whose behavior appeared to assure parental love. Her fear of loss of power at puberty was also related to her equation of anality and female genitality. In addition, Dee confronted her terror of feeling empowered, a previously suppressed aspect of her perception of female development. Insights with respect to defenses, in the context of transference, and oedipal and preoedipal issues, elaborated both in displacement and in the transference, permitted further integration, which became part of new organizations that emerged with each successive developmental phase. In this way, developmental pathways, from which there had been earlier departure, could resume a more even progression. This patient's sustained use of insight, markedly discontinuous in our early work, enabled her to work analytically in an independent manner.

PRELATENCY CONSIDERATIONS

From my perspective, use of insight in prelatency children requires a delicate balance of cognitive (including, of course, imaginative) and affective components in examining psychic processes. As insight increases, the use of unconscious defenses against unwanted impulses decreases. Given the sometimes fragile state of emerging defenses in the very young, responsible use of insight requires attunement to stages of maturation and careful coordination of analytic and developmental goals. Acquisition of insight requires, above all, a capacity for self-observation. While prelatency children do not typically present themselves with an awareness of pathology, they appear capable of astute self-observations, some of which may lead to insight, at least in its broadest definition. So our task may be to ascertain under what circumstances self-observations in the very young flourish and under what circumstances they lead to insight, both in treatment and in normal development. While it is true that the insights of the very young are not enduring in most cases, their presence suggests the question of whether our emphasis ought to be on the persistence of particular insights or, rather, on finding creative ways to extend the pathways (grids, perhaps) that are required to establish such connections. Such networks may remain in place even while the repression following the oedipal phase appears to eradicate the specific insights achieved earlier.

With respect to self-observations, a two-year, nine-month-old girl, involved in relaxed play with her mother, asserted, "Mommy, I love you so much that I miss you even when I am with you." A three-year, four-month-old girl whose grandmother laughed over her astute observations but rarely inquired further stated, "Grandma, I don't like when people laugh because I don't understand and feel left out."

Why are we surprised when young children verbalize observations (of self and other) and insights that appear to us "beyond their years"? I think that just as there was once an inattentiveness to the sexual wishes and feelings of young children, so we adults may permit ourselves to be oblivious to the insights of which young children are capable. We may even maintain this posture by holding, at times too rigidly, to our criteria of what structural components appear to be absolute necessities for insight to be present. For example, a three-year-old boy with a newborn sister drew a face with "eyes, nose, mouth and *very angry, jealous, eyebrows.*" We may choose to let this pass, assuming that no insight is available or that the ego is too fragile to bear interpretation. Alternatively, we might intervene by acknowledging the wide range of feelings that we have toward people whom we love and then interpreting in this way: "Sometimes it feels safer to tell about some of our feelings with our eyebrows than with our words." If the child replies, "I hate when Mom stops telling me a story just because the baby cries," do we refer to this as insight? proto-insight?

When we help prelatency children to establish pathways from self-observation to insight, we find the need for developmental assistance, such as extending the pathways for externalization.[2] A four-year-old boy in analysis, whose mother had died in childbirth, lived with his father and stepmother, whom his father had married when the boy was fifteen months old. Father and stepmother were warm, devoted, and available to this child. When he asked, repetitively, for me to pretend that we were experiencing volcanos and earthquakes, and the material had been explored from a wide variety of perspectives, I asked if he wanted me to pretend to *feel* something during these natural disasters. He said, "Sure, pretend you are scared. Very scared." This material

2. I have referred to this material in *Child Analysis,* June 1999. Published by Cleveland Center for Research in Child Development, ed. Denia Barrett.

evolved for some days, the affective component became firmly rooted in the play, and then I asked, "Might I have some pretend thoughts to think while I'm pretending to be so scared?" With great enthusiasm, he told me to pretend to think that I had been lost on a beach and was unable to find my parents. During the succeeding weeks, affect and associated ideas became linked, rooted, thus expanding our operative field. Sometime later, returning to the theme of loss that took place symbolically with disasters of weather, I wondered if I might pretend to remember something from long ago that might help as I pretended to feel afraid and pretended to think my assigned thoughts. The boy said he felt very cold, shivered, wondered if we might turn up the heat, and then said with unprecedented intensity: "My Mommy who died would buy me new toys five times every day."

The essential issue is that each matter that I introduced in a gradual, gentle manner (over weeks) became incorporated into his general communications. He played with toy cars or puppets and assigned them not simply roles but on occasion feelings as well, thoughts to accompany the feelings, memories, and even occasionally a dream. I consider this a form of introduction to child analysis, equivalent to explaining the free-associative method to an adult, except that in the analysis of children the form occurs in displacement and may take weeks or months to become established firmly.

I think that one further area of productive study is the moment at which prelatency children stop sharing thoughts with their parents. For the preoedipal child, one might say that thoughts are withheld in response to fear of the child's expression of anger of the parent, and for the oedipal child, one might attribute withholding to guilt over incestuous wishes. Yet the explanation may extend further. The young child may have an insight regarding what the parent can tolerate in terms of painful affects. Additionally, he or she may have used insight in determining what can be withheld, contained, without undue distress. Clearly, the issue of insight in children presents a wide variety of areas that might reward productive study.

BIBLIOGRAPHY

BULLETIN OF THE HAMPSTEAD CLINIC, Vol. 3, Part 3, 1980.
FREUD, ANNA. (1981). "Insight," in *Psychoanalytic Study of the Child,* 38: 241–249.
——— (1979). "The Role of Insight in Psychoanalysis and Psychotherapy—Introduction," *J. Amer. Psychoan. Assoc.,* 27, Supplement: 3–7.
FREUD, SIGMUND. (1933). New Introductory Lectures. *S.E.,* 101.
——— (1905). Three Essays on Sexuality. *S.E.,* 187.

HOLY BIBLE. (1962). Rev. Standard Ed., Meridian Books. (Cleveland: World Publishing). Leviticus 12.

KENNEDY, HANSI. (1979). "The Role of Insight in Child Analysis: A Developmental Viewpoint," *J. Amer. Psychoan. Assoc.* 27. Supplement: 9–28.

MAYES, LINDA C., & COHEN, DONALD J. (1995). "Constitution." In *Psychoanalysis: The Major Concepts.* eds. Burness E. Moore and Bernard D. Fine (New Haven: Yale University Press).

NEUBAUER, PETER. (1979). "The Role of Insight in Psychoanalysis," *J. Amer. Psychoanal. Assn.* 27, Supplement: 29–40.

SHENGOLD, LEONARD. (1992). *Halo in the Sky: Observations on Anality and Defense.* (New Haven: Yale University Press).

Index

Abraham, K., 263
Abrams, S., 19–24, 87–89, 265
Acting out, 113, 292–95
Adam and Eve story, 209–10
Adaptation, 97
Adler, A., 126
Adler, G., 143
Adolescent analysis: analysts as "new"
  objects in, 88, 89; coordination of, with
  developmental process, 19–24, 87–89;
  detours in female adolescent development, 22, 47–67; idealization of analyst
  in, 58, 64–65; identification with analyst
  in, 53–56, 88; and popular culture,
  324–28; questions and issues in, 88–89;
  resistance in, 320; sexual relationships,
  51, 53–59, 63–64, 66; termination in,
  351; transference in, 51, 53–63, 65–67,
  352
Adolescents: challenges of, 87–88; clothing
  worn by, 324–25, 328–333; and menarche, 345–46; and popular culture, 319–
  37; and popular music, 320–28, 331; and
  tattoos and piercings, 330, 333–37. See
  also Adolescent analysis
Affect intolerance, 230–32
Affective distancing, 229
Aggression, 29, 37, 42, 292, 297–98, 305–9
Agoraphobia, 328–29
Alexander, F. G., 126
Almansi, R. J., 262
Amsden, Dr., 144
Anality, 44, 345–46, 352
Anal-sadistic desire, 33, 42
Analysis. See Adolescent analysis; Child
  analysis; Psychoanalysis; Transference;
  other psychoanalytic concepts
"Analyzing instrument," 106
Anger: of boy with atypical ego develop-
  ment, 28–38, 42; of boy with deviational
  development, 69, 75–77; of diabetic
  woman, 298, 305, 306–09; of fathers at
  children, 209; of female about termination, 162–63; of male toward father at
  abandonment, 206; of obsessional patients, 223, 231; of preadolescent girl

with compulsive symptoms, 342–43, 349;
  of sixteen-year-old girl, 48, 53–54, 55
Anonymity of analyst, 121–22
Anxiety: of boy with atypical ego develop-
  ment, 29–30, 32, 39–42, 44, 45; of boy
  with deviational development, 79; castra-
  tion anxiety, 42, 73, 263, 264, 267, 273,
  275, 278; integration anxiety, 292–95; of
  sixteen-year-old female, 54–59, 61–63.
  See also Fears
Anzieu, D., 196, 198
Arlow, J. A., 101–3, 108, 109, 112, 117–18,
  263n1
Artists, S. Freud on, 4–5
Asperger, H., 28
Asperger's Syndrome, 28–46
Assassination of Rabin, 205–14
Astington, J., 236
Attention cathexis, 101–2, 104n
Austin, J. L., 234
Ausubel, D. P., 173
Autonomy, 3, 3n
Avery, R., 321

Badaracco, J. E. G., 205
Balter, L., 93–126
Barbey d'Aurevilly, J., 246
Barrett, D., 353n2
Baum, J. D., 296
Beck, J., 321
Becker, E., 2
Behavioral minimalism, 121
Bene-Moses, A., 197
Berendt, J., 9
Berg, S., 11
Bergman, P., 176
Bernays, M., 6
Bernstein, A., 11
Berry, W., 8, 8n, 15
Bettelheim, B., 320
Bibring, E., 136
Bick, E., 196
Bion, W. R., 196
Bipolar disorder, 329
Birth fantasy, 43
Bisexuality, 57

Bladder control, 44
Blanton, S., 141, 143–45
Blind peer reviews, 14n
Blos, P., 321
Blum, H. P., 116, 118 ·
Bodily ego, 196
Body-dissolution fears, 42–43, 45
Body-phallus equation, 263–64
Bollas, C., 195, 196
Borderline personality disorder, 326
Boundaries of the self, 299–302
Bowel control, 44
Boyd, M., 10
Boys. *See* Males
Brain, R., 333, 337
Breastfeeding, 70, 301–2
Breasts, 82, 262, 268, 281, 282, 344
Brenner, C., 94–97, 122–23
Breuer, J., 7
Brill, Dr., 144
British School, 150
Bruecke, E., 6
Bruner, J., 235–36
Buhrich, N., 333
Burgner, M., 45
Burlingham, D. T., 176, 310
Butterworth, G. E., 236

Calvino, I., 245–46
Caplan, R., 333
Carver, R., 11–14, 13n13
Castration anxiety, 42, 73, 263, 267, 273, 275, 278
Change as constant, 94–99
Charcot, J.-M., 7
Charlemagne, 245–46
Charlesworth, W. R., 173
Chatman, S., 249
Child analysis: analysts as "new" objects in, 88, 89; boy with atypical ego development, 23–46; boy with deviational development, 22–23, 68–85; coordination of, with developmental process, 19–24, 87–89; developmental fantasies in, 182–88; identification with analyst in, 83–84, 88; insight used in, 339–54; interpretations and clarifications in, 69–70, 89; and mother's death, 353–54; obsessional manifestations in children, 219–32; questions and issues in, 88–89; termination of, 82–83; transference in, 81–82, 84–85
Chronic illness, 289–313
Chused, J., 64, 219–32
Cicchetti, D., 181

Clarifications, with boy with deviational development, 69–70
Clothing of adolescents, 324–25, 328–333
Coates, S., 85
Cobain, K., 321–22
Cochran, E., 236
Coen, S., 6
Cohen, D., 27, 39
Cohen, D. J., 178–79, 181, 340
Coleman, D. J., 233–56
Coleman, L., 254
Collaborations, creative, 1–15
Compromise formation: of boy with atypical ego development, 45; Brenner on, 95–97; centrality of, 94–99; S. Freud on, 107. *See also* Transference neurosis
Compulsive symptoms: in preadolescent girl, 340–52. *See also* Obsessional manifestations
Conflict: centrality of, 94–99; definition of, 94
Conroy, P., 9
Consciousness, 99–102, 117–18
Constant psychic change, 94–99
Correlations, 245
Couch, A. S., 130–65
Countertransference, 112, 132, 150–51, 299–300
Crawford, C., 81
Creativity: collaborations in, 1–15; and consciousness of mortality, 3n; of S. Freud, 6–8; S. Freud on, 4–5; Gardner on, 5–6, 5n; of psychoanalysts, 3–4, 6–8; as response to feelings of powerlessness, 2–3; writer-editor partnerships, 9–15, 9–10n6, 13n, 14–15n
Crow, 325
Crystal, D., 238

Dallenbach, L., 235
Daniolos, P., 319–37
Dann, O. T., 265
Darwin, C., 173
Day, M., 156
Daydreaming, 4–5, 102–3
Death: fear of, 298; of mother, 353–54; of relatives of preadolescent girl with compulsive symptoms, 341; of siblings, 70, 248
Defenses: of boy with atypical ego development, 44, 45; of boy with deviational development, 69, 73; and sixteen-year-old female, 62
Defensive processing, 201
Deictics, 242–43, 246–47, 251–52

Déjà vu experience, 263, 263n
Demorest, A., 254
Denial, of boy with obsessional manifestations, 223
Dennett, D. C., 178n4
DEPM. *See* Dramatic Enactment Performance Mode (DEPM)
Depression, 48–49, 53, 329
DeSousa, R., 237, 247
Deutsch, F., 126, 262
Deutsch, H., 141
Developmental fantasies of children and adults, 171, 182–90
Developmental object, analyst as, 55–56
Developmental process: adaptationist approach to, 178–82, 178n4; approaches to regulation of psychological development, 173–82, 176–78nn; in boy with atypical ego development, 23–46; of boy with deviational development, 22–23, 68–85; caveats on, 171–73; contemporary models of, 170–71, 173–82, 176–78nn; coordination of, with psychoanalytic process, 19–24, 87–89; definition of, 172n, 173; detours in female adolescent development, 47–67; fantasies of children and adults about, 171, 182–90; A. Freud on primary developmental disturbances, 26; gene-environment interaction models of, 178–82; metapsychological functions of developmental fantasies, 171, 187–90; overview of dynamics of, 169–73, 172n; questions and issues in, 88–89
Deviational development of boy, 22–23, 68–85
Diabetes, 289–313, 295n
Dickinson, E., 170
Discourse. *See* Narrative performance mode (NPM) of discourse
Displacement, 223
Divorce, 30–31, 35–38, 72, 75–76
Doolittle, H., 141
Dorsey, J., 145
Dowling, S., 223n1
Dramatic Enactment Performance Mode (DEPM), 234, 240–44, 246–49, 251, 252
Drawings, of boy with deviational development, 73, 75, 78, 81
"Dream screen," 262
Dreams: of boy with deviational development, 71; S. Freud on, 260–61; Gray on, 242; of man with regressive ego functioning, 266, 270, 275; of preadolescent girl with compulsive symptoms, 343, 345,

350; of sixteen-year-old female, 59–60; on successful resolution of problems, 161

Easson, W. M., 264
Edelman, G., 237, 242
Edelson, M., 172
Edgecumbe, R., 310
Editor-writer partnerships, 9–15, 9–10n, 13n, 14–15n
Ego development: bodily ego, 196; boy with atypical ego development, 23–46; boy with deviational development, 22–23, 68–85
Ego erection. *See* Regressive ego phenomena
Ego synthesis, 164
Eidelberg, L., 293
Eissler, K., 134, 156
Eliot, T. S., 13, 13n13
Emde, R., 6, 8, 196, 197, 236
Empathy, 43–44, 111
Erikson, E., 126, 254–55, 332
Erikson, J., 255
Escalona, S. K., 176
Esman, A. H., 196
Evenly suspended attention of analyst, 106–8, 111, 120–22, 126
Extra-analytic determinants of analytic data, 112–20, 125

Fairy tales, 320
Fantasies: birth fantasy, 43; of boy with atypical ego development, 29–32, 34–37, 39, 42–43; of boy with deviational development, 81–82, 83; of children with obsessional manifestations, 222, 226, 227; developmental fantasies of children and adults, 171, 182–90; "Golden Fantasy," 148; Gulliver fantasies, 263; of man with regressive ego functioning, 266; masturbatory fantasy, 262; metapsychological functions of developmental fantasies, 171, 187–90; Oedipal fantasies, 31, 42; oral-aggressive fantasies, 29, 30, 42, 303; of sixteen-year-old female, 52, 62, 63, 65; Stein on, 102. *See also* Daydreaming
Farrow, J. A., 333
Fashion choices of adolescents, 324–25, 328–333
Fathers: absence of and abandonment by, 206, 304; of adolescent with panic disorder, 328–29; anger of, at children, 209; of boy with atypical ego development, 26–27, 30–31, 33–38, 39, 41–44; of boy with deviational development, 72, 74, 81,

Fathers (continued)
82; of boy with obsessional manifestations, 222; of diabetic female, 295–96,
304, 305, 307–9; illness of, 211–12; males
and paternal object relation, 205–14; of
man with regressive ego functioning,
278–79; of preadolescent girl with compulsive symptoms, 342, 344; reaction of,
to five-year-old daughter's urination outside, 63; of sixteen-year-old female, 51–
55, 60, 62–63, 66
Fears: and body-phallus equation, 264; of
boy with atypical ego development, 29–
30, 32, 39, 42, 45; of death, 298; of girl
with obsessional manifestations, 223; in
recognizing boundaries of the self, 299–
302. *See also* Anxiety
Feder, S., 323
Feldman, G., 9
Females: clinical example of narrative performance mode (NPM) of discourse,
247–49; clinical material on detours in
female adolescent development, 47–67;
clinical vignette on "real relationship"
in psychoanalysis, 160–63; developmental fantasies of, 182–89; insight in analysis of preadolescent girl, 339–54; inte
grative processes in woman with diabetes, 289–313; masturbation by girl,
226–27; and narcissism, 201–3; obsessional manifestations in girls, 223–29;
sexual relationships of sixteen-year-old
female, 51, 53–59, 63–64, 66. *See also*
Mothers
Fenichel, O., 98, 108, 113, 121, 126, 136,
137, 154, 249
Ferenczi, S., 126, 136, 263
Fink, G., 262
Finn, M. H. P., 262
Fitzgerald, F. S., 10, 13n13
Fliess, W., 6, 7
Fluss, E., 6
Fonagy, P., 26, 296
Francis, P. L., 177n2
Fredu, S., on id, 310
Free association, 106, 107, 108, 110, 111,
126, 140
Freud, A.: on developmental process, 175,
177; on id, 310; on identification with ag-
gressor, 305; on insight, 339–40; on inte-
gration, 291; on mother's role in integra-
tion, 311–12; on neutrality of analyst,
120; on obsessional neurosis, 226; on pri-
mary developmental disturbances versus
neurotic disturbances, 26; on "real rela-

tionship" in psychoanalysis, 137, 138,
139–40; on transference, 139–40, 339
Freud, E. L., 6
Freud, S.: on "affective change," 255; on
anal pleasures, 345–46; biographical information on, 6–8; on body-phallus
equation, 263; on child at play, adult daydreamer, and creative artist, 4–5; on
compromise formation, 107; on consciousness, 99–101, 105–6; on countertransference, 150, 151; on dreams, 260–
61; on ego synthesis, 164; on fetish, 246;
Gardner on creative breakthroughs of,
6–8; on insight, 340; on "kernel of
truth," 313; and Lucy R. case, 242; on
"material" truth, 311; on *nachträglichkeit*
(deferred effect), 118; on narcissism,
194, 195–96, 197, 199; on neurosis, 126;
on obsession, 219, 229; on Oedipus complex, 126; on peace process, 213; on pleasure principle, 291; psychoanalytic
method of, 105–6, 109, 119, 121, 131,
133–34, 138–46, 158, 244; psychoanalytic technique versus technical "rules"
of, 141–43; on psychosexual stages, 174;
"Rat Man case of, 142, 234–35, 248, 249;
on rational framework of analysis, 156–
57; on regression, 261; reports of analyses with, 143–46; on repression, 250; on
sadomasochism, 105n; on transference,
105n, 107, 114–15, 126, 133, 140–41,
148; on transference neurosis, 116–17;
on unconscious, 99–101
—works: *Ego and the Id*, 94; "Etiology of
Hysteria," 7; *Inhibitions, Symptoms and
Anxiety*, 94; *Interpretation of Dreams*, 250,
260–61; *New Introductory Lectures*, 346;
"Note upon 'the mystic writing pad,'"
100–101; *Studies in Hysteria*, 7
Friedman, R. C., 85
Furman, E., 291–92, 310, 311
Furman, R. A., 292

Gaddini, E., 290–91, 292, 294, 302, 306
Galatzer-Levy, R., 120
Gardner, H., 5–8, 5n
Gender identity disorder, clinical material
on, 22–23, 68–85
Genette, G., 239
Gesell, A., 174
Gide, A., 235
Gill, M. M., 104n1, 265
Girls. *See* Females
Gitelson, M., 137–38, 153
Glenn, J., 264, 265

Glover, 136
Goldberg, R., 322
"Golden Fantasy," 148
Gosse, E., 236–37
Gottlieb, G., 174, 177, 179, 180
Gray, P., 98–99, 107–8, 112, 241–48, 255
Greenacre, P., 126, 246, 311
Greenough, W. T., 179
Greenson, R., 132–35, 137, 140, 147, 151, 152, 156, 159, 160
Grief, 206–14
Grinker, R., 141
Grumet, G. W., 334
Grunberger, B., 195, 197

Hall-Smith, P., 333
Harley, M., 85
Harrison, A., 293
Hartmann, H., 86, 97, 110, 119–20, 176, 265, 310, 312
Havens, L., 332
Heimann, P., 150
Heisenberg uncertainty principle, 120
Hellman, I., 176
Helplessness, 225–26, 231
Hemingway, E., 10, 13n
Hickock, W. B., 336
Hierarchical principle of therapeutic interventions, 154–55
Hierarchy of basic human needs, 154–55
Hills, O. F., 259–86
Hitchcock, A., 246
Hockaday, T. D. R., 295n1
Hoffer, A., 121
Hoffman, I., 118
Homosexuality, 266, 304–5
Housman, A. E., 238
Houzel, D., 196, 197
Huttenlocher, P. R., 179
Hypnagogic hallucinations, 262
Hysteria, 7

Id, 310
Idealization of analyst, 58, 64–65
Identification: in adulthood generally, 230; with analysts, 53–56, 83–84, 88; of boy with atypical ego development, 38–39, 41; of boy with deviational development with analyst, 83–84; in childhood generally, 230; projective identification, 112; of sixteen-year-old female with analyst, 53–56; of sixteen-year-old girl with parents, 54
Illness: diabetes, 289–313, 295n; as way of avoiding mental integration, 297–98

"Indiana Jones and the Last Crusade," 78–80, 84
Individuation, in adolescent development, 47–67
Infant-mother relationship, 235–36
"Influencing machine," 263
Insight: in child analysis, 339–54; clinical material on, 340–51; definition of, 340; discussion of clinical material on, 351–54; and prelatency considerations, 352–54
Integration: acting out as consequence of integration anxiety, 292–95; avoidance of integration of libidinal and aggressive drives toward paternal figure, 305–9; bodily illness as way of avoiding, 297–98; clinical material on, 295–309; discussion of clinical material on, 309–13; dread of, in woman with diabetes, 289–313; fear/inability to recognize boundaries of the self, 299–302; mother's role in, 291–92, 311–12; separation and fear of, 309–10; theoretical views of, 291–92
Internalization, 38–41
Interpretations: with boy with deviational development, 69–70; S. Freud on, 109; with obsessional patients, 231; questions on use of, 89
Intrapsychic defenses. *See* Defenses
Introspection, 99, 104–5, 109, 111
Isakower, O., 106, 260, 261, 262, 263, 264, 265, 283, 285
Isakower phenomenon, 259–86
Isolation, of boy with deviational development, 69

Jagger, M., 321, 322
Jakobson, R., 246, 252
Joffe, W., 45, 199, 229
Johnson, M., 237
Johnson, T. H., 170
Jones, E., 126, 144
Joseph, B., 98–99, 113
Joseph, E. D., 262
Journals, psychoanalytic writing for, 14–15n
Junctures, 241, 245, 247–49
Jung, C., 126, 143
Juvenile (brittle) diabetes, 289–313, 295n

Kardiner, A., 141, 145
Kass, N., 319–37
Katan, A., 34
Kay, P., 254
Kennedy, H., 298, 310, 340

Kepecs, J. G., 262
Kernberg, O., 195, 197, 243, 305
Kessen, W., 172n1
King, P., 150
Kinmonth, A. L., 296
Kleinian psychoanalysts, 111–12
Kligerman, C., 5
Kohut, H., 111, 195
Koller, C., 6
Krafft-Ebing, R., 7
Kris, A., 245
Kris, E., 101, 102–3, 108, 119–20, 237, 265
Kris Study Group, 262–63, 263n
Kruger, L.-M., 247

Lampl-De Groot, J., 141, 340
Language, of boy with atypical ego development, 28, 33–34, 35, 39–40, 44
Laor, N., 197
Latency: of boy with atypical ego development, 44–45; challenges of, 87; patients' use of analysts during, 88
Lear, J., 236, 250
Leary, K., 119
Leckman, J. F., 178–79
Leekam, S., 254
Leonard, H., 219
Leslie, A., 254
Lewin, B. D., 262, 263, 264
Lewy, E., 262
Lipton, S., 133–35, 142–43, 148, 153, 156, 159
Lish, G., 11–14
Little, M., 150
Loewald, H., 137, 157, 190, 284
Lothane, Z., 106–7, 108
Louis, J., 249
Lucy R. case, 242

Mahler, M., 175, 263n1
Males: analysis of boy following mother's death, 353–54; atypical ego development in boy, 23–46; clinical example of narrative performance mode (NPM) of discourse, 242–45; clothing of adolescent males, 324–25, 328–33; deviational development in boy, 22–23, 68–85; narcissistic immunization process in, 205–14; obsessional manifestations in a boy, 221–23, 225–26, 228, 229; popular music in adolescent analysis, 324–28, 331; regressive ego phenomena in, 265–86. *See also* Fathers
Manson, C., 325
Manson, M., 325

Martin, A., 319–37
Maslow, A., 154
Masturbation, 226–27, 262
Max, D. T., 11–13, 12n, 13n13
Mayes, L., 27, 39, 169–90, 340
McCord, Dr., 143
McDevitt, J., 86
Meares, R., 236
Menaker, E., 137
Metallica, 327
Meyer, B., 5
Meyer, W., 10
Meyerson, P. G., 154
Michel, R., 124–25
Miller, J. H., 238
Minor Threat, 331
Mitchell, B., 9
Mitchell, S., 123–25
Modell, A. H., 196, 242
Mogliano, X., 141
Monday crust, 114–15
Moran, G., 26
Moran, G. S., 298, 310
Moran, M. G., 99, 104
Morrison, A. P., 195
Moses, R., 197
Mothers: absence of and abandonment by, 48–49, 51, 58, 65, 222, 223, 307, 326; of adolescent male with panic disorder, 329, 330, 331; with bipolar disorder, 329; with borderline personality disorder, 326; of boy with atypical ego development, 26–27, 29–31, 33–38, 39, 41–43; of boy with deviational development, 70–74, 82; of children with obsessional manifestations, 222, 223, 224; death of, 353–54; depression of, 48–49, 329; of diabetic female, 295–96, 302, 307, 311–12; girl's erotic fantasies about, 226; infants' relationship with, 235–36; and integrative processes, 291–92, 311–12; and man with regressive ego functioning, 267, 272–73, 275, 278–79; of preadolescent girl with compulsive symptoms, 341, 343–48, 350; with schizophrenia, 295–96, 311; of sixteen-year-old female, 48–49, 51, 53–54, 57–58, 62, 65, 66
Movies, 78–81, 84, 325
Murphy, W. F., 262
Music, 320–28, 331

Nacht, S., 137, 148
Nachträglichkeit (deferred effect), 118, 242, 248
Narcissism: and analyst/analysand relation-

ship, 203–5; clinical implications of narcissistic envelope, 203–5; clinical vignettes on, 194–95, 201–2, 204, 205–14; S. Freud on, 194, 195–96, 197, 199; and interaction between self and others, 198–214; origin of term, 193–94; and regressive ego phenomena, 280–82; theoretical bases of current views on, 195–98
Narcissistic envelope, 198–205
Narcissistic immune processing, 198–214
Narrative performance mode (NPM) of discourse: clinical examples of, 242–45, 247–49; and junctures, 241, 245, 247–49; minimal requirements of narrative, 238–40; narrative acquisition, 253–56; nature of narrative, 234–35; overview of, 233; and prenarrativity, 235–37; purpose of narrative, 237–38; and rhymes of events, 245–46; stories in psychoanalytic situation, 240–47; technical elements of, 250–52; therapeutic action by recognition scenes, 249–50
Neubauer, P. B., 19–24, 87–89, 340
Neurosis: A. Freud on, 26; S. Freud on, 126; obsessional neurosis, 226, 229
Neutrality of analyst, 120–22, 136
Newman, G., 333
Nielsen, A., 245, 249
Nirvana (music group), 322
Non-integration phase, 292
NPM. *See* Narrative performance mode (NPM) of discourse
Nunberg, H., 136, 310

Object constancy, 43, 50, 52, 65, 197
Object relations: in adolescent development of sixteen-year-old female, 52–53; and integration, 311; and narcissistic envelope, 198–205; paternal object relation and males, 205–14
Obsessional manifestations: for affective distancing, 229; in boy, 221–23, 225–26, 228, 229; in children, 219–32; clinical material on, 221–27; discussion of clinical material on, 228–32; etiology of, 220; in girls, 223–29; limitations of psychoanalysis for, 219; pharmacological treatment of, 219; in preadolescent girl, 341. *See also* Compulsive symptoms
Obsessional neurosis, 226, 229
Oedipal fantasies, 31, 42
Oedipus, meaning of, 283
Oedipus complex: and boy with deviational development, 73, 81–82, 84–85; and *déjà vu* experience, 263; S. Freud on, 126; as

insight of psychoanalysis, 110; and Isakower phenomenon, 263; in man with regressive ego functioning, 269–70, 275, 278; and narcissism, 202–3; and sixteen-year-old female, 66, 67
Ogden, T. H., 196
Olesker, W., 23–46
Oppenheim, R. W., 177, 180
Oral-aggressive fantasies, 29, 30, 42, 303
Oral deprivation, 262
Orality, 262, 263–64

Pacella, B. L., 263n1
Paley, V. G., 5
Panic disorder, 328–29
Paolino, T. J., 139
Parents. *See* Fathers; Mothers
Penis, 81–82. *See also* Body-phallus equation
Penn, P., 254
Perelberg, R., 305
Perkins, M., 9, 10–11, 10–11nn7-10, 12, 13n13
Person, E. S., 1–15
Physical handicaps of sibling, 70–71, 76–77
Piaget, J., 175, 177
Piercings. *See* Tattoos and piercings
Pine, F., 34
Plato, 254
Play: of boy with atypical ego development, 28, 32, 44; of boy with deviational development, 72, 73, 74–75; S. Freud on, 4–5; and narrative acquisition in children, 254–56; self-observations during, 353
Pleasure principle, 104, 291, 292
Plomin, R., 179
Poland, W., 120
Pomorska, K., 252
Popular culture: clothing of adolescents, 324–25, 328–333; music, 320–28, 331; tattoos and piercings, 330, 333–37
Popular music, 320–28, 331
Posegrove, C., 13
Pound, E., 13, 13n13
Powerlessness, strategies to counteract, 2–3
Prechtl, H. F. R., 172, 177
Prelatency children, 352–54
Prenarrativity, 235–37
Projective identification, 112
Promiscuity, 58–59
Protective maneuvers, 312
Psychic envelopes, 196, 198
Psychoanalysis: cautions about "by-paths" in, 119–20; changes in, 123–26; and constant change in mental life, 94–99;

Psychoanalysis (continued)
    effects of analyst's interventions in,
    120–25; extra-analytic determinants of
    analytic data, 112–20, 125; frequency
    and duration of, 115–16, 115n; hierar-
    chical principle of therapeutic interven-
    tions, 154–55; Kleinian psychoanalysts,
    111–12; literature review on, 132–40;
    and narcissistic immune processing,
    200–205; rational framework of, 156–57;
    real relationship in, as therapeutic, 130–
    65; and resolution of analytic dilemma,
    147–48; standard criteria for, 115–16;
    stories in, 240–47; therapeutic alliance
    and physician's role in, 151–52, 160, 163;
    and therapeutic barrier, 146–47; and un-
    conscious mental processes, 99–112,
    125; unique and characteristic insights
    of, 110; unknowability in, 93–126; widen-
    ing scope of, 155–56. *See also* Adolescent
    analysis; Child analysis; Transference;
    other psychoanalytic concepts
Psychoanalytic Research and Development
    Fund, 19
Psychoanalytic writing for journals, 14–15n
Psychosexual stages, 174

Rabin, Y., 205–14
Rado, S., 234
Rafeal-Leff, J., 305
Rank, O., 126
Rapaport, D., 265
Rasmussen, S. A., 219
Rat Man case, 142, 234–35, 248, 249
"Real relationship" in psychoanalysis: clini-
    cal aspects of, 146–63; clinical manifesta-
    tions of, 157–60; clinical vignette on,
    160–63; communication between analyst
    and patient, 131, 157–59; conclusion on,
    165; contrast between S. Freud's tech-
    nique and technical "rules," 141–43;
    countertransference versus, 150–51; ear-
    lier literature on, 136–40; feelings of an-
    alyst and patient toward each other, 159–
    60; A. Freud on, 138; S. Freud on, 133–
    34, 138–46; Greenson on, 132–33; hier-
    archical principle of therapeutic inter-
    ventions, 154–55; and interweaving with
    transference imagoes, 152–54; introduc-
    tion to, 130–32; Lipton on, 133–35; liter-
    ature review on, 132–40; negative feel-
    ings between analyst and patient, 159–
    60; personality of analyst, 131; and physi-
    cian-client relationship, 151–52; relation
    of, to rational framework of analysis,

156–57; relation of, to widening scope of
    analysis, 155–56; reports of analyses with
    S. Freud, 143–46; and resolution of ana-
    lytic dilemma, 147–48; and termination,
    160–65; and therapeutic alliance, 151–
    52, 160, 163; and therapeutic barrier,
    146–47; therapeutic functions of, 163–
    65; transference neurosis in, 164; trans-
    ference versus, 148–50; Viederman on,
    135–36
Reality, acceptance of, 164
Recognition scenes, 249–50
Regression: of boy with deviational devel-
    opment, 69, 73, 74; S. Freud on, 261; and
    music, 323
Regressive ego phenomena: clinical mater-
    ial on, 265–79; discussion of clinical ma-
    terial on, 279–86; literature review on,
    260–65; overview of, 259–60
Reich, W., 126, 136
Renik, O., 121–22, 237
Representations of interactions that have
    been generalized (RIG), 196–97
Repression, 250
Rescheduling of session, 271–72
Resistance: in adolescent analysis, 320; of
    boy with deviational development, 73;
    Gray on, 98, 107–8; in obsessional
    patients, 230
Reston, V. A., 321
Reverse engineering, 178n4
Reznor, T., 321
Rhymes of events, 245–46
Richards, A. D., 265
Richards, K., 321
RIG, 196–97
Rimmon-Kenan, S , 254
Ritvo, S., 86
Rock and roll. *See* Popular music
Rolling Stones, 322
Rosaldo, M., 238
Rose, R. J., 179
Rosen, J., 126
Rosenblum, D. S., 319–37
Rosenfeld, S. K., 292
Rosenfield, I., 197
Ross, L., 13
Rudnytsky, P. L., 283, 284
Ruitenbeek, H. M., 141
Rycroft, C., 262

Sadism, 65
Sadomasochism, 105n
Salinger, J. D., 333
Salome, 346

Sandler, A.-M., 299, 340

Sandler, J., 45, 149, 152, 195, 196, 197, 199, 229, 249, 264, 299, 310

Sarton, M., 3

Scaife, M., 235–36

Schafer, R., 111, 112

Schizophrenia, 295–96, 311

Schmukler, A. G., 22, 23, 47–67, 339–54

School issues, 48, 50, 53, 58, 60, 82, 328–29, 344–45, 347, 350–51

Secrets, 348

Self, boundaries of, 299–302

Self-control, 3

Self-identity, interaction between self and others, 193–214

Self-observations, 353

Self-regulation, 3, 39–40

Semrad, E., 156

Separation, in adolescent development of sixteen-year-old female, 47–67

Sexual relationships: of diabetic woman, 303; of sixteen-year-old female, 51, 53–59, 63–64, 66

Shakespeare, W., 150

Shame, of boy with atypical ego development, 44

Shapiro, T., 121

Sharpe, E., 136, 158

Shawn, W., 13

Shengold, L., 6

"Shifters," 246–47, 251–52

Siblings: child's jealousy and anger at new-born sibling, 353; death of, 70, 248; of diabetic girl, 296; physical handicaps of, 70–71, 76–77; of preadolescent girl with compulsive symptoms, 341–43, 348, 349, 352

Silberstein, E., 6

Simon, B., 237

Sleep, 261–62, 264

Smith, S., 148

Social constructivism, 118

Solan, R., 193–214

Solnit, A. J., 19–24, 87–89, 197, 198, 201

Sorce, J. F., 236

Spencer, J. H., 106–7, 108, 111

Sperling, O. E., 262

Spitz, R., 175, 176, 262, 263n1, 264

Sprince, M. P., 292

Stein, M. H., 101–3

Stepparents, 72, 73, 82, 353

Sterba, R., 141, 145, 151, 154

Stern, D. N., 196, 197

Stern, M., 262

Stolorow, R. D., 199

Stone, L., 137, 138, 139, 147, 152, 159

Stories. *See* Narrative performance mode (NPM) of discourse

Strachey, J., 119

Suicide and suicidal feelings, 306, 322

Superego, 43, 59, 208, 228, 262, 273, 275, 284, 308, 351–52

Talese, N., 9

Tallandini, M. A., 289–313

Tarachow, S., 146–47, 156

Tattoos and piercings, 330, 333–37

Tausk, V., 263

Termination: in adolescent analysis, 351; of child analysis, 82–83; of diabetic woman, 306–9; and "real relationship" in psychoanalysis, 160–65

Thass-Thienemann, T., 283

Therapeutic alliance, 151–52, 160, 163

Therapeutic barrier, 146–47

Thomson, W., 335

Toilet training, 49, 341

Townshend, P., 321

Transference: of boy with deviational development, 81–82, 84–85; of children with obsessional manifestations, 223, 224; and constant psychic change, 98–99, 113; of diabetic woman, 301–2; differentiation of, from "real relationship" in psychoanalysis, 148–50; extra-analytic derivatives of, 113–15; and feelings of powerlessness, 2; A. Freud on, 139–40, 194; S. Freud on, 105n, 107, 114–15, 126, 133, 140, 148; Greenson on, 132–33; interweaving with transference imagoes, 152–54; and Monday crust, 114–15; of preadolescent girl with compulsive symptoms, 345, 352; of sixteen-year-old female, 51, 53–63, 65–67; Strachey on, 119; between writers and editors, 14–15

Transference neurosis: definition of, 116n; S. Freud on, 116–17; in "real relationship" in psychoanalysis, 153, 160, 164

Turpin, Archbishop, 245–46

Tustin, F., 196, 312

Tyson, P., 170, 173

Tyson, R., 170, 173

Unconscious: Arlow on, 101–2, 108, 109, 117–18; S. Freud on, 99–101, 105–6; Jung's collective unconscious, 126; and unknowability in psychoanalysis, 99–112, 125

Unknowability in psychoanalysis: conclusions on, 125–26; and constant change

Unknowability in psychoanalysis (continued)
in mental life, 94–99; and effects of analyst's interventions, 120–25; and extraanalytic determinants of analytic data, 112–20, 125; overview of, 93–94; and unconscious mental processes, 99–112, 125
Urination: of boy with atypical ego development, 44; father's reactions to daughter's urination outside, 63

Vagina, 81–82, 345–46
Vaillant, G., 333
Viederman, M., 135–36
Violence. *See* Assassination of Rabin

Waddington, C. H., 177
Waelder, R., 94, 96, 243
Walker, P., 234
Weil, A. P., 310
Weintrobe, S., 293
Welles, J., 247

Wexler, M., 137, 140, 156
Wharton, E., 8, 8n, 15
Will-power, 3
Winner, E., 254
Winnicott, D. W., 137, 150, 196, 197, 292, 322, 324
Wolf, D. P., 247
Wolf, J. M., 176
Wolfe, S., 85
Wolfe, T., 10–11, 10–11nn, 12, 13n
Wolff, P. H., 172, 177, 181
Wolpert, L., 172
Wortis, J., 141
Writer-editor partnerships, 9–15, 9–10n, 13n, 14–15n
Wrye, H., 247

Yorke, C., 45, 296

Zetzel, E. R., 137, 138–39, 151, 152, 156
Zients, A. B., 22–23, 68–85